Comprehensive Review
for the Radiology Registry

A Centralized Resource

Comprehensive Review
for the Radiology Registry
A Centralized Resource

MARK F. PIERCE, RT (R) (CT)
Hot Springs, Arkansas

with

RICHARD CARNOVALE, MD
San Antonio, Texas

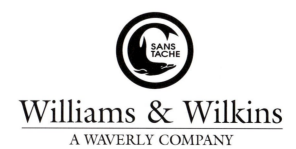

Williams & Wilkins
A WAVERLY COMPANY

BALTIMORE • PHILADELPHIA • LONDON • PARIS • BANGKOK
BUENOS AIRES • HONG KONG • MUNICH • SYDNEY • TOKYO • WROCLAW

Editor: Elizabeth A. Nieginski
Manager, Development Editing: Julie Scardiglia
Managing Editor: Darrin Kiessling
Marketing Manager: Peter Darcy
Development Editor: Rosanne Hallowell
Production Coordinator: Danielle Hagan
Text/Cover Designer: Shephard, Inc.
Illustration Planner: Ray Lowman
Typesetter: Maryland Composition Co., Inc.
Printer/Binder: Mack Printing Group

Copyright © 1998 Williams & Wilkins

351 West Camden Street
Baltimore, Maryland 21201-2436 USA

Rose Tree Corporate Center
1400 North Providence Road
Building II, Suite 5025
Media, Pennsylvania 19063-2043 USA

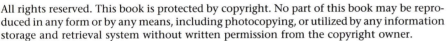

Printed in the United States of America

Library of Congress Cataloging-in-Publication Data

Pierce, Mark F.
  Comprehensive review for the radiology registry : a centralized
resource : Mark F. Pierce, with Richard Carnovale.
     p.   cm.
  Includes index.
  ISBN 0-683-30145-4
  1. Radiologic technologists—Examinations, questions, etc.
I. Carnovale, Richard. II. Title.
  [DNLM: 1. Radiology—examination questions.   WN 18.2 P617c   1998]
RC78.15.P53   1998
616.07'57'076—dc21
DNLM/DLC
for Library of Congress   97-42655
                                                        CIP

The publishers have made every effort to trace the copyright holders for borrowed material. If they have inadvertently overlooked any, they will be pleased to make the necessary arrangements at the first opportunity.

To purchase additional copies of this book, call our customer service department at **(800) 638-0672** or fax orders to **(800) 447-8438.** For other book services, including chapter reprints and large quantity sales, ask for the Special Sales department.

Canadian customers should call **(800) 665-1148,** or fax **(800) 665-0103.** For all other calls originating outside of the United States, please call **(410) 528-4223** or fax us at **(410) 528-8550.**

Visit Williams & Wilkins on the Internet: http://www.wwilkins.com or contact our customer service department at **custserv@wwilkins.com.** Williams & Wilkins customer service representatives are available from 8 30 am to 6 00 pm, EST, Monday through Friday, for telephone access.

98 99 00 01 02
1 2 3 4 5 6 7 8 9 10

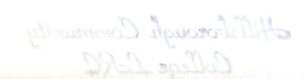

For my mom and dad, from whom
I inherited a legacy of words,
and
in loving memory of Stanley Loeffler—
he would've liked this book.

Contents

Preface

Throughout my career in radiologic technology, I've witnessed grim-faced student technologists lamenting, "I wish there were one book I could use to study for the Registry. But look at this mess! There's so much stuff here, I don't know what to study next!" Senior technologists respond with a knowing smile and a sympathetic shaking of the head: We've all been there.

While the students' plea is partly due to the anxiety commonly associated with comprehensive examinations such as the Radiology Registry, their dilemma serves to emphasize the situation confronting student technologists everywhere.

The study of radiologic technology is a complex endeavor, involving in most cases 2 years of a voluminous mixture of academic and clinical preparation. Throughout the course of study, the student naturally acquires a formidable assemblage of textbooks, each of which addresses a portion of the aggregate whole. Along with the texts, the student compiles reams of notes and handouts. The aspiring student preparing for the American Registry of Radiologic Technologists (ARRT) Registry Examination must synthesize this data into a meaningful body of knowledge.

The difficulty with this approach is that there is simply so much information to sort out. Each text, each lecture, treats its subject matter from the standpoint of its own unique microcosm—that is to say, exhaustively. So, there is a great deal of chaff to go along with the wheat. The problem from the students' point of view is: which is which?

It is the purpose of ***Comprehensive Review for the Radiology Registry: A Centralized Resource*** to solve this dilemma. It does so by providing a unique centralized examination resource, a type of reference previously unavailable to the student radiologic technologist. In other words, this text provides all the information you need—a kind of one-stop shopping place—for successfully completing the ARRT Registry Examination. It achieves this goal by integrating several approaches.

First, the scope of the text is confined to material pertinent to the Registry Examination. We assume that, if you purchased the book, you have already completed or are about to complete a rigorous course in radiologic science; information that was necessary in the classroom setting but which is extraneous to the examination, is of little value to you now. We therefore have excluded any material we determined to be only tangentially relevant to the Registry Examination, saving you an enormous amount of time and effort.

The ARRT divides the examination into five major categories:

Category	Percent of Test	Number of Questions
Patient Care	15%	30
Radiographic Procedures	30%	60
Radiation Protection	15%	30
Image Production and Evaluation	25%	50
Equipment Operation and Maintenance	15%	30
Totals:	100%	200

This book contains five chapters, one for each category of the text. The 1996 ARRT examinee handbook lists content specifications, further subdividing each of the five primary categories into sets of subclassifications. Our book treats each of these subdivisions on an individual basis in an outline format.

To illustrate: The category "Patient Care" is outlined into five major Roman-numeral headings:

I. Legal and Professional Responsibilities
II. Patient Education, Safety, and Comfort
III. Prevention and Control of Infection
IV. Patient Monitoring
V. Contrast Media

Each of these sections is then further subdivided using capital-letter headings, as reflected in the Table of Contents preceding this Preface. In each of these capital-letter subdivisions, the pertinent information is provided in brief expository manner, followed by a mini-exam of 4 to 6 questions, followed by the answers to those questions. At the end of each chapter, there are questions and answers related to all of the material in that chapter. Finally, a complete Simulated Examination of 200 questions is provided at the end of the book; it recreates as closely as possible the actual Registry Examination.

In planning the format of this book, we examined all the existing study aids. In addition, we solicited input from radiology communities all over the world, by way of the Internet. The final form of this book was conceived as a hybridization of known approaches, in addition to our own ideas. We believe our systematic method will yield the best results yet achieved in the long history of such endeavors.

Good luck!

Mark F. Pierce, RT(R)(CT)
Richard Carnovale, M.D.

Patient Care

I. LEGAL AND PROFESSIONAL RESPONSIBILITIES
A. Scheduling and Sequencing Examinations

Successful outcome of routine and fluoroscopic examinations is dependent on appropriate examination sequencing. Preparatory considerations are most crucial when scheduling examinations using **barium** sulfate.

The intravenous pyelogram (IVP), barium enema (BE), and **upper gastrointestinal (UGI)** and **small bowel series** must be scheduled in a specific order. The IVP is done first, because water-soluble contrast media is rapidly excreted. Next, the barium enema is done. These two examinations are often performed the same day. Last, the UGI tract may be studied. If these three examinations are performed in close proximity, generally a 1-day lapse between the IVP/BE and the UGI is required, and the patient is given a mild laxative in the interim. Any residual barium from the BE will generally not interfere with imaging the esophagus, stomach, and proximal small bowel, although in this instance an abdominal radiograph is generally taken before the examination.

Although the preceding is generally accepted as the correct sequencing protocol, it is important to note that some authors have advocated performing the UGI examination first. Supporters of this approach note the direct relationship between effectiveness of colon preparation and accuracy of diagnosis. Fecal material may not be appreciated on a routine abdominal scout view, whereas the lack of residual contrast medium found on a scout radiograph obtained subsequent to UGI examination is an obvious indicator of colon cleanliness.

Residual barium from prior examinations may obscure bone detail for conventional dorsal, lumbar spine, or pelvic examinations, as well as for abdominal computed tomographic (CT) and some nuclear medicine examinations.

Length of routine and fluoroscopic examinations varies from department to department, and is dependent upon the requirements of the radiologist performing and interpreting the examination, as well as condition of the patient, and technical expertise of the radiographic technologist. When scheduling, the technologist must consider these factors, so as not to overload department resources.

UGI, esophagram, small bowel follow-through (**SBFT**), BE, and IVP examinations usually require the patient to refrain from eating for a predetermined interval before examination; this time period usually consists of an overnight fast. This policy is flexible for fragile patients such as diabetics. Non–insulin-dependent diabetics should withhold their morning meal, but must be given scheduling priority by being examined in the early morning. Departments may keep a supply of juices and snacks on hand for these patients after their examinations are completed. Patients who take insulin must be instructed not to take insulin the morning of the examination, and these patients also must be scheduled first in the morning.

Health maintenance organization patients must obtain authorization for radiologic examinations. Therefore, it is important to inquire about the patient's insurance when scheduling, so necessary permission is verified.

QUESTIONS FOR SCHEDULING AND SEQUENCING EXAMINATIONS

select the best answer

1. In which order should the following examinations be performed?
    1. Lumbar spine
    2. BE
    3. UGI
   (A) 1, 2, 3
   (B) 3, 1, 2
   (C) 2, 3, 1
   (D) 2, 1, 3

2. Which of these examinations should be performed first?
   (A) SBFT
   (B) IVP
   (C) BE
   (D) UGI

3. A diabetic patient is to be scheduled for a UGI examination. You should:
   (A) fit him in the first available slot.
   (B) check the insurance.
   (C) remind the patient to take his/her insulin.
   (D) schedule him for the first examination in the morning.

4. Having had a barium enema, the patient returns to your department the following day for a UGI examination. You should:
   (A) prepare the barium mixture.
   (B) contact the radiologist.
   (C) take an abdominal scout view.
   (D) prepare the fluoro tower.

▶▶ ANSWERS TO SCHEDULING AND SEQUENCING EXAMINATIONS

1. The correct answer is (A). The lumbar spine should be imaged without the interfering influence of barium, followed by the BE, and the UGI on the following day.
2. The correct answer is (B). The correct sequence is IVP, BE, UGI, SBFT.
3. The answer is (D). Although insurance information should be verified, and convenience of the first available appointment should also be considered, the most important factor of these is the maintenance of the diabetic patient's sugar levels.
4. The correct response is (C). Although room and supply readiness is important, this patient may have too much residual barium to permit an optimal examination.

B. Legal Aspects of Radiography

A **radiograph request form** must be submitted on all patients **(Figure 1-1)**. Information included on the form typically consists of examination requested, patient name, date of birth, requesting physician, patient location [i.e., emergency room (ER), floor, intensive care unit (ICU), or outpatient], and pertinent clinical history.

There will be occasions when, for technical reasons, the requested examination will not reflect the most appropriate means for providing the radiologist with the best imaging information possible. In this instance, after obtaining an accurate patient history, the technologist should discuss the requested examination with the radiologist on duty or, if not possible, with the requesting physician.

At all times the patient's **right to confidentiality** should be considered. As members of the health care team, technologists must comply with the same standards concerning the patient's personal history that clinicians and radiologists abide by.

No detail of the patient's history or condition must be discussed with other patients or outside of the hospital. The technologist should refrain from speculating as to the patient's condition in conversations with the patients themselves. Inquiries from the patients should be handled tactfully and with respect, and the patient should be informed that questions pertaining to his/her medical condition are best discussed with the primary care physician.

Procedures such as **biopsies** and **angiography** carry with them some degree of risk. Therefore, it is common practice to obtain **informed consent** from the patient. In the case of the incapacitated patient, an authorized family member must sign the form. The consent itself is generally a standardized form that describes the procedure and risks involved. The technologist must take time to answer any questions patients may have regarding the procedure before having them sign the consent form. Because the physician is ultimately responsible for issues of liability relevant to the procedure, all questions beyond those that are concerned with the technologist's duties (i.e., results of the biopsy, differential diagnoses) should be referred to the physician.

Some facilities require that patients undergoing examinations using **iodinated contrast material**

NAME
M.R.#: RAD #.
DOB 12/18/19 AGE: 77
DATE 05/12/97
SAN ANTONIO COMMUNITY HOSPITAL
8026 FLOYD CURL DRIVE
SAN ANTONIO, TX 78229 210-692-8155

FLASH CARD

ACCT. #
RAD #

TRANSPORTATION

NAME:
ACCT.#
LOC. N.3W ROOM/BED N.308-02 02
SEX F D.O.B. 12/18/19
HT 5/1 WT 100/8
EXAM TYPE RADIOLOGY
How is patient transported P - PORTABLE
000046166 CHEP - CHEST AP

RADIOLOGY
000046166 CHEST AP ONLY PORTABLE

_____ EXAM COMPLETED - MAY EAT

_____ PATIENT TO RETURN FOR FOLLOW UP AT _____

_____ EXAMS NOT DONE - CANCELED

ATTENDING M.D. VanCleave,Stephen J
ORDERING M.D. VanCleave,Stephen J (REPRINT) (REPRINT

NAME DOB: 12/18/19 HT 5/1
ACCT.# SEX F WT 100/8
M.R.# N00537055 RAD # ENTERED BY NSEC.AFA
EXAM DATE: 05/12/97 AT: ENTRY DATE 05/12/97
LOCATION: N.3W ROOM/BED N.308-02 02
ALLERGIES: NKA, PCN, PCN CODEIN, PCN, CODEINE, PCN, CODIENE
DIAGNOSIS: CHF

EXAM TYPE: RADIOLOGY
How is patient transported? P - PORTABLE
Is patient pregnant?
Clinical History: CHF

EXAM: 000046166 CHEST AP ONLY PORTABLE R (05/12/97-1443)
Reason for Exam?
Is patient prepped?
Area of interest?
Comments: FTF

FILMS		TECH
14 X 17	_____	_____
14 X 14	_____	_____
11 X 14	_____	_____
10 X 12	_____	_____
9 X 9	_____	_____
8 X 10	_____	_____
OTHER	_____	_____

REPEAT REASON

LIGHT _____
DARK _____
POSITION _____
MOTION _____
EQUIPMENT _____

OTHER _____

PREVIOUS EXAM:

RAD/ABDOMEN AP & W/UP
04/28/97

(REPRINT)

TECHNOLOGIST COPY

NAME LOC N.3W ROOM/BED N.308-02 02
ACCT.# SEX F DOB 12/18/19 (77)
M.R.# N00537055 RAD # EXAM DATE 05/12/97 AT:
ATTENDING M.D. VanCleave,Stephen J ORDERING M.D. VanCleave,Stephen J
ALLERGIES NKA, PCN, PCN CODEIN, PCN, CODEINE, PCN, CODIENE
DIAGNOSIS: CHF

EXAM TYPE: RADIOLOGY
How is patient transported? P - PORTABLE
Is patient pregnant?
Clinical History: CHF

EXAM: 000046166 CHEST AP ONLY PORTABLE R (05/12/97-1443)
Reason for Exam?
Is patient prepped?
Area of interest?
Comments: FTF

CONTROL COPY

SAN ANTONIO COMMUNITY HOSPITAL
8026 FLOYD CURL DRIVE
SAN ANTONIO, TX 78229 210-692-8155

EXAM EXPLAINED _____

FIGURE 1-1. A typical x-ray request form. This particular request also serves as a flash card for the film identification system.

sign a consent form. The form will contain questions regarding the patient's medical history, with emphasis on whether any of the following exist: prior history of iodinated contrast-agent administration, known iodine allergies, or asthma.

Patients do not own the radiographs; they are part of the patient's record. Radiographic services cover procedure and interpretation, and radiographs are available for use, should they be requested by medical professionals elsewhere.

Patients' rights are defined by the American Hospital Association's **Patient Bill of Rights.** The rights are: To refuse treatment to the extent permitted by law, to confidentiality of records and communication, to informed consent, privacy, respectful care, access to personal records, refusal to participate in research, an explanation of hospital charges, and continuing care.

Torts are **intentional** or **unintentional** acts that result in damage or wrongful injury. **Invasion of privacy,** that is, the unnecessary reading or public discussion of a patient's record, and **false imprisonment,** the restraining of a patient unnecessarily, or purposefully refusing to shield a patient, are examples of intentional misconduct. Were a patient to sustain an injury while the technologist performed another job-related task, such as getting a radiograph or setting technique at the control panel, the radiographer would be considered guilty of unintentional misconduct.

QUESTIONS FOR LEGAL ASPECTS OF RADIOGRAPHY

select the best answer

1. Which of the following information should be contained on a radiography request form?
   1. Name
   2. Date of birth
   3. Requesting physician
   4. Examination requested
   (A) Choice 1 only
   (B) Choices 1 and 2
   (C) Choices 2 and 3
   (D) All of the aforementioned

2. Besides the information contained in question 1, which other information should be on the radiography request?
   1. Patient location
   2. Insurance information
   3. Clinical history

   4. Information on persons living with the patient
   (A) Choice 1 only
   (B) Choices 1 and 3
   (C) All of the aforementioned
   (D) None of the aforementioned

3. Which examination requires that a consent form be signed by the patient?
   (A) UGI
   (B) IVP
   (C) Cerebral arteriogram
   (D) Preoperative chest radiograph

4. A tort is:
   (A) a viral infection.
   (B) a hospital policy.
   (C) an act that results in injury.
   (D) a patient right.

5. The patient has a right to:
   1. a diagnosis from the technologist.
   2. confidentiality.
   3. the lowest reasonable price for treatment.
   4. refuse the examination.
   (A) All of the aforementioned
   (B) None of the aforementioned
   (C) Choices 1 and 3
   (D) Choices 2 and 4

6. A patient comes to the radiology department from the emergency room and presents a request for a left knee examination. Upon investigation, the radiographer discovers that the right knee is injured, not the left. He should:
   (A) send the patient back to the emergency room.
   (B) discuss the situation with another technologist.
   (C) radiograph the right knee.
   (D) inform the radiologist.

▶▶ ANSWERS TO LEGAL ASPECTS OF RADIOGRAPHY

1. The answer is (D). All of this information would be pertinent to the request form.
2. The answer is (B). The patient's location and history should be known by the technologist.
3. The answer is (C). The arteriogram has a higher degree of risk than do the other procedures listed.

4. The answer is (C). The tort may be considered intentional or unintentional.
5. The answer is (D). The patient bill of rights includes the right to: refuse treatment to the extent permitted by law, confidentiality of records and communication, informed consent, privacy, respectful care, access to personal records, refusal to participate in research, an explanation of hospital charges, and continuing care.
6. The answer is (D). The patient should not be inconvenienced, but a radiographer may not independently determine the correct examination. If a radiologist is not available, the ordering physician should be apprised of the situation.

C. Patient Identification

To minimize occurrences of mistaken identity and the attendant risk of performing the wrong examination on the wrong patient, the technologist must always ensure that the radiographic request, patient identification (commonly a wrist band), and the order for radiograph in the patient's chart are in accord.

In most cases, investigation of the patient identification should be supplemented with questioning the patient as to his/her identity and the nature of the visit to the radiology department. In some instances, the patient may exhibit decreased mental capacity; if this is the case, he/she may not be considered a reliable historian.

In the event of a discrepancy among the requested examination, the patient record, and the patient, the technologist must vigorously pursue the source of the inaccuracy by whatever means are at his/her disposal. These methods would include telephoning the ordering physician, questioning the nursing service to which the patient is assigned, questioning the patient, or discussing the situation with the radiologist. The most appropriate response will vary according to the clinical situation.

QUESTIONS FOR PATIENT IDENTIFICATION

select the best answer

1. What is the best method of ensuring that you are about to perform the correct examination on the correct patient?
   (A) Call the nurse
   (B) Ask the patient
   (C) Look at the request form
   (D) None of the aforementioned

2. You receive a request for a thoracic spine examination. The order in the chart reads lumbar spine, complete. You should:
   1. ask the patient where it hurts.
   2. telephone the nurse who is taking care of the patient.
   3. perform the thoracic spine examination.
   4. perform the lumbar spine examination.
   (A) Choice 3 only
   (B) All of the aforementioned
   (C) Choices 1 and 2 only
   (D) None of the aforementioned

3. You receive a request for a posterior, anterior, and lateral (PAL) radiograph on a patient. The orderly informs you of the patient's location, and you discover that the patient is comatose. In order to make sure you have the correct patient, you should:
   (A) attempt to revive the patient.
   (B) check the arm band identification.
   (C) perform the radiograph and check for matching anatomy on previous examinations.
   (D) check the chart.

▶▶ ANSWERS TO PATIENT IDENTIFICATION

1. The answer is (D). The best way to be certain in this situation is to check for matching information on the request and the chart as well as questioning the patient.
2. The correct answer is (C). The technologist should use whatever means are at his/her disposal to ensure accuracy in the clinical situation.
3. The answer is (B). The patient arm band identification is generally a reliable method of determining patient identification.

D. Verification of Requested Examination

The primary sources of information regarding the requested examination are the **patient chart and the radiograph request.** The **written order** is often conveyed by brief phrases and abbreviations that the technologist must be familiar with. A listing of common medical abbreviations and phrases appears in **Appendix A.** Familiarity with these common terms is a requirement for successful completion of the registry examination.

Occasionally, errors are made in transcription of the physician's order. You may, for example, receive a request for a radiograph of the left forearm, and the patient will actually have an injured right arm. Situations such as these highlight the importance of obtaining a patient history. This does not mean that the technologist should understand in detail the patient's course of treatment, but rather that thoughtful consideration be given to ensuring the requested examination is appropriate for the clinical situation. If the technologist feels that a mistake has been made, the examination should be verified by the attending physician, radiologist, or nurse assigned to the care of the patient.

Pathology (a positive finding as determined by the radiologist, such as fracture or pneumonia) or suspected pathology that is found on initial radiographic examination may require further investigation. The radiologist determines the need for additional examination **(Figure 1-2).**

The injured patient may be limited in his/her ability to comply with the necessary positions for standard examinations. For example, a patient who has a fractured elbow may not be able to extend the arm completely. In this case, the technologist must consult with the radiologist or attending physician, and a plan of action should be determined **(Figure 1-3).** In general, limited examinations are comprised of two views obtained at right angles. Standard modifications of some examinations exist, and are discussed in Chapter 5.

QUESTIONS FOR VERIFICATION OF REQUESTED EXAMINATION

select the best answer

1. An emergency room patient is seen for examination with an injured left ankle. The requested examination is for the right foot. You should:
   1. ask the patient where it hurts.
   2. perform the right foot examination.
   3. consult with the radiologist.
   4. assess the patient and perform the examination that you think is appropriate.
   (A) Choice 3 only
   (B) Choices 1 and 3
   (C) Choice 2 only
   (D) Choices 2 and 4

2. A patient who has severe low back pain undergoes a lumbar spine examination. The patient is unable to lie supine. You should:

   1. perform a modified prone study.
   2. send the patient back to his/her room.
   3. call the nurse to assist you.
   4. consult with the radiologist.
   (A) Choices 1 and 4
   (B) Choice 2 only
   (C) Choices 1 and 3
   (D) Choice 4 only

3. A patient's chart reads: BPH/U/S in AM/NPO. The most likely examination to be performed is which of the following?
   (A) Barium enema
   (B) UGI
   (C) Ultrasound of the prostate
   (D) Bone survey

4. A patient with coxa plana has:
   (A) an enlarged coccyx.
   (B) flat feet.
   (C) club feet.
   (D) flattened femoral head.

5. A compound fracture:
   (A) is incomplete.
   (B) is displaced.
   (C) penetrates the skin.
   (D) has multiple parts.

▶▶ ANSWERS FOR VERIFICATION OF REQUESTED EXAMINATION

1. The answer is (B). The technologist should always obtain a patient history. In the case of a mistaken request, the radiologist should be informed, and instructions concerning the examination should be taken from him/her.
2. The answer is (D). It is not appropriate for the technologist to determine the correct examination.
3. The answer is (C). BPH is an abbreviation that means benign prostate hypertrophy, an inflammatory process often studied with ultrasound. NPO means nothing by mouth. See appendix A for a more complete listing of common medical abbreviations.
4. The answer is (D). Coxa plana, also known as Legg-Calvé-Perthes syndrome, is a disease of the femoral head caused by lack of blood supply.
5. The answer is (C). A compound fracture is one that penetrates the skin. A comminuted fracture is bone that is splintered or crushed into parts. A displaced fracture is one that affects the natural alignment of the bone.

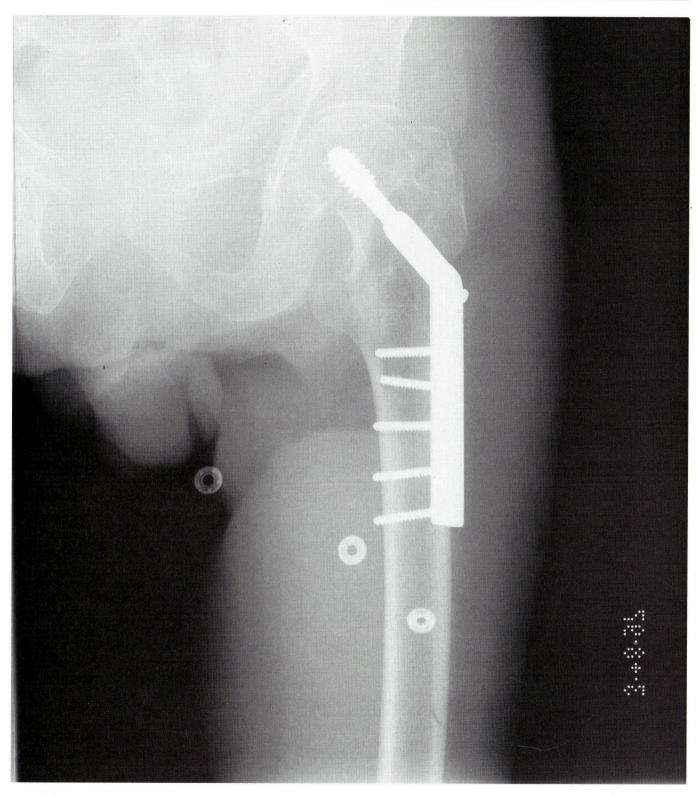

FIGURE 1-2.   Additional projection of left hip taken on 14 × 17 film, instead of the normally used 10 × 12 size. The patient had undergone surgical reduction and internal fixation. In order to include the entire length of surgical instrumentation, a larger film was required.

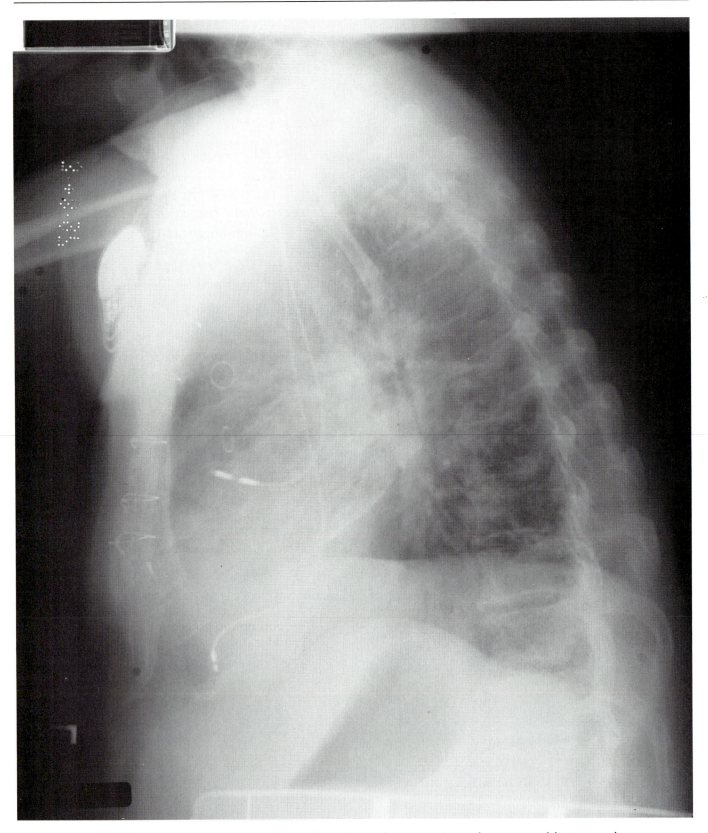

FIGURE 1-3. Lateral chest radiograph performed on a patient who was unable to stand. Note the outline of the wheelchair armrest at the bottom of the film.

II. PATIENT EDUCATION, SAFETY, AND COMFORT
A. Communication With Patients

The first step toward successful completion of any radiographic examination is communication with the patient. The interaction may take place in the following ways: **verbally,** as when you introduce yourself, or explain the examination; **nonverbally,** as with body language or facial expressions; **touch,** as when you reassure the patient; and **by appearance,** that is, how you present yourself in the work environment.

The medical record and the patients themselves are important resources in determining pertinent clinical history. The medical chart should be reviewed concerning name, age, location, diagnosis, and general condition. These factors should be correlated with the requested examination. Often the patient will reveal key information that is not contained in the chart, so careful interview of the patient whenever feasible is of paramount importance. The radiologist should be made aware of pertinent medical history. For example, you have observed the patient coughing. This information should be passed along to the radiologist so it is taken into consideration when the patient is examined.

Patients are often anxious and confused about procedures. The technologist should provide the patient with a thorough explanation concerning the test that he/she is about to undergo. In this matter, the technologist's personal observation of the patient should serve as a guide concerning the quantity and content of the explanation. The patient should not be given too much technical information; however, it should not be assumed that the patient is incapable of understanding important facts related to the examination.

Technologists must be able to respond effectively to commonplace inquiries concerning other modalities within the radiology department **(Figure 1-4).** Responses should consist of basic information regarding the nature of the examination, along with any preparatory requirements. Examples of such requirements include female patients refraining from the use of deodorant, makeup, or jewelry when having a mammogram, or instructing patients to arrive in the department with a full bladder before pelvic ultrasound. Most departments have pamphlets available that explain the rudiments of various procedures, with titles such as "MRI and You." The radiologic technologist should be familiar with these publications.

QUESTIONS FOR COMMUNICATION WITH PATIENTS

select the best answer

1. Forms of patient communication include which of the following?
   (A) Verbal
   (B) Facial expressions
   (C) Appearance
   (D) All of the aforementioned

2. The magnetic resonance image (MRI) unit:
   1. uses image-producing ionizing radiation.
   2. is safe for operators and patients alike.
   3. uses image producing magnetic fields.
   4. is used for examinations that are not covered by most insurance.
   (A) Choice 3 only
   (B) Choice 4 only
   (C) Choices 2 and 3
   (D) None of the aforementioned

3. Suppose that you are working at night, and no radiologist is available. While performing an acute abdominal series, the patient has an episode of hematemesis. You should:
   (A) inform the ordering physician.
   (B) do nothing.
   (C) hurry up with the examination.
   (D) perform a UGI examination.

4. An elderly woman is seen for a barium enema examination. She is alert and oriented, but frail and anxious. You should:
   (A) explain colon anatomy so that she understands it.
   (B) outline the procedure.
   (C) inform the radiologist.
   (D) begin the enema.

▶▶ ANSWERS TO COMMUNICATION WITH PATIENTS

1. The answer is (D). Other forms are touching and body language.
2. The answer is (C). The MRI unit uses high-power magnetic fields to produce images. It is extremely safe.
3. The answer is (A). The ordering physician should be apprised of the situation.
4. The answer is (B). In general, an outline summa-

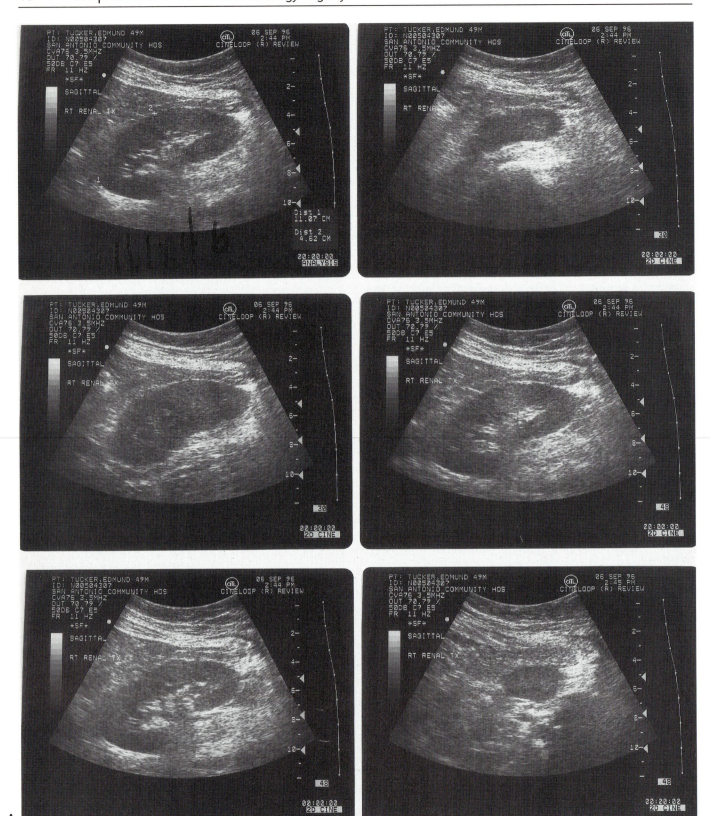

FIGURE 1-4. Examples of other modalities in the radiology department. **(A)** Renal ultrasound. **(B)** Nuclear medicine Cardiolite scan. **(C)** CT brain scan. **(D)** MRI, right shoulder.

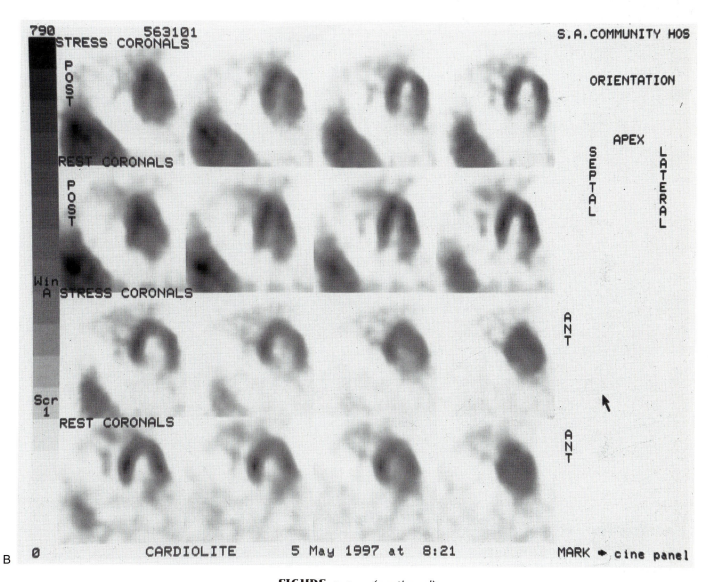

FIGURE 1-4.   *(continued)*

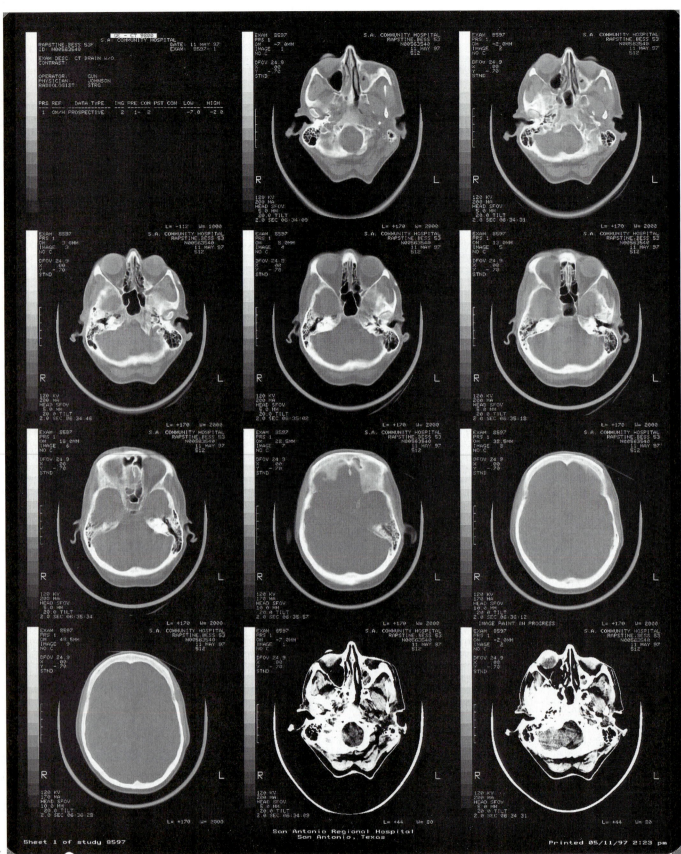

FIGURE 1-4. *(continued)*

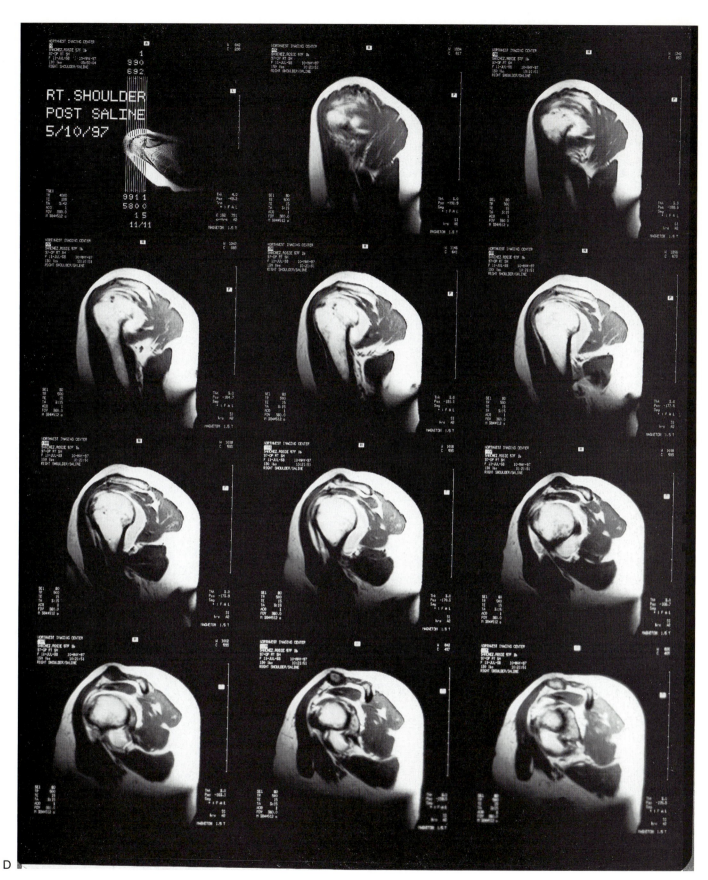

FIGURE 1-4. *(continued)*

tion is enough to allay anxiety. The radiologist depends on the technologist to explain the procedure; unless you encounter a situation that you feel will infringe upon the efficacy of the examination, you need not inform the radiologist of every detail.

B. Assessment of Patient Condition (e.g., Motor Control, Severity of Injury)

Careful assessment of the patient's condition is a crucial first step in your interaction with him. The severity of the patient's condition and his ability to ambulate, express discomfort, and comply with the demands of the examination must all be evaluated before proceeding. Never force a patient to assume a position that he states is unassumable. Modify positioning with the guidance of the radiologist, when possible.

The patient must be properly attired in order to produce radiographs free of artifact resulting from clothing, jewelry, or personal effects. The technologist should note how the patient is dressed and then give the patient dressing instructions in accordance with the needs of the examination. The part under examination must be free of any material that produces density on the radiograph **(Figure 1-5).** For example, a PAL chest examination for a female requires the patient to remove all clothing and jewelry from the waist up, and to don an examination gown with the opening to the back. Improper examination attire is a frequent cause of repeat examination; therefore, it is vital that the technologist give clear, concise instructions regarding dressing procedure.

The personal needs of the patients must be attended to. A patient may have a specimen bag of urine or feces that needs to be collected, or the ambulatory patient may want to use the restroom. Be aware that some patients are being monitored for output of such specimens, and a mistaken disposal could invalidate the findings of a 24-hour collection.

Assuring the physical comfort of the patient will aid you in achieving a successful examination. Thin patients get cold easily and find hard tables difficult. Provide blankets and a pad, when possible. Patients with a productive cough or nausea should have appropriate receptacles within easy reach. Glasses, hearing aids, wallets, dentures, purses, jewelry, and other personal belongings are essential to the patient's everyday life. Special consideration should be given to these possessions, and their whereabouts made known to the patient.

Clinical observations made by the radiographer compare the actions and appearance of the present patient to previous patients she has encountered. An easily recognizable sign is skin color. The cyanotic patient exhibits a bluish skin coloration, which indicates lack of oxygen in the tissues. This symptom is most easily observed in the lips, lining of the mouth, or nail beds. Although chronically ill cardiac or pulmonary patients may exhibit these symptoms in their usual state, a patient who becomes cyanotic needs immediate medical attention

The condition of the skin must also be assessed. Elderly, bedridden patients often have decubitus ulcers, commonly called bedsores, which are the result of decreased circulation from lying in one position for too long a time. Decubitus ulcers may be minimized by turning the patient often.

Patients may have seizures while in the radiology department. The technologist should gently restrain the patient until the seizure passes, and then turn the patient on her side to prevent aspiration of vomitus or oral secretions.

Because of the redirection of air past the vocal cords, tracheotomy patients have difficulty speaking. A gurgling or rattling sound is an indication to the technologist of the need for suction. The utmost care must be applied when working with tracheotomies, because moving or dislodging them could result in an obstructed airway.

QUESTIONS FOR ASSESSMENT OF PATIENT CONDITION

select the best answer

1. A patient arrives in radiology on a stretcher, and is apparently unconscious. You are to obtain PAL chest radiographs. You should:

   (A) attempt to revive the patient.
   (B) assist the patient to a standing position.
   (C) modify the requested examination.
   (D) obtain assistance from another technologist.

2. A patient arrives for lumbar spine examination on a busy day and informs you that he/she needs to use the restroom. You should:

   (A) allow him/her to use the facilities.
   (B) inform the patient that the department is very busy and ask him/her to wait.
   (C) tell the patient nothing and assist him/her onto the table.
   (D) check with the patient's nurse.

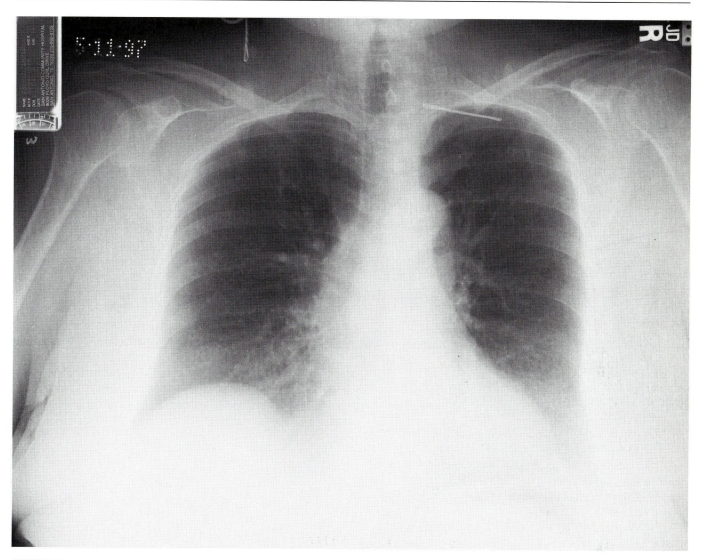

FIGURE 1-5. This PA chest exam had to be repeated because the patient had hairpins overlying the area of interest.

3. A patient's tracheostomy tube makes a rattling sound. This indicates:

   (A) the need for suction.
   (B) the tracheostomy is dislodged.
   (C) the tube must be changed.
   (D) the physician must be alerted.

4. Cyanosis is an indication of:

   (A) osteoporosis.
   (B) end-stage renal disease.
   (C) lack of oxygen to the tissues.
   (D) hypovolemia.

5. Decubitus ulcers:

   (A) may be minimized by frequent turning.
   (B) are commonly called bedsores.

   (C) are caused by lack of oxygen to tissue.
   (D) are all of the aforementioned.

───────────────────────

▶▶ **ANSWERS FOR ASSESSMENT OF PATIENT CONDITION**

1. The answer is (C). An unconscious patient will never stand or be able to cooperate for standard PAL views. Typically, the examination will be modified in a manner that is correlated with the clinical situation, at the direction of the department supervisor. This individual will notify the radiologist of the change.

2. The answer is (D). Although the technologist should be aware of the workload and the need

for an orderly flow of patients, the needs of the patient must come first. Some patients are undergoing monitoring of urinary output; therefore, the need to take an appropriate measurement, or send the specimen back with the patient, must be evaluated.

3. The answer is (A). A rattling or gurgling sound is an indication of accumulated secretions that should be suctioned.

4. The answer is (C). A bluish tint, especially in the area of mucous membranes, is a sign of cyanosis, a condition brought on by lack of oxygen to the tissues. Long-term cardiac or pulmonary patients may exhibit this symptom chronically.

5. The correct answer is (D). The technologist should be aware of patients who have decubitus ulcers so that appropriate protective measures, such as increased padding and gentle positioning, may be used. The ulcers are a result of decreased oxygen flow to an area due to pressure. When this condition exists, the centers of the affected cells die first, and then ulcers form.

C. Proper Body Mechanics for Patient Transfer

The principles of body movement, alignment, and balance are known as body mechanics. In order to assure the personal safety of both patient and radiographer, the proper application of these principles is essential.

Body mechanics may be broadly summarized by a few simple rules:

- Establish a stable base of support by standing with feet apart and one foot slightly forward.
- Keep loads well balanced and reduce strain to a minimum by maintaining carried items as close to the body as possible.
- Keep the back straight, avoid twisting or turning when lifting. Bend your knees and lift by using the muscles in your thighs (quadriceps) and abdomen (rectus abdominis and external obliques).
- Reduce overhead lifting by maintaining work at a comfortable level. Use stools and ladders when necessary.
- Push rather than pull heavy objects.

Before transferring any patient, ensure that the pertinent information on the radiographic request form matches the patient wrist identification bracelet. Next, speak with and assess the patient, in order to determine the extent to which the patient will be able to assist with the transfer. Moving extremely heavy or unstable patients may require another person.

For a bed-to-wheelchair transfer, lower the bed to the level of the chair, if possible. Raise the head of the bed. Place the chair parallel to the bed, with wheels locked and footrests raised. Placing one arm behind the patient's shoulders and the other under the knees, raise the patient to a sitting position in a single smooth motion. Allow the patient a moment to adapt to the new position.

Next, stand facing the patient. Place both hands on his/her scapulae, allowing his/her hands on your shoulders. Give the patient a signal, usually a 1-2-3 count, and raise him/her to a standing position. Pivot a quarter turn, so that the seat of the wheelchair touches the patient's knees. Ease the patient to a sitting position.

To transfer from the chair to the radiographic examination table, begin with the chair parallel to the table, wheels locked, and footrests raised. Stand the patient as explained previously. Next, have the patient place one hand on your shoulder and another on a stool handle. Assist the patient to step up on the stool and pivot him/her simultaneously. Once the patient is seated, place one arm behind the shoulders and one under the knees as previously described and lay him/her down in a single motion.

A stretcher should be used to transport patients who are unable to stand. Again, assessing the patient in advance of the transfer will aid the radiographer in determining the amount of assistance required. The transfer should begin with the stretcher being placed parallel with the bed and at the same height, with the wheels locked. The patient should be instructed to flex his/her knees and place the feet flat. For the technologist working alone, lean across the stretcher with one hand under the patient's head, and the other under the pelvis. On the technologist's signal, usually a 1-2-3 count, the patient pushes with his/her elbows and feet as the technologist lifts and pulls. When this maneuver is accomplished with two technologists, one person handles the head, neck, and shoulders, and the second is responsible for the pelvis and knees.

A variation of this technique uses the draw sheet, a single sheet folded in half, which is placed under the patient's midsection. The sides of the draw sheet are rolled and used as handholds to maneuver the patient into position. When three individuals are available to help with this type of transfer, generally two will stand on the destination side, either the bed or radiograph table, with the third lifting and guiding the opposite side. It is imperative that the patient be instructed to lift his/her head and feet so that these body parts are not injured during the move. If he/she is not able to lift, more help should be sought to assist with these areas.

first, and then the remainder of the body is moved.

QUESTIONS FOR PROPER BODY MECHANICS FOR PATIENT TRANSFER

select the best answer

1. The principles of body movement, balance, and alignment are known as:

   (A) kinetics.
   (B) patient transfer rules.
   (C) body mechanics.
   (D) none of the aforementioned.

2. The best way to move a stretcher-bound paraplegic onto a radiograph table is using:

   (A) more than one person.
   (B) draw-sheet techniques.
   (C) a single smooth motion to sit the patient up.
   (D) the strong muscles in your legs.

3. You encounter an unconscious patient for an abdominal examination. The first thing you should do is:

   (A) get a lot of help to move the patient.
   (B) see if a draw sheet is available.
   (C) attempt to revive the patient.
   (D) check the patient's wrist identification band.

4. In order to transfer a patient to a wheelchair, the chair should:

   1. be parallel with the bed.
   2. have the wheels locked.
   3. be in good working order.
   4. have the footrests raised.

   (A) All of the aforementioned
   (B) Choices 2 and 3
   (C) Choice 1 only
   (D) Choice 4 only

5. When two persons are moving a patient from bed to stretcher:

   (A) one guides the head, and the other guides the feet.
   (B) two persons are not enough for stretcher transfer.
   (C) one guides the head, neck, and shoulders; the other guides the pelvis and knees.
   (D) they pull the head of the patient across

▶▶ ANSWERS FOR PROPER BODY MECHANICS FOR PATIENT TRANSFER

1. The answer is (C). Collectively, these standards are known as body mechanics.
2. The best answer is (B). Although the other answers are important rules to remember, a stretcher-bound patient is usually best moved via a draw sheet or Plexiglas sliding board.
3. The answer is (D). You should always check the patient's identification band before proceeding with anything.
4. The answer is (A). All of these conditions should be met before using a wheelchair to move a patient.
5. The correct answer is (C). With two individuals, the best way to divide the patient is into roughly equal halves, with all portions being supported equally.

D. Patient Privacy, Safety, and Comfort

The use of strategically positioned radiolucent sponges and positioning devices will promote patient cooperation, because they allow the patient a higher degree of comfort. Unless it interferes with the examination, place a pillow or sponge under the patient's head in order to reduce neck strain and allow the patient to view what you are doing. A raised head also permits easier breathing. Additionally, sponges placed underneath the knees reduce lordotic curvature, thereby minimizing lower back pain, particularly in elderly and arthritic patients. Sponges placed under various bony prominences like the heels or ischial tuberosities are also of value.

Disoriented or unstable patients may require restraints that generally consist of cloth and Velcro wrist and ankle devices, generally tied to the stretcher, and applied before arriving in radiology. Restraints must be ordered by a physician. The radiographer may never leave a restrained patient unattended.

Uncooperative children may occasionally need to be restrained, although it is preferable to obtain their confidence before resorting to physical immobilization. Prefabricated devices exist for this purpose, such as the pig-o-stat, an apparatus used for pediatric chest radiographs. Other well-known methods, such as the papoose wrap, which uses a baby blanket to wrap the child, are used also. Stockinette may also be used to confine the child's arms above the head, or hold the legs in place.

Wheelchairs are equipped with footrests, armrests, and wheel locks, and as a point of safety these features should be employed without exception. Similarly, stretchers have safety straps or belts as well as side rails that must be used during patient transport.

The patient's sense of modesty must be considered. Patients are supplied with adequately sized gowns to cover the body. Obese individuals may require two gowns, one for the front, and one for the back. Patients should be kept covered with a sheet or blanket whenever practical. Keep in mind that radiographic rooms tend to be cold, especially to scantily clad patients.

The patient's right to privacy must be given consideration. There may be situations, for example, when an immobilized patient may need a bedpan or urinal during the course of the examination. The radiographer should inquire whether the patient needs assistance, and if not, the radiographer should discreetly leave the room for a few moments. There may also be times when a patient will receive distressing news regarding his/her health while in your care. Your ability to evaluate the situation will grow with experience, but radiographers should realize that there will be occasions when the patient's mental status, comfort, and right to privacy will take priority over speedy completion of the examination.

QUESTIONS FOR PATIENT PRIVACY, SAFETY, AND COMFORT

select the best answer

1. Which of the following would you consider the best policy regarding the restraint of pediatric patients for radiographic examination?

    (A) Always restrain them
    (B) Never restrain them
    (C) Use only approved restraint devices
    (D) Restrain only when other alternatives fail

2. The radiologic technologist can facilitate a lumbar spine examination by increasing the patient's comfort level by:

    (A) requesting pain medicine for the patient.
    (B) placing a pad or sponge under the patient's knees.
    (C) limiting the examination to anteroposterior (AP) and lateral views.

    (D) performing the examination as rapidly as possible.

3. What must be present in order for an adult patient to be restrained?

    (A) A stated or perceived threat to the patient or hospital staff
    (B) A request from a family member
    (C) A physician's order
    (D) Approved restraining equipment

4. A stretcher with only one working side rail:

    (A) must be repaired before use for patient transport.
    (B) may be used for moderately impaired patients.
    (C) may be used as a substitute for a wheelchair.
    (D) must be thrown out.

5. A young woman comes into radiology via the ER, having been in a motor vehicle accident. She is conscious but has a fractured left femur. She experiences the onset of her menstrual cycle during the course of your examination and does not have needed supplies. As a male technologist, you should:

    (A) explain that the nurse in the ER will take care of her when she returns.
    (B) find the appropriate supplies and female personnel to assist.
    (C) explain that the seriousness of her injury outweighs a small discomfort.
    (D) attempt to assist her yourself.

▶▶ ANSWERS FOR PATIENT PRIVACY, SAFETY, AND COMFORT

1. The answer is (D). It is always preferable to try to gain the child's confidence and cooperation whenever possible.

2. The best answer is (B). A pad underneath the knees reduces the lordotic curvature, thus lessening the strain on the patient. The technologist may not independently limit the examination or order medicine, and an examination done too rapidly will be prone to error, and may be difficult for a patient to tolerate.

3. The answer is (C). Adults may only be restrained by order of a physician.

4. The answer is (A). For use with patients, a stretcher must be completely functional.

5. The answer is (B). The patient's needs and right to privacy must be taken into account.

III. PREVENTION AND CONTROL OF INFECTION
A. Transmission of Infection

Microorganisms are infectious organisms too small to be seen with the naked eye. Bacteria, fungi, and viruses are all examples of microorganisms. **Pathogens** are organisms capable of causing disease.

For infection to occur, four conditions must be present. The presence of the organism is the first condition. Second, a reservoir, or source, in which the organism can thrive and multiply must be present. Third, there must be a host organism that is susceptible to the infection. Last, there must be a means of transmitting the infection. These four conditions may be collectively referred to as the **cycle of infection (Figure 1-6).**

There are four primary routes for the transmission of an infectious organism:

- **Direct contact:** This route of transmission occurs when the host organism is touched by the carrier. In hospitals, skin infections are one common manifestation of direct contact transmission, occurring when the hospital worker comes in contact with a patient who has staphylococcus or streptococcus infection.
- **Fomites:** A fomite is an object that has had direct contact with a pathogenic organism. Common fomites in the hospital include the radiograph table, Foley catheters, chest tubes, or bandages.
- **Vectors:** A vector is any animal whose body acts as a reservoir for the multiplication or

maturation of an infectious organism. For example, dogs are vectors who carry rabies, and mosquitoes are vectors that carry malaria.
- **Airborne contamination:** Airborne contamination occurs via droplets, as in the case of a sneezing or coughing patient, or by means of dust, onto which spore-forming organisms may attach themselves until the opportunity arises to invade a host organism. Spore-type organisms are responsible for many potentially lethal conditions, including tetanus, gangrene, and septicemia.

An infection acquired in the hospital environment is called a **nosocomial** infection. Common examples of nosocomial infections include urinary tract, wound, and respiratory tract infections.

QUESTIONS FOR TRANSMISSION OF INFECTION

select the best answer

1. During the course of a portable chest examination for a patient who has a diagnosis of viral pneumonia, the most likely means of infection transmission to the radiographer would be:
    1. vector.
    2. fomite.
    3. direct contact.
    4. air contamination.
   (A) Choice 4 only
   (B) Choices 2 and 4
   (C) Choice 2 only
   (D) Choice 3 only

2. An example of a microorganism is a:
   (A) virus.
   (B) fungus.
   (C) bacteria.
   (E) all of the above.

3. The place where an infection may thrive and multiply is known as a:
   (A) host.
   (B) reservoir.
   (C) vector.
   (D) pathogen.

4. A nosocomial infection is one that:
   (A) is acquired from a friend or loved one.
   (B) is non communicable.

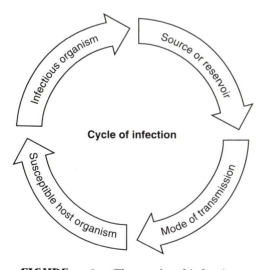
FIGURE 1-6.   The cycle of infection.

(C) is acquired in the hospital setting.
(D) presents no danger to the patient.

▶▶ ANSWERS TO TRANSMISSION OF INFECTION

1. The answer is (B). The likelihood of contamination from a patient who has this diagnosis via coughing is great; however, during the course of a portable chest examination, the radiographer must come into contact with a great many fomites (e.g., the patient's bed, linen, and clothing) in order to accomplish the examination. The likelihood of direct contact with infectious mucus or mucous membrane is possible, but not probable. Therefore, air contamination and fomites best fulfill the conditions of this question.
2. The answer is (D). Viruses, bacteria, and fungi are all examples of microorganisms.
3. The answer is (B). There are absolute conditions necessary for infection to occur. They are: The infectious organism must exist; there must be a host organism susceptible to the infection; there must be a means of transmittal; and there must be a place for the organism to thrive and multiply, which is known as a reservoir.
4. The answer is (C). A nosocomial infection is obtained in the hospital setting.

B. Universal Precautions

Radiographers have daily direct patient contact and are considered to be at high risk for occupational exposure to infectious microorganisms. Of particular concern are human immunodeficiency virus (**HIV**), autoimmune deficiency syndrome (**AIDS**), and hepatitis B virus (**HBV**) infection.

Studies have indicated that HIV may be transmitted only via direct contact with body fluids of the infected individual. Infection occurs through direct sexual contact, the sharing of contaminated needles, transfusion of contaminated blood, or transmission from an HIV–infected mother to her child. HIV assaults the immune system, and may live in dry blood for 1 to 4 hours.

HBV is a bloodborne pathogen that primarily affects the liver. It may live in dry blood for up to 1 week. **Table 1-1** lists the various body fluids that may contain bloodborne pathogens.

Patients afflicted with infectious microorganisms may not exhibit symptoms, making it impossible for health care workers to determine whether a patient is infected or not. For this reason, health care facilities

▶ TABLE 1.1. Various Body Fluids that May Contain Bloodborne Pathogens

Blood	Synovial fluid
Urine	Pericardial fluid
Saliva	Tears
Semen	Mucous secretions (nasal, oral)
Vaginal secretions	
Sweat	Breast milk
Cerebrospinal fluid	Feces
Peritoneal fluid	

now practice **universal precautions (Table 1-2)** to prevent the spread of disease to other patients and health care workers. Universal precautions is a concept that treats all body fluids or substances as if they were infectious. A radiographer practicing universal precautions considers every patient a potential source of infection.

The Occupational Health and Safety Administration (**OSHA**) is the federal regulatory agency responsible for setting and maintaining workplace standards for health care workers. The statute that governs occupational exposure of health care workers to toxic and hazardous substances, specifically blood and other potentially infectious materials, is **Federal Register 1910.1030**, often called the **bloodborne pathogens standard.** This standard provides that: "Universal precautions shall be observed to prevent contact with blood or other potentially infectious

▶ TABLE 1.2. Guidelines for Universal Precautions

- Provide face shields when the possibility of blood or fluid splash to the area of the face exists
- Wear gloves when touching body fluids or contaminated surfaces
- Wear protective aprons when splash hazard to clothing exists
- Change gloves and wash hands after every patient interaction
- Body fluid spills are cleaned with a solution of 1:10 bleach and water solution
- CPR equipment must include mouthpieces and resuscitation bags
- Needles are never recapped or separated from the syringe, and are disposed of in appropriately marked sharps containers

materials. Under circumstances in which differentiation between body fluid types is difficult or impossible, all body fluids shall be considered potentially infectious materials . . . ."

Important employer responsibilities governed by standard 1910.1030 include: Determining if an employee is **high risk** for occupational exposure; enforcing **universal precautions**; providing **employee training, HBV inoculations,** and **personal protective equipment;**, and maintenance of an **exposure control plan.**

QUESTIONS FOR UNIVERSAL PRECAUTIONS

select the best answer

1. All of the following are employer responsibilities to health care workers under the bloodborne pathogens statute (OSHA document 1910.1030) except:
   (A) risk determination.
   (B) monthly HIV testing.
   (C) exposure control plan.
   (D) HBV inoculation.

2. Which of the following personal protective items should a radiographer wear when performing a barium enema examination?
   (A) Gloves only
   (B) Gloves and protective gown
   (C) Gloves, protective gown, mask
   (D) Gloves, protective gown, mask, and protective eyewear

3. HBV has its primary effect on the:
   (A) blood.
   (B) respiratory system.
   (C) immune system.
   (D) liver.

4. HIV may be transmitted in all of the following ways except:
   (A) transfusions.
   (B) giving birth.
   (C) sharing drinking water.
   (D) sharing needles.

5. Which of the following radiographic procedures carry the risk of exposure to bloodborne pathogens?
   1. Arthrography
   2. Myelography
   3. Endoscopic retrograde cholangiopancreatography (ERCP)
   4. UGI
   (A) Choices 1 and 3
   (B) Choices 2 and 4
   (C) All of the aforementioned
   (D) None of the aforementioned

6. While in the radiology department, a patient has an episode of hematemesis. The body fluids are on the floor and radiograph table. The proper material to use for cleanup is which of the following?
   (A) 1:10 solution of bleach and water
   (B) 1:10 solution of povidone-iodine and water
   (C) Disinfectant spray
   (D) Rubbing alcohol

▶▶ ANSWERS TO UNIVERSAL PRECAUTIONS

1. The answer is (C). An employee who sustained occupational exposure to known HIV-positive body fluids would be tested, and an occupationally exposed employee may request and then receive testing even if the exposure source tests negative. However, the statute does not provide for monthly HIV testing for employees. Risk determination, the availability of HBV vaccine, and a known exposure control plan are required by law.

2. The answer is (B). Although the remote possibility exists of exposure to the mucous membranes of the eyes, nose, and mouth, the radiographer's primary concern in this situation is to keep his/her hands from direct contact with body fluids, and to protect his/her clothing from contamination.

3. The answer is (D). Although transmitted by blood, the hepatitis B virus damages the liver. Studies indicate over 1 million Americans have chronic hepatitis B, and are therefore potential transmitters of the disease.

4. The answer is (C). Inanimate objects such as glasses, water fountains, toilet seats, and telephones will not transmit HIV.

5. The answer is (C). Arthrography is associated with exposure to synovial fluid; myelography is associated with cerebrospinal fluid; and ERCP and UGI examinations are associated with mucous secretions from the biliary and gastrointestinal tract.

6. The answer is (A). The proper material for cleanup of body fluid spills is a solution of 1 part bleach to 10 parts water.

C. Disinfection and Sterilization: Asepsis and Sterile Technique

Antiseptics are materials that retard the growth of bacteria. Isopropyl alcohol is an example of an antiseptic.

Medical sepsis is a method that both reduces the number of infectious microorganisms being transmitted to a susceptible host and intervenes in the process by which they spread.

Surgical asepsis is the complete removal of all organisms and their spores from equipment used to perform patient care.

Radiographers can avoid transmitting infection by simple **cleanliness** measures. These measures include hand washing, proper handling of linen, cleaning equipment, and dusting. **Hand washing** is the single most important measure of aseptic technique. **Disinfection** is the process of destruction of pathogenic organisms by chemical means. Common disinfectants are hydrogen peroxide, boric acid, and bleach. **Sterilization** is the process of making items germ-free by treatment with gas, heat, or chemicals, and then storing these items in a manner that prevents contamination.

Medical asepsis is always required for radiography in general, but surgical asepsis must be employed for radiographic invasive procedures, such as myelography or angiography. **Table 1-3** presents the five methods of sterilization.

Radiographers must be acquainted with sterile technique. To assemble the needed materials for a surgical procedure such as a biopsy, the radiographer must:

- Place the surgical pack on a clean surface, usually a designated stand.
- Break the seal, opening the first fold away from you. Next, unfold the two sides. Last, open the fold toward you, and drop it. Take care to avoid touching the inner surface. If there is an inner wrap, open it in the same manner. The sterile field is now established.
- To add double-wrapped items to the field, hold the item in the non-dominant hand, open the first fold away from you, grasp the free edges with the other hand, and drop the item onto the tray.
- To add items like gloves in peel-down wraps, grasp the top of the package and peel down. Invert the package and drop it onto the tray.
- To add liquid, such as povidone-iodine, dispose

TABLE 1.3. Five Methods of Sterilization

Chemical: Immersion of clean objects into germicidal solution. Effectiveness dependent on solution concentration, temperature, and length of time in solution. Contamination of solution is difficult to determine. Not recommended for instruments that require surgical asepsis.

Boiling: Sterilization by complete immersion in boiling water for 12 minutes. Rarely used, except when instruments are needed in a hurry. Certain microorganisms are resistant to this method, making it unacceptable for use in surgery.

Dry heat: Used when moist heat is inadvisable. Time required varies from 1 to 6 minutes; temperature range varies from 329° to 338°F (165°–170°C).

Gas: Usually a mixture of ethylene oxide and Freon. Used primarily for electrical, plastic, and rubber items, such as scopes, BP cuffs, telephones, and stethoscopes. Gas must be dissipated by means of aeration in a controlled environment, which is a time-consuming process.

Autoclaving: Steam sterilization under pressure. Quickest and most convenient of methods. Color-coded indicators are used inside and outside of packages to ensure that sterile conditions have been achieved.

of the first few drops, thus washing the lip of the bottle, and then pour the needed amount into the receptacle on the tray. If the physician is present, show him the bottle.

Technologists who assist with sterile procedures are required to work within the sterile field itself, and therefore must wear sterile gloves in order to handle the equipment without compromising the field. Gloving procedures are as follows:

- Wash your hands.
- Open the outer wrapper.
- Open the inner wrap, touching only the outside portion, with the cuff ends facing you.
- Put on the first glove, touching only the inner surface of the cuff.
- Grasp second glove under the cuff.
- Put on second glove and unfold cuff.
- Unfold first cuff.

These standard rules apply to all sterile procedures:

- Any sterile field or object touched by a nonsterile person or object is contaminated.
- Never reach across a sterile field.
- Any object suspected of contamination should be discarded.
- Never pass between the physician and sterile field.
- The area between the draped patient and the instrument table is known as the sterile corridor, which should be occupied by only the physician and the primary assistant, who are properly gloved and gowned.
- Never leave the sterile field unattended.

QUESTIONS FOR DISINFECTION AND STERILIZATION: ASEPSIS AND STERILE TECHNIQUE

select the best answer

1. Which kind of solution is considered an antiseptic?

    (A) Isopropyl alcohol
    (B) Povidone-iodine
    (C) Sterile water
    (D) 1:10 bleach and water solution

2. Which of the following best describes the complete removal of pathogenic organisms from an object?

    (A) Sterile corridor
    (B) Surgical asepsis
    (C) Scrubbing in
    (D) Medical asepsis

3. The single most important measure of aseptic technique is which of the following?

    (A) Hand washing
    (B) Scrubbing in
    (C) Establishing the sterile corridor
    (D) Wearing sterile gloves

4. While opening various materials for a sterile biopsy tray, you notice that one of the biopsy needles has been partially opened. You should:

    (A) inform the physician.
    (B) check the date on the package.
    (C) discard the needle in a sharps container.
    (D) send the item to central supply for re-sterilization.

5. The major drawback of gas sterilization is which of the following?

    (A) Expense
    (B) Time
    (C) Number of personnel required
    (D) None of the aforementioned

6. Autoclaving a surgical instrument can be best described as:

    (A) complete immersion in boiling water for 12 to 15 minutes.
    (B) steam sterilization under pressure.
    (C) the use of dry heat at extreme temperatures.
    (D) a mixture of freon and ethylene oxide under pressure.

▶▶ ANSWERS TO DISINFECTION AND STERILIZATION: ASEPSIS AND STERILE TECHNIQUE

1. The answer is (A). Isopropyl alcohol is an example of an antiseptic, a material that retards the growth of bacteria. Povidone-iodine and 1:10 bleach and water solutions are disinfectants, materials that destroy pathogenic organisms. Sterile water has neither antiseptic nor disinfectant properties.
2. The answer is (B). The complete removal of pathogenic organisms and their spores from an object is surgical asepsis, whereas medical asepsis is a method that reduces the number of infectious microorganisms being transmitted to a susceptible host as well as intervening in the process by which they spread.
3. The answer is (A). The single most important factor of aseptic technique is hand washing. The technologist's job requires a series of brief contacts with a series of patients; he/she must always wash hands before and after each interaction.
4. The answer is (C). Never use an item on a sterile tray that has been opened. Although some larger instruments—biopsy guns, for example—are reused, needles are used only once.
5. The answer is (B). Gas sterilization, while effective, requires dissipation of the material by aeration, which is a time-consuming process.
6. The answer is (B). The most convenient and frequently used method of sterilization is autoclaving—steam sterilization under pressure.

D. Handling Biohazardous Materials

Biohazardous materials can be described as objects or substances encountered in the health-care workplace that may endanger the health of the health-care worker. There are two types of biohazardous materials: The first type is biomedical waste, including body substances and associated equipment, such as sharps, chest tubes, intravenous (IV) tubes, and urinary catheters. Universal precautions must be used in handling these materials. Gloves should be worn when handling urinals, bedpans, bandages, or dressings. Urinals and bedpans should be emptied at once, and then either disposed of or returned to the patient after cleaning. Bandages and dressings must be placed in waterproof biohazard bags.

Sharps must be disposed of in approved sharps containers, preferably without recapping. The majority of reported finger punctures occur during needle recapping. If a needle must be recapped, use a one-handed technique, placing the needle cover on a hard surface, and guide the syringe into it. Other biomedical waste is packaged in specially marked, impermeable bags and removed from the premises by a biomedical waste company.

Contaminated linen is handled in a similar manner. Never use any linen for more than one patient. The linen should be handled as little as possible, folding it carefully and never shaking it before placing it in a marked, reinforced linen bag.

The second type of biohazardous materials are non-biomedical substances such as developer and fixer, as well as common office supplies such as toner, white-out, and glass cleaner. A health care worker may expect to come into contact with these materials in the course of his/her duties, and a potential for health risk exists as a result.

Interactions with these types of substances by workers are governed by OSHA Hazard Communication Standard 1910.1200, which is commonly known as the **Emergency Planning and Community Right to Know Act.** The central idea of this legislation is that workers have a right to information about potentially dangerous substances they may come into contact with at work. The information must be posted in an easily accessible location in the workplace, called the **right to know station.**

Material safety data sheets found within the station provide information about substances in the workplace that are potentially harmful. **Table 1-4** shows a portion of one of these sheets, which identifies 2.4% aqueous glutaraldehyde solution (CIDEX so-

> **TABLE 1.4.** Portion of a Material Safety Data Sheet for Hydroquinone

Common Name: Hydroquinone
CAS Number: 123-31-9
DOT Number: UN 2662
Date: January, 1989

HAZARD SUMMARY
* Hydroquinone can affect you when breathed in.
* Because this is a MUTAGEN, handle it as a possible cancer-causing substance WITH EXTREME CAUTION.
* Exposure can irritate and may burn the eyes. Contact can irritate the skin, and may cause a rash.
* Repeated exposure can cause discoloration of the skin, eyes, and inner eyelids. Over years this can cause clouding of the eyes and permanently damage vision.
* Hydroquinone is a very toxic poison if swallowed; poisoning does not seem to occur from exposure to dust or vapor.

IDENTIFICATION
Hydroquinone is a white, tan to gray crystalline material. It is used in photographic developers, in making dyes, and in paints, motor fuels, soil, polymers, and medicines.

REASON FOR CITATION
* Hydroquinone is on the Hazardous Substance List because it is regulated by OSHA and cited by ACGIH, DOT, NIOSH, DEP, NFPA and EPA.
* This chemical is on the Special Health Hazard Substance List because it is a MUTAGEN.
* Definitions are attached.

lution) as one of these hazardous substances. Hydroquinone is a white or tan to gray crystalline material. It is used in photographic developers, paints, motor fuels, soil, polymers, and medicines, and also in making dyes.

QUESTIONS FOR HANDLING OF BIOHAZARDOUS MATERIALS

select the best answer

1. Body fluids obtained from medical equipment can be best described as which of the following?

(A) Mutagens
(B) Carcinogens
(C) Contaminated
(D) Biomedical waste

2. The Emergency Planning and Community Right to Know Act is primarily concerned with:

(A) disposal of contaminated waste.
(B) disposal of nuclear waste.
(C) providing information about emergencies.
(D) providing information about hazardous materials.

3. The proper protective attire to be worn when cleaning up after a lumbar puncture would be:

(A) gloves only.
(B) gloves and gown.
(C) nothing.
(D) gloves, gown, and mask.

4. Where would a technologist find biohazard information about glutaraldehyde?

(A) Processor manual
(B) Material safety data sheet
(C) Infection control nurse
(D) Risk manager

▶▶ ANSWERS FOR HANDLING OF BIOHAZARDOUS MATERIALS

1. The answer is (D). The two types of biohazardous material are biomedical and non-biomedical.
2. The answer is (D). The primary purpose of the Emergency Planning and Community Right to Know Act is to make information regarding potentially harmful materials accessible to workers.
3. The answer is (A). Once the technologist is acquainted with universal precautions procedures, correct attire is largely a matter of common sense. Cleaning after a lumbar puncture is a simple affair, requiring disposal of the tray, cleaning the table, and changing linen.
4. The answer is (B). Although either the hospital risk manager or the processor manual may have information regarding glutaraldehyde, the important fact for the technologist to remember is that material safety data sheets are a central resource for biohazard information.

E. Isolation Procedures

Interaction with patients isolated from the general patient population requires specific knowledge about the type of isolation involved, and which protective measures to take as a result. There are five main categories of isolation.

Respiratory isolation is required for patients who are infected with a disease spread by **droplet contact,** that is, disease transmitted by means of coughing or sneezing. The patient must be placed in a private room. Measles, mumps, and meningitis are examples of diseases spread via droplet contact. Technologists should wear a mask, gown, and gloves when interacting with these patients.

Acid-fast bacillus (AFB) isolation is used with patients who are infected with tuberculosis (TB). AFB isolation patients require a private, specially ventilated room. With AFB isolation, a mask should be worn, but gown and gloves are required only if flagrant contamination is likely.

Methicillin-resistant *Staphylococcus aureus* (MRSA) isolation is used with patients who are infected with pathogens resistant to standard antibiotic therapy. Contact with MRSA patients requires diligent hand washing and glove wearing. **Vancomycin-resistant enterococcus** is another organism in this category.

Diseases such as conjunctivitis, herpes zoster, scabies, and impetigo are spread by direct or close contact; thus, these conditions require **contact isolation.** Masks, gowns, and gloves are required to interact with this patient group.

Protective, reverse, or neutropenic isolation are names for a type of isolation whose purpose is to protect the patient. Immunosuppressed patients, such as patients who have AIDS or bone marrow transplantation patients who are receiving immunosuppressant drugs, as well as burn patients, are more susceptible to infection; these patients are sometimes placed on this type of isolation.

Special consideration must be given to radiography of the isolation patient. When transporting contact isolation patients, two sheets must be used to cover the wheelchair or stretcher. The inner sheet is placed around the patient, which thus contaminates the sheet, and the outer sheet is used to move the patient.

The radiography room should be available immediately for isolation patients, thus avoiding the spread of infection by having such a patient wait in a hallway or waiting area. Two technologists should be available. The first, dressed in protective attire, will position the patient, and the second technologist adjusts the controls to make the exposure. The patient is returned to his room by wrapping him in the same manner as previously described. All linen should be disposed of in designated bags; the radiograph table should be disinfected; and hands should be thoroughly washed after completing the procedure.

Mobile radiography of some selected isolation patients also necessitates a two-man approach. As discussed previously, one technologist positions the patient, and one operates the controls, but both are gowned and gloved. The cassette is dropped inside a protective plastic bag or pillowcase; one technologist positions it, and the other operates the portable unit. After the exposure is made, the positioning technologist opens the protective cover and allows the control technologist to remove the cassette. All protective attire is disposed of in appropriate containers just inside the doorway. Once outside the room, hands should be washed, and the mobile unit should be thoroughly disinfected. Hands should be washed again after finishing this task.

QUESTIONS FOR ISOLATION PROCEDURES

select the best answer

1. Which type of isolation may require that the patient be placed in a specially ventilated room?

    1. Respiratory
    2. Contact
    3. Protective
    4. AFB

    (A) Choice 1 only
    (B) Choice 2 only
    (C) Choices 1, 3, and 4
    (D) All of the aforementioned

2. The highest incidence of infection transmission can be attributed to which of the following?

    (A) Hands
    (B) Improper sterilization
    (C) Droplet contact
    (D) Improper linen disposal

3. Which type of isolation has as its primary purpose the protection of the patient?

    (A) Burn
    (B) Reverse
    (C) Universal
    (D) Contact

4. When is the best time of day to bring an isolation patient to the radiology department for a procedure?

    (A) First thing in the morning
    (B) Last patient of the day
    (C) Slowest part of the day
    (D) Lunch time

5. Performing portable chest radiography of isolation patients can be best described as:

    (A) best done with two technologists, one operating the controls, the other positioning the patient.
    (B) best done with one technologist, which minimizes the number of health care personnel to whom the patient is exposed.
    (C) best done with two technologists, one wearing protective attire, the other operating the controls.
    (D) best done when the patient is placed in a specially ventilated room.

▶▶ ANSWERS TO ISOLATION PROCEDURES

1. The answer is (C). All methods except contact may require a specially ventilated room.
2. The answer is (A). The most common means of spreading infection is via human hands. Hand washing is the most effective method of reducing the spread of infection.
3. The answer is (B). Reverse or protective isolation measures are taken primarily to protect an immunocompromised patient from infection.
4. The answer is (C). An isolation patient should always be brought to the department when there is an available room, in order to minimize his/her time in the department, thus reducing the chance of spreading infection.
5. The answer is (A). When strict isolation patients must be examined with a mobile unit, only one technologist should have physical contact with the patient, and he/she must not operate the unit. Another technologist makes the exposure; then protective attire is left in the appropriate container just inside the door of the room, hands are washed, and the machine is disinfected immediately after the technologists have left the room.

IV. PATIENT MONITORING
A. Routine Monitoring

Monitoring of the patient has traditionally been regarded as the province of nursing, but the technologist must be able to perform routine monitoring of the patient as well.

▶ **TABLE 1.5.**   Average Normal Adult
Temperatures

Oral	Rectal	Axillary	Esophageal	Forehead
37°C	37.5°C	36.5°C	37.3°C	34.4°C
98.6°F	99.5°F	97.6°F	99.2°F	94°F

Measurements of a patient's temperature, pulse, respiration, and blood pressure are known as **vital signs.** The term **cardinal signs** may also be used. Changes in vital signs reflect the functioning of key body systems; therefore, accurate assessment of vital signs is essential.

A patient's temperature is generally assessed by placing a **thermometer** in one of four locations. By placing the thermometer in the patient's mouth, **oral temperature** is obtained; in the rectal canal, **rectal temperature;** in the axilla, **axillary temperature;** and in the esophagus, **core temperature.** Body temperature is maintained by the **hypothalamus,** a structure located at the base of the brain. Elevation of normal body temperature is known as **pyrexia. Hyperpyrexia** is an extremely high temperature, usually above 105.8°F. Pyrexia is a common sign of illness, and evidence indicates that pyrexia helps the body fight disease. **Table 1-5** demonstrates average normal adult temperatures.

The patient who has a fever is said to be febrile. Symptoms of fever include flushed face; hot, dry skin; loss of appetite; thirst; headache; and general malaise. Potentially dangerous signs associated with fever are dehydration, rapid heart rate, and decreased urinary output. Survival of patients who have fever over 110°F is rare.

Body temperature below normal is called **hypothermia.** Death generally occurs when core temperature falls below 93.2°F; however, survival has been reported in isolated incidences at temperatures as low as 82.4°F.

The **glass thermometer** has two parts: the bulb, which contains liquid mercury, and the stem, along which measurements are taken. This type of instrument may be calibrated in either Celsius or Fahrenheit. Celsius thermometers are subdivided into increments of 0.1°, and Fahrenheit thermometers have gradients of 0.2°. Various **electronic thermometers** are also available. Most thermometer models measure the temperature in 25 to 50 seconds and give a digital readout of the finding, as do **automated monitoring devices,** which give continuous information regarding the patient's vital signs. Also available are **disposable, single-use thermometers** and **temperature-sensitive tape or patches.**

The **pulse rate** is the number of heart pulsations felt in a minute. The range for normal pulse varies with patient age and condition. A rapid heart rate is known as **tachycardia.** A slow rate is referred to as **bradycardia. Palpitation** means that the patient is aware of his own heart beating without having to feel for it over an artery. Stimulation of the **parasympathetic nervous system** slows the heart rate, whereas stimulation of the **sympathetic nervous system** will increase it.

The following conditions increase the pulse rate:

- Pain
- Strong emotion
- Exercise
- Prolonged exposure to heat
- Decreased blood pressure
- Elevated temperature
- Low blood oxygen concentration

Assessment of pulse is achieved by compressing an artery close to the skin surface against an underlying bone with the tips of the fingers. The most common site is the radial artery, located laterally in the wrist.

Other factors to consider are **pulse amplitude,** which is the fullness of the pulse that reflects the strength of ventricular contraction, and **pulse rhythm,** which is the pattern of pulsations and the rests between them. Irregular pulse rhythms are known as **arrhythmias** or **dysrhythmias. Table 1-6** presents average normal pulse rates for various age-groups.

Inspiration is the act of breathing in, and **expiration** is the act of breathing out. The number of respirations per minute is the **respiratory rate.** The average adult has a respiratory rate of 16 to 20 breaths

▶ **TABLE 1.6.**   Average Normal Pulse
Rates

Age	Approximate Range (bpm)	Approximate Average Rate (bpm)
Newborn to 1 mo	120–160	140
1–12 mo	80–140	120
1–2 yr	80–130	110
2–6 yr	75–120	100
6–12 yr	75–110	95
13 to adult	60–100	80

per minute. **Apnea** is the condition of no breathing, whereas **dyspnea** refers to labored breathing. Patients who have dyspnea generally breathe in a rapid, shallow manner. **Orthopnea** indicates the ability to breathe easier when an individual is in an upright position. **Cheyne-Stokes** breathing is an abnormal pattern of respiration—characterized by gradually increasing, then gradually decreasing, depth of respirations—followed by a period of apnea.

Adventitious sounds are abnormal breath sounds; there are several types. A **rale** is a crackling breathing sound, not unlike the sound of rice cereal in milk. A **rhonchus** is a gurgling breath sound, caused by secretion accumulation. A **wheeze** is a high-pitched labored breath sound, caused by constricted respiratory passages. A **friction rub** is a highly characteristic grating sound made by a dry pleural membrane moving over a lung.

The respiratory rate is obtained by observing the number of rises and falls (each rise and fall is considered one respiration) of a patient's chest for a period of 30 seconds, and multiplying that number of rises and falls by the number 2. If abnormal respirations are present, it is recommended that the patient be observed for a full minute. The procedure is usually done while the health care worker is taking the patient's pulse, which prevents awareness on the part of the patient that his/her respirations are being monitored (which could possibly alter the rate). A normal patient breathes 16 to 20 respirations per minute.

Blood pressure is the measure of force exerted on artery walls. Systolic pressure is a measurement of ventricular contraction, whereas diastolic pressure is a measurement of the heart at rest. Blood pressure is measured in millimeters of mercury (mm Hg) and expressed as a fraction; systolic pressure is the numerator, and diastolic pressure is the denominator. **Table 1-7** presents factors that influence blood pressure.

The condition of elevated blood pressure for a sustained period is known as **hypertension.** If the cause of hypertension is not known, it is called **primary, or essential hypertension;** when the hypertension is due to a known pathology, it is referred to as **secondary hypertension.** Blood pressure below

TABLE 1.7. Factors That Influence Blood Pressure

Age	Exercise
Time of day	Emotions
Gender	Posture (standing,
Nutritional status	sitting, and so on)

TABLE 1.8. Average Blood Pressures for Different Age-Groups

Age	Average Pressure
Newborn	40 mm systolic
1 mo	85/54 mm Hg
1 yr	95/65 mm Hg
6 yr	105/65 mm Hg
10–13 yr	110/65 mm Hg
14–17 yr	120/80 mm Hg
≥18	120/80 mm Hg

normal is called **hypotension.** Hypotension may be associated with weakness or fainting when an individual rises to an erect position, and in this case is referred to as **postural, or orthostatic, hypotension. Table 1-8** presents average blood pressures for different age-groups.

A **sphygmomanometer,** consisting of a **cuff** and a **manometer,** and a **stethoscope** are used to obtain blood pressure. The cuff contains an airtight rubber bladder encased in cloth, and attaches around the arm with Velcro, usually at the site of the brachial artery. There are two primary types of manometers: the mercury-filled tube calibrated in millimeters, and the circular, dial type, also calibrated in millimeters.

Auscultation is the process of listening for sounds within the body. The stethoscope is used to auscultate sound over the artery as pressure in the cuff is released and blood is permitted to flow. The sounds produced by this process are known as **Korotkoff sounds.**

QUESTIONS FOR ROUTINE MONITORING

select the best answer

1. An adult patient who has a systolic pressure of 160 could best be described as which of the following?
   (A) Hypertensive
   (B) Hypotensive
   (C) Orthostatic
   (D) Dysrhythmic

2. Which of the following medicines would be used to treat hyperpyrexia?
   (A) Penicillin
   (B) Acetylsalicylic acid
   (C) Vitamin C
   (D) NACL

3. The most comfortable position for a patient who has orthopnea would be which of the following?
   - (A) Sims'
   - (B) Fowler's
   - (C) Trendelenburg's
   - (D) Erect

4. An otherwise healthy patient experiences diaphoresis during the course of his UGI examination. You call the radiologist, and he instructs you to obtain the patient's pulse. The most appropriate sight would be which of the following?
   - (A) Popliteal artery
   - (B) Superior vena cava
   - (C) Radial artery
   - (D) Carotid artery

5. The systolic figure of blood pressure is properly expressed as the _____ in a fraction, and is an expression of _____.
   - (A) numerator, ventricular relaxation
   - (B) numerator, ventricular contraction
   - (C) denominator, ventricular fibrillation
   - (D) denominator, atrial contraction

▶▶ ANSWERS TO ROUTINE MONITORING

1. The answer is (A). The average adult systolic pressure is 120. The condition of elevated blood pressure is known as hypertension.
2. The answer is (B). Hyperpyrexia is the condition of extremely high fever, usually treated with acetylsalicylic acid, or aspirin.
3. The answer is (D). Patients who have dyspnea sometimes experience relief from symptoms when assuming an upright position. The condition is known as orthopnea.
4. The answer is (C). The most common site for palpation of the pulse is the radial artery in the wrist. The carotid, femoral, or popliteal arteries may be used as alternative site, but generally not in a healthy patient.
5. The answer is (A). Systolic pressure is a measurement of ventricular contraction and is written as the numerator in the fraction.

B. Support Equipment (IV Equipment, Chest Tubes, Catheters, and Other Devices)

Patients often require the assistance of biomedical support equipment during the course of treatment.

Intravenous equipment, consisting of IV solutions, needles, IV tubing, IV catheters, heparin locks, infusion sets, and IV poles, are used for the infusion (administration via the bloodstream) of medication and fluids.

A **heparin lock,** consisting of either a catheter with a resealable injection pad or a winged infusion needle with a short catheter, is used when the patient requires intermittent medication. The patient is connected to medication for the duration of the infusion, and then disconnected when the infusion is completed, which allows the patient greater freedom than that associated with continuous infusion, and prevents scarring, which can occur with repeated injection to the same site. The site is flushed with dilute heparin, a medication that prevents clotting, in order to assess placement and patency before and after infusion of medication.

Intermittent medication may also be placed in a **central intravenous line,** a catheter placed in the subclavian vein. One type of central line is called a **Hickman catheter,** which is often used to infuse chemotherapy. Aseptic technique must be observed when administering medication through a central line.

The IV bag itself should be placed at a level 18 to 24 inches above the vein. Placing the bag below the vein will result in the stoppage of flow, and blood will back up into the IV tubing. Placing the bag or bottle too high will cause the medication to run too quickly. The position of the needle or catheter relative to the vein will affect the rate of flow. The catheter may become lodged against the wall of the vein, stopping flow, or it may become dislodged completely. A displaced catheter will cause extravasation, the collection of infused fluid in the tissue surrounding the vein.

IV needles and catheters are sized according to their diameter. The measurement of diameter is referred to as the **gauge.** As the diameter of the needle or catheter increases, the gauge decreases; thus, a 23-gauge needle is smaller than an 18-gauge needle.

Various devices are used to deliver oxygen to the patient; they are classified as either low- or high-flow. A **nasal cannula** is a low-flow oxygen device used to supplement room air. It consists of plastic tubing that connects to the oxygen source, usually a wall outlet with a **flowmeter,** which measures the amount of oxygen to the patient, and a cannulated end, which has prongs that fit in the patient's nostrils. Oxygen delivered in this manner is often humidified by forcing the oxygen through a water reservoir. Humidifying the O_2 prevents dehydration of the patient's mucous membranes.

A simple **oxygen mask** is connected in the same manner as the nasal cannula. The mask has vents that allow room air to leak in, diluting the pure oxygen. A flowmeter rate of 6 to 10 liters per minute delivers 35% to 60% oxygen. The mask can become sticky and uncomfortable for the patient and must be removed for meals; therefore, this type of mask is generally used for periods of less than 12 hours.

Partial rebreather masks are equipped with reservoir bags that collect the first portion of the patient's expired air. The air is mixed with 100% oxygen, and the patient breathes approximately one third of the expired air through the bag, with the remainder being expelled through vents in the mask. Partial rebreather masks facilitate the conservation of oxygen.

Of all mask types, **nonrebreather masks** provide both the highest concentration of oxygen and the most precise means of oxygen administration to a spontaneously breathing patient. This mask is similar in design to the partial rebreather mask, but has a two-way valve that permits exhaled air to escape.

Total rebreather masks have a reservoir bag, but no opening to room air. Carbon dioxide is absorbed by chemical means, and the bag may supply other gases.

Venturi masks allow precise delivery of oxygen concentration. The mask has a large tube with an oxygen inlet. Narrowing of the tube causes pressure to drop and air to be inspired through the side ports. The ports are adjusted according to the O_2 needs of the patient.

Clear plastic **oxygen tents** deliver cool, humidified air via a motor-driven unit. Oxygen tents do not deliver precise oxygen concentration and are therefore not often used, with the exception of treatment for pediatric pneumonia patients who require a cool, humidified airflow.

An **endotracheal tube** is an airway inserted through the mouth or nose into the trachea to administer oxygen in conjunction with a **mechanical ventilator.** The tube facilitates suctioning of secretions and keeps the tongue clear of the airway. Ventilators may either assist or completely control respiration.

A **tracheostomy** is a surgical opening into the trachea. A tube measuring 5 to 7.5 cm is inserted into the opening, and is used in conjunction with a ventilator or to bypass upper airway obstruction.

An **Ambu bag** is a respiratory assistive device, generally used in emergency situations. The patient's head is tilted back, the jaw thrust forward, and the airway cleared; then the mask portion is fitted over the patient's nose and mouth. Ambu bags are also used to temporarily supply oxygen to ventilator-dependent patients who must be temporarily taken off the ventilator, usually to transport the patient to another department. In this instance, the mask portion is removed, and the bag is fitted over the tracheostomy or endotracheal tube.

Urinary catheterization introduces an **indwelling urinary catheter,** commonly called a **Foley catheter,** into the bladder through the urethra. Sterile technique is used for catheterization; improper catheterization technique is the leading cause of nosocomial infections. Urine is collected in a bag or graded plastic container.

In patients who have rectal incontinence, fecal impaction, or uncontrolled diarrhea, **rectal catheters,** or modified Foley catheters, are used. Sometimes a surgical opening called an **ostomy** is performed to allow fecal elimination through the abdominal wall. The intestinal mucosa is brought out through the abdominal wall and sutured to the skin, forming a **stoma.** An **ileostomy** allows fecal content to be eliminated from the ileum through the stoma, whereas a **colostomy** permits feces to exit from the colon.

Nasogastric and **nasointestinal tubes** are employed for the removal of gastric fluid and air. The tubes are approximately 4 ft in length and are passed through the nose and into the desired area. **Single-lumen tubes** (the lumen is the open, inner space) may not be suctioned because they lack a venting system. With **double-lumen sump tubes,** one lumen empties the gastric fluid, while the other provides airflow. Placement of gastric-type tubes is generally confirmed with a thoraco-abdominal radiograph.

Chest tubes are employed following thoracic surgery as well as to reinflate the lung following pneumothorax by drawing air out of the pleural space. Chest tubes consist of the rubberized tube, sutured in place, and the drainage system, which has three parts: the suction control chamber; the collection chamber, for collection of serous secretions; and the water-seal chamber, which prevents the flow of air into the pleural space and chest cavity. The chest tube must be placed below the level of the patient and should be disturbed as little as possible.

QUESTION FOR SUPPORT EQUIPMENT

select the best answer

1. A patient who has chest tubes is being transferred to the radiology department for examination. Where is the ideal location for

the drainage system during transport via stretcher?

(A) Hung on an IV pole above the patient
(B) On the guardrail beside the patient
(C) At the foot of the bed, below the level of the chest
(D) Carried by a transporter, below the level of the chest

2. The smallest catheter is which of the following?

(A) 18 gauge
(B) 19 gauge
(C) 21 gauge
(D) 23 gauge

3. The ideal location to hang a bag of intravenous solution of 5% dextrose in water is:

(A) 5 feet above the patient.
(B) as high as the IV pole will allow.
(C) 18 to 24 inches above the patient.
(D) on a level with the IV site.

4. A Foley catheter is used for treatment of which of the following?

(A) Incontinence
(B) Bladder obstruction
(C) Diarrhea
(D) All of the aforementioned

5. A patient whose respirations are controlled via ventilator may also have a(n)_____ in place.

1. partial rebreather mask
2. endotracheal tube
3. Venturi mask
4. tracheostomy

(A) All of the aforementioned
(B) Choices 1 and 3 only
(C) Choices 2 and 4 only
(D) Choice 4 only

▶▶▶ ANSWERS TO SUPPORT EQUIPMENT

1. The answer is (B). The chest tube should not be stretched, as would happen by placing it at the end of the bed; nor should there be a risk of the tube becoming dislodged, as may happen when it is hand carried. The guardrail permits the drainage to collect when hung below the level of the chest.
2. The answer is (D). The diameter of a catheter decreases as the number increases.
3. The answer is (C). The ideal height is 18 to 24 inches above the IV site.

4. The answer is (D). Although primarily used in conjunction with treatment of the urinary tract, Foley catheters may also be used as a rectal tube.
5. The answer is (C). A ventilated patient will have either an endotracheal tube or tracheostomy in place. A patient with long-term ventilator dependence is more likely to have a tracheostomy.

C. Common Medical Emergencies

An emergency may be defined as an abrupt change in the patient's condition that requires immediate medical attention. The radiology technologist must be familiar with common medical emergencies and know which actions are appropriate to a given situation.

Epistaxis is the medical term for nosebleed. It may have varying etiologies; the most common are hypertension, dry mucous membranes, trauma, or sinusitis. Epistaxis may be treated by the radiographer with cold compresses to the nose and back of the neck and by placing the patient in a seated or Fowler's position.

Vomiting is the reflex emptying of the stomach by a different route, usually caused by the presence of irritants such as alcohol, bacterial toxins, or excessively spicy food. Sensory impulses from the irritated site reach the **emetic center** in the medulla, initiating the motor responses that cause vomiting. The primary concern for a vomiting patient is aspiration of the **emesis** or **vomitus.** An emesis basin should be provided, and care should be taken to ensure that the recumbent patient is turned on his/her side.

Postural or **orthostatic hypertension** is a sudden decrease of blood pressure secondary to rising to an erect position. The patient who has this condition feels faint and usually should be assisted to a seated or recumbent position. Similarly, **vertigo** is the sensation of feeling the room spinning, which is generally caused by an inner ear disturbance, whereas **syncope** is the term for fainting. Fall precautions should be taken with these patients, and an emesis basin should be nearby; patients who have vertigo in particular often experience accompanying nausea.

A patient who has a suspected **spinal injury** should never be moved without supervision from a physician. One of the most common clinical scenarios a radiographer encounters is radiography of the cervical spine following a motor vehicle accident. In this situation, AP and cross-table lateral radiographs are obtained before removing any restraints that have already been applied by emergency medical services personnel to ensure the safety of the patient. Sometimes odontoid views are also obtained.

Obtaining clinical radiographs sometimes necessitates moving a patient who has a **fracture or dislocation.** Any movement of an injury of this nature is extremely painful for the patient. Whenever possible, the proximal and distal ends of the injury should be supported. The least amount of movement of the affected area is best; therefore, cross-table techniques should be applied, if possible. Do not remove any cast or splint devices unless directed to do so by the physician. Displacement of fractures may occur easily, particularly in the first days following injury.

Grand mal seizures are characterized by involuntary muscle contractions, loss of consciousness, and falling; these seizures are associated with epilepsy. The radiographer should ensure that any objects in the area that could be harmful to the patient are removed and that tight clothing is loosened. The patient's head is turned to the side, and a padded blade is inserted between the teeth to discourage tongue biting. **Febrile convulsions** are common in children and mimic the grand mal seizure, but these convulsions are caused by high fever.

Shock is the condition of diminished peripheral blood flow and accompanying decrease in oxygen supply to tissue. It has a number of causes, including trauma, allergic reaction, blood loss, or infection. The shock patient is pale; has a rapid, weak pulse; and may be cyanotic. Breathing is shallow and rapid, and blood pressure is low. The patient should be kept warm and in either recumbent or Trendelenburg's position.

Patients may experience **loss of consciousness** while in your care. The unconscious patient should not be left unattended. The patient's level of consciousness is an important marker of his clinical situation; it is the radiographer's responsibility to monitor this situation carefully while interacting with the patient.

Respiratory failure may be characterized as acute or chronic. In the acute setting, the radiographer should be prepared to perform the **Heimlich maneuver** to clear an airway obstruction, or to call for help and initiate cardiopulmonary resuscitation (CPR) in the instance of complete respiratory arrest. In a like manner, **cardiopulmonary arrest** is the sudden cessation of circulation and productive respiration. Most hospitals have definite protocols for instigating a response to life-threatening emergencies, which are usually referred to as a "code." The radiographer must be thoroughly acquainted with these measures and initiate them quickly when the situation arises.

A **cerebrovascular accident (CVA)** is the proper term for a **stroke,** which is the single most common nervous system disorder. Strokes are caused by interruption of the blood flow to part of the brain, and may result from either occlusion or rupture of a cerebral vessel. Deprivation of blood supply to tissue is called **ischemia.** A CVA may be recognized by cool, sweaty skin; aphasia; dysphasia; hemiparesis; or hemiplegia.

QUESTIONS FOR COMMON MEDICAL EMERGENCIES

select the best answer

1. While in your care, a child suddenly exhibits uncontrollable muscle spasms and loses consciousness. The most likely cause is which of the following?
   (A) Fever
   (B) Epilepsy
   (C) Astrocytoma
   (D) Allergic response

2. A patient who has extensive blood loss secondary to trauma will most likely suffer:
   (A) respiratory arrest.
   (B) cardiac arrest.
   (C) shock.
   (D) CVA.

3. What is the most important action a technologist should take regarding a patient who is vomiting and unresponsive?
   (A) Provide an emesis basin
   (B) Call the nurse
   (C) Turn the patient into a prone position
   (D) Turn the patient into a lateral recumbent position

4. Which condition may cause epistaxis?
   (A) Hypertension
   (B) Trauma
   (C) Sinusitis
   (D) All of the aforementioned

5. Which blood pressure indicates shock?
   (A) 110/80
   (B) 160/110
   (C) 80/60
   (D) None of the aforementioned

▶▶ ANSWERS TO COMMON MEDICAL EMERGENCIES

1. The answer is (A). Although all of these conditions may cause seizure, febrile convulsions are relatively common in children.

2. The answer is (C). Shock is the condition of diminished peripheral blood flow and resulting decreased oxygen levels to tissue.
3. The answer is (D). The primary concern of the technologist regarding the vomiting patient is to prevent aspiration.
4. The answer is (D). All of these conditions may result in nosebleeds.
5. The answer is (C). Shock is characterized by low blood pressure. Breathing is shallow and rapid; the patient may be cyanotic; and the pulse is rapid and weak.

D. Management of Common Medical Emergencies

As a rule, the radiologic technologist is not the primary caregiver during life-threatening medical emergencies. However, it is critical that the technologist has the ability to accurately evaluate the emergency situation, and is aware of whom to call and what stabilizing help to administer until assistance arrives.

Many hospitals require radiologic technologists to be certified in **CPR,** which is the process of oxygenating the lungs via mouth-to-mouth breathing (or through an airway to the victim's mouth) and circulating blood with chest compressions. CPR should always be administered whenever there is an absence of breathing or heartbeat.

CPR is often described with the mnemonic ABC: **A**irway: tilt the head backward, check for respiration. **B**reathing: if no spontaneous breathing exists, give two slow, deep breaths. **C**irculation: check for pulse at the carotid artery; if no pulse, begin CPR.

CPR may be administered by either one or two trained individuals. There are slight variations in technique with the two approaches; also, minor differences apply to CPR of the pediatric patient.

The basic steps for one-man, adult victim CPR are as follows:

- Assess responsiveness. Ask, "Are you OK?" Call for help.
- Position the victim supine, preferably on a flat, smooth surface.
- Tilt the head backward, hand on forehead, fingers under jaw, opening the airway.
- Determine respiratory status, listen with ear over mouth, and observe chest movements.
- Remove loose dentures.
- If there is no breathing, pinch nose with the hand that is already on forehead. Seal mouth with either your mouth or an artificial airway,

and give two breaths. Lift your face away between breaths, and observe the chest rise and fall.
- Determine status of pulse and palpate carotid artery for 5 to 10 seconds.
- If there is no pulse, begin chest compressions. Kneel at the victim's side. Hands are placed interlocked, heel of hand on top of the other, approximately 2 inches above the xiphoid process. Place shoulders over hands and arms straight. Hands remain in place between compressions.
- Compress at the rate of 80 to 100 beats per minute.
- Complete four cycles of 15, counting aloud, and two ventilations.
- Reassess cardiopulmonary status.

Patients who have complete airway obstruction will exhibit the universal distress signal, which is clutching at the throat with both hands. In order to clear the obstruction, an abdominal thrust technique known as the Heimlich maneuver is applied. The steps for this maneuver are as follows:

- Ask, "Are you choking?"
- If yes, stand behind the victim.
- Arms are wrapped around the victim's waist.
- Make a fist and place the thumb side against the victim above the navel and below the xiphoid process.
- Grasp the fist with the other hand.
- Initiate quick firm thrusts upward until object is expelled, or victim becomes unconscious.

With an unconscious victim, the Heimlich maneuver may be applied with the victim in the supine position. After 6 to 10 thrusts, a finger sweep of the mouth is performed to check for expelled objects.

Patients may experience postoperative wound complications in a sudden manner. It is not uncommon for a patient to comment that something has suddenly given way following sneezing, coughing, or vomiting. **Dehiscence** is a total or partial disruption of the surgical wound layers, whereas **evisceration** is the protrusion of viscera through the incisional area. Either of these two situations constitutes an emergency and should be addressed by covering the area with sterile towels soaked in saline, and then contacting the physician immediately.

Hemostasis is the cessation of bleeding or blood flow. If a blood vessels wall breaks, the body responds with a series of reactions in three phases. These phases are **vascular spasm, platelet plug,** and **coagulation.** Eventually, fibrous tissue will grow at the site, preventing further blood loss, but the technologist can aid the process by the application of **direct pressure** on the wound site. Ice can reduce inflammation and pain. Patients may suffer from **thrombocytopenia,** a deficit of platelets, or **hemophilia,** a deficit of certain coagulation factors, making them more prone to acute bleeding difficulties. Liver disease, such as **cirrhosis** or **hepatitis,** may also cause bleeding disorders, because many of the coagulation proteins are manufactured in the liver.

QUESTIONS FOR MANAGEMENT OF COMMON MEDICAL EMERGENCIES

select the best answer

1. The mnemonic ABC is a shorthand expression for which of the following emergency procedures?
   (A) Heimlich maneuver
   (B) CPR
   (C) Hemostasis
   (D) Mouth-to-mouth resuscitation

2. For a patient who has thrombocytopenia, the emergency measure a radiologic technologist would be most likely to take would be which of the following?
   (A) CPR
   (B) Direct pressure
   (C) Wound precautions
   (D) Heimlich maneuver

3. The correct sequence for CPR in an adult victim with one rescuer is:
   (A) 15 respirations, 2 compressions.
   (B) 15 respirations, 15 compressions.
   (C) 15 compressions, 2 respirations.
   (D) 2 respirations, 15 compressions.

4. Which common medical emergency requires the use of sterile towels and saline?
   (A) Dehiscence
   (B) Hemorrhage
   (C) Respiratory arrest
   (D) Cardiac arrest

5. The universal distress signal is:
   (A) 911.
   (B) clutching at the chest.
   (C) clutching at the throat.
   (D) head held in the hands.

▶▶ ANSWERS TO MANAGEMENT OF COMMON MEDICAL EMERGENCIES

1. The answer is (B). ABC is shorthand for airway, breathing, and circulation, the three primary components of CPR.
2. The answer is (B). Thrombocytopenia is lack of platelets, an important blood component in clotting. Although in this patient population wound precautions are advisable, they are not considered to be an emergency measure.
3. The answer is (D). Ventilate; then circulate at this rate.
4. The answer is (A). A patient with dehiscence has suffered a partial or total disruption of the surgical wound. Immediate treatment requires covering the wound with sterile towels soaked in saline.
5. The answer is (C). The universal distress signal of both hands held at the throat is a sign that the victim cannot breathe.

V. CONTRAST MEDIA
A. Types and Properties

The purpose of **contrast media** is to artificially increase the contrast of body tissues where little contrast exists. Contrast media may be described as **positive (radiopaque)** contrast material, or **negative (radiolucent)** contrast material.

Positive contrast media introduce into a body area an element with a higher atomic number than that of the surrounding tissue, whereas negative contrast media, usually air or carbon dioxide, instill an element of a lower atomic number.

Some studies, barium enemas, and arthrograms, for example, use both positive and negative contrast media. These studies are referred to as **double-contrast** examinations. The positive media act as a coating agent, while the air fills the remaining space.

Iodinated contrast material may be either **oil-** or **water-based.** Oil-based contrast material is not readily absorbed, and therefore remains in the body for a longer period than is desirable.

Before the advent of iodinated intrathecal agents like **iopamidol (Isovue),** oil-based dye was removed after completion of myelography. The most common oil-based contrast material used for myelography was **iophendylate.** Iophendylate has high **viscosity** (degree of stickiness caused by friction between molecules of an element) and low **miscibility** (ability of an element to mix into solution). These characteristics reduce detailed visualization of intraspinal structures, and prevent wide filling of nerve root sleeves. **Iohexol (Omnipaque)** and **iopamidol** are the contrast agents of choice for myelography today, providing superior visualization with relatively low toxicity **(Figure 1-7).** These agents are readily absorbed and excreted.

Advances in imaging techniques and improvement in contrast agent technology have rendered oil-based contrast agents nearly obsolete. They are, however, still used infrequently for lymphangiograms (**Ethiodol**) and bronchograms (**propyliodone**).

Water-soluble iodinated contrast material is used chiefly to examine the urinary tract, vascular systems, biliary tract, and GI tract when barium sulfate is contraindicated. This type of contrast material also is used in conjunction with computed tomography examinations.

Water-soluble contrast material may be described as **ionic** or **non-ionic**, labels that refer to the structural composition of the molecules contained in the contrast agent. Ions are electrically charged (positively or negatively) molecules.

Osmolality refers to the number of particles in solution. In general, ionic contrast agents are **high-osmolality contrast media (HOCM),** and non-ionic agents are **low-osmolality contrast media (LOCM).**

Excluding enteric (oral, rectal) water-soluble media, there are three primary types of water-soluble media to consider: Conventional ionic contrast media such as **iothalamate meglumine** and **Renografin** have a ratio of three iodine atoms to two particles in solution, and are thus referred to as ratio 1.5 media. These are high-osmolality contrast media. Non-ionic contrast media such as **iopamidol** and **iohexol** use three iodine atoms to one particle in solution, yielding a ratio 3 contrast media **(Figure 1-8).** These agents are low-osmolality contrast media. A third type of media, **Hexabrix,** is a ratio 3 media (low-osmolality), but is ionic.

When a study that normally uses **barium** cannot be performed because of suspected GI perforation, a water-soluble iodinated contrast agent, generally **meglumine diatrizoate,** is used instead. In the case of enemas, the meglumine diatrizoate is generally diluted; the concentration varies, but is generally approximately 25%. These studies are generally performed with fluoroscopy, to prevent massive filling of the peritoneum. Meglumine diatrizoate may also

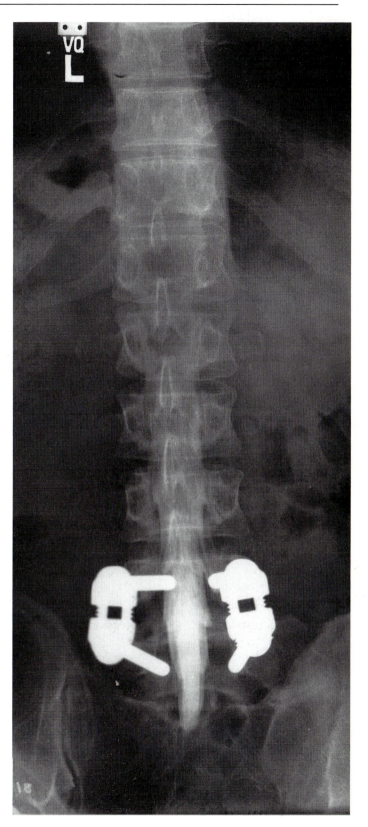

FIGURE 1-7. PA radiograph of lumbar spine myelogram using iopamidol (Isovue). The patient has undergone internal fixation of L4 and L5.

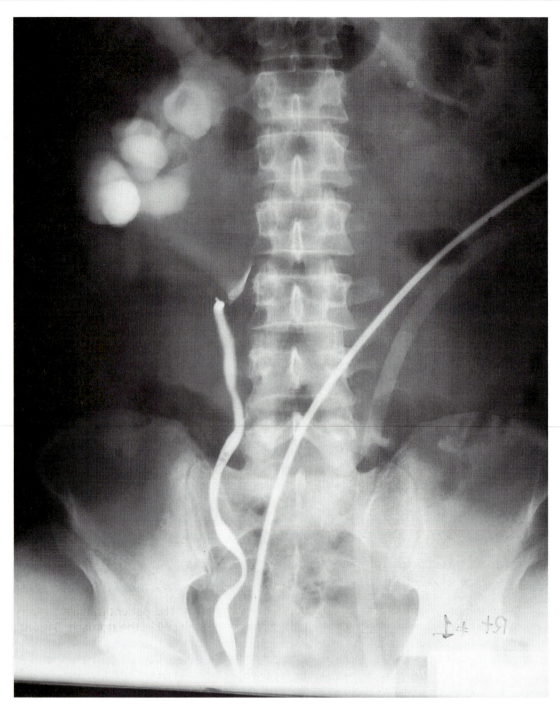

FIGURE 1-8. A retrograde pyelogram performed using iopamidol (Isovue). The examination was carried out in the cystoscopy suite of the operating room. Note the polycystic kidney.

be used to study fistulas, sinuses, and stub wounds. Because of its low toxicity, some authors have advocated the use of enteric-coated metrizamide for high-risk patients.

Barium sulfate is the non–water-soluble agent of choice for evaluation of the GI tract. Although the literature is somewhat hazy regarding its early use, it was probably used as early as 1896. Over the years, many improvements have been made in its composition, and there are now a wealth of commercial products available specific to each portion of the GI tract. The ideal mixture of barium is dense, yet will flow

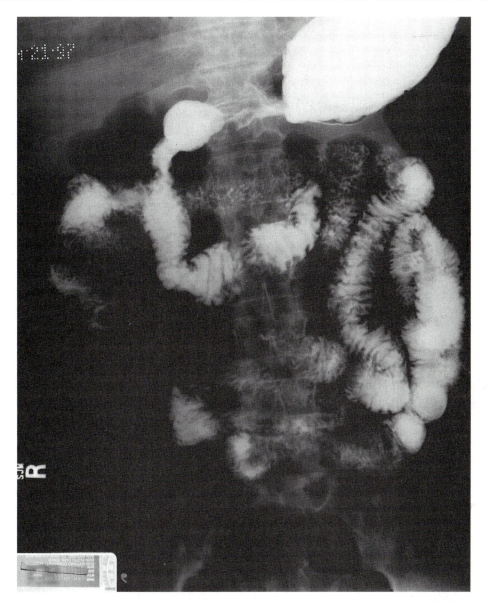

FIGURE 1-9. Thirty-minute follow-up film of a UGI and SB examination. The patient is initially given barium and effervescent crystals, and the UGI films are performed. Note the residual air still in the stomach. Barium and air used together is an example of a double contrast study. Following completion of the UGI, the patient is given another cup of barium and 100 cc undiluted Gastrografin. Films are taken every 30 minutes until the contrast material reaches the terminal ileum. The radiologist generally takes a spot film documenting the terminal ileum.

easily under the influence of gravity. Barium is the least toxic contrast medium **(Figure 1-9).**

QUESTIONS FOR TYPES AND PROPERTIES

select the best answer

1. Barium sulfate is an example of which of the following types of contrast media?

1. Enteric
2. Intravenous
3. Positive
4. Negative

(A) Choice 1 only
(B) Choices 2 and 4 only
(C) Choices 1 and 3 only
(D) All of the aforementioned

2. All of the following are characteristics of Iohexol except which of the following?

   (A) Approved for intrathecal use
   (B) HOCM
   (C) Positive contrast media
   (D) LOCM

3. A patient who has a suspected perforated duodenal ulcer would most likely be examined with which of the following?

   (A) Meglumine diatrizoate
   (B) Iothalamate meglumine
   (C) Renografin
   (D) Barium sulfate

4. Which would be an example of an examination that would use double-contrast?

   (A) Myelogram
   (B) ERCP
   (C) Arthrogram
   (D) IVP

5. Which contrast medium is both ionic and low osmolality?

   (A) Renografin
   (B) Iothalamate meglumine
   (C) Barium
   (D) Hexabrix

▶▶ ANSWERS TO TYPES AND PROPERTIES

1. The answer is (C). Barium is used in the examination of the GI tract, and is administered via the oral or rectal routes. It may also be given through a nasogastric (NG) tube.
2. The answer is (B). Iohexol is a low-osmolality contrast agent.
3. The answer is (A). A water-soluble enteric contrast agent, usually meglumine diatrizoate, is used to examine the GI tract of patients who have suspected GI tract perforation. Barium is not used; if spilled into the peritoneum, it may cause peritonitis.
4. The answer is (C). Arthrography is generally performed using both positive and negative contrast media.
5. The answer is (D). Hexabrix has a unique chemical composition, making it both an ionic and low-osmolality contrast agent.

B. Appropriateness of Contrast Medium to Examination and Patient Condition

The type, amount, and route of administration of contrast media selected by the radiologist depend on the patient's condition. An extremely fragile or critically ill patient is likely to suffer dire consequences from an extended stay in the radiology department; therefore, the requested examination is limited in such a way that only the crucially needed diagnostic information is obtained.

A patient who is unable to swallow or is unresponsive is likely to have a contrast agent administered through an NG tube when scheduled for a UGI examination. A procedure called **enteroclysis,** sometimes called a small bowel enema, is done when a more sensitive study of the small bowel is necessary; whereby an NG tube is positioned beyond the duodenum, and a contrast agent, usually meglumine diatrizoate, is introduced.

The toxicity of contrast agents is of particular clinical significance in pediatric patients. Neonatal patients may have seizures following entry of contrast agents into the brain, and pulmonary hemorrhage may occur in instances of contrast agent overdose. Recommendations regarding dose and patient weight vary, but in general are in a range between 2 and 5 cc per kg.

Renal function may also be adversely affected by contrast agent injection. In patients who have end-stage renal disease, a history of **renal transplantation** or **nephrectomy,** or elevated levels of **blood urea nitrogen (BUN)** or **creatinine,** the administration of contrast material is always a matter for serious concern.

Non-ionic contrast agents are much less toxic than conventional ionic contrast medium; however, they are also markedly more expensive. The exclusive conversion to non-ionic agents may place an undue financial burden on some facilities, as well as the patient. Therefore, certain guidelines are recommended for the use of these agents. Non-ionic contrast material is preferable for use in the following:

- Patients less than 1 year of age
- Patients who have a history of adverse contrast agent reaction
- Patients who have significant cardiovascular or cerebrovascular disease
- Patients who have asthma or histories of severe allergies
- Severely debilitated patients
- Patients who have multiple myeloma or sickle cell anemia
- Patients who have impaired renal function

select the best answer

1. Elevated BUN and creatinine levels are markers of which of the following?
(A) Patient age
(B) Renal function
(C) Small bowel obstruction
(D) All of the aforementioned

2. All of the following conditions are indicators for the use of non-ionic contrast material except:
(A) patients who have a history of asthma.
(B) patients who have AIDS.
(C) patients who have a history of adverse contrast agent reaction.
(D) patients less than 1 year of age.

3. A patient who has suspected perforated duodenal ulcer would most likely have an examination using which of the following?
(A) Meglumine diatrizoate
(B) Metrizamide
(C) Iopamidol
(D) Barium sulfate

▶▶ ANSWERS TO APPROPRIATENESS OF CONTRAST MEDIUM TO EXAMINATION AND PATIENT CONDITION

1. The answer is (B). BUN and creatinine are markers of renal function. In patients who have elevated levels, the possibility of limiting the dose or not performing the examination is considered.
2. The answer is (B). AIDS is not a factor in contrast agent selection.
3. The answer is (A). Meglumine diatrizoate is used instead of barium in patients who have suspected perforation; barium spilled into the peritoneum may cause peritonitis.

C. Contraindications

Contraindications are symptoms or conditions that make it inadvisable to proceed with normal treatment. In the case of contrast media, there are occasions when contrast material will not be given at all, and other occasions when its administration will be modified by substitute contrast material, decreased dose, or route of administration.

Because not all patients are good candidates for standard examinations using intravascular contrast media, it is vital that the technologist obtain a thorough history from the patient. Most hospitals use a release form the patient must sign, which includes questions regarding the patient's history of allergy and prior contrast-agent administration.

As previously discussed, a patient who has suspected bowel perforation will receive a dilute water-soluble iodinated contrast agent, usually meglumine diatrizoate, instead of barium sulfate. Barium spilled into the peritoneum may cause peritonitis, sometimes called **barium peritonitis** (*get a radiograph of extravasated contrast material, if possible*). Gastric and colorectal perforations have been reported in roughly 1 in 12,000 patients, which occur secondary to poor technique during the examination. In the case of the stomach, these perforations have been attributed to too vigorous compression and palpation, and in the case of the rectum, tears may be attributed to the insertion of the enema tip, or inflation of the balloon. Tears of the vaginal wall by incorrect placement of the enema tip have also been reported.

Because water-soluble oral contrast material is **hyperosmolar** (remember, osmosis is the tendency of fluid to flow from an area of lesser concentration to an area of greater concentration until the two solutions are equalized in pressure), there are times when its use is contraindicated. When an esophagobronchial fistula exists, for example, aspiration of meglumine diatrizoate into the lungs may lead to pulmonary edema and even death. In this case, cautious use of barium with fluoroscopy is recommended. Likewise, when a patient being examined for small-bowel obstruction is hypovolemic (has low fluid volume), the tendency of the contrast media to draw interstitial fluid into the bowel lumen may lead to shock and possibly death if fluid is not replaced.

Intravenous water-soluble contrast media are also contraindicated in some cases. Studies indicate a range of reactions from 1 in 5,000 to 1 in 40,000 for ionic contrast material, and roughly 1 in 200,000 for non-ionic contrast material.

Contraindications for intravascular administration of iodinated contrast media include compromised renal function, history of asthma or severe allergies, history of prior reaction to contrast material, multiple myeloma, and sickle cell anemia. If a contrast agent must be administered in these cases, the use of non-ionic contrast material is suggested.

The use of iophendylate in myelography is contraindicated if CT or MRI is to be done following myelography, because the contrast material is too dense to be visualized on CT, and residual contrast material on MRI may be misinterpreted as small lesions.

The same contraindications that hold true for lumbar puncture (i.e., bloody spinal tap, arachnoiditis) also are true for the application of water-soluble myelography agents. In addition, patients who have known seizure disorder, alcoholism, chronic obstructive pulmonary disease, or known history of iodine reaction are also considered high risk. Patients receiving medication that lowers the threshold for seizures should have medication withdrawn 48 hours before myelography.

QUESTIONS FOR CONTRAINDICATIONS

select the best answer

1. Which examination would most likely require the patient to sign an allergy history form?

    (A) Barium swallow
    (B) Meglumine diatrizoate enema
    (C) Barium enema
    (D) IVP

2. Which of the following conditions would prohibit the performance of a standard UGI series?

    (A) Perforated ulcer
    (B) Gastric cancer
    (C) Cholecystitis
    (D) Crohn's disease

3. In the case of a patient who has suspected esophagobronchial fistula, what would be the most likely choice for a contrast agent in a fluoroscopy-directed examination?

    (A) Meglumine diatrizoate
    (B) Barium sulfate
    (C) Air
    (D) Gadolinium

4. Which of the following are contraindications for the use of conventional ionic contrast media?

    (A) History of asthma
    (B) History of prior contrast agent reaction
    (C) Multiple myeloma
    (D) All of the aforementioned

5. Which characteristic makes meglumine diatrizoate a poor choice of contrast agent for hypovolemic patients?

    (A) High viscosity
    (B) Low osmolality
    (C) Hyperosmolarity
    (D) Low viscosity

▶▶ ANSWERS TO CONTRAINDICATIONS

1. The answer is (D). Patients generally sign an allergy history form when undergoing examinations using iodinated contrast media.
2. The answer is (A). In cases of suspected perforation, barium is not used; meglumine diatrizoate is used instead.
3. The answer is (B). Although meglumine diatrizoate aspiration may lead to pulmonary edema, the small amount of barium aspiration necessary to demonstrate the fistula is generally not harmful to the patient.
4. The answer is (D). A patient who has any of these conditions would be a poor candidate for ionic contrast media.
5. The answer is (C). Meglumine diatrizoate is hyperosmolar. The tendency of meglumine diatrizoate to draw interstitial fluid into the bowel lumen, causing electrolyte imbalance, makes it a poor choice for the hypovolemic patient.

D. Patient Education

Patients may experience constipation following UGI or BE examinations. Barium can become thickened in the bowel as a result of fluid absorption, a process called **inspissation.** To prevent constipation, fecal impaction, or possible bowel obstruction, patients should be instructed to increase their fiber and fluid intake and take a mild laxative following the examination.

Intravascular water-soluble contrast agents have a diuretic effect; however, patients may also be instructed to increase fluid intake following administration of such agents in order to speed excretion further.

Distention of the joint space following double-contrast arthrography may cause patient discomfort. Patients may be instructed to exercise the area to hasten absorption of the media.

Although this examination has been largely replaced by ultrasound, the **oral cholecystogram (OCG)** is still performed. Patients are allowed a fat-free meal the evening before the examination. The patient ingests **iopanoic acid** approximately 14 hours before the examination, and ingests nothing by mouth after that. A double dose of **ipodate** may also be used in the 25% of patients who have nonvisualized gallbladders after ingesting a single dose of ipodate. Bowel movements or vomiting should be reported by the patient to assure that the contrast agent has not been lost. If no stones are found on the initial radiographs, the patient is given a commercially prepared fatty meal to demonstrate contraction (emptying) of the gallbladder. If stones are seen, the fatty meal is not given, because emptying of the gallbladder may release a stone into the biliary system.

The diagnostic quality of many examinations is directly dependent on patient preparation. A colon poorly prepared for barium enema examination can lead to degraded image quality and increased discomfort during the examination for the patient. Although protocols vary between institutions, preparation for most fluoroscopic examinations involves **restricting diet,** usually for a period of 12 hours; use of a **purgative** such as magnesium citrate; and insertion of a **suppository** several hours before the examination.

The diabetic patient may have to refrain from the use of insulin if he/she must be kept strictly on an NPO status. The use of insulin without eating may lead to insulin shock. Whenever possible, a diabetic patient should be scheduled as the first patient in the morning. (See section IA for more detailed information regarding scheduling.)

Some diabetic patients are treated with metformin (Glucophage,) an oral hypoglycemic agent excreted by the kidneys. Administration of Glucophage is usually suspended for 48 hours before intravascular contrast agent injection so that patients who have decreased renal function do not become hypoglycemic.

Following myelography, the patient is typically confined to bed for a period of 18 to 24 hours, with the head elevated 30 to 45 degrees for the first 8 hours. The patient is then placed flat, or with the head elevated slightly, which reduces the risk of cerebrospinal fluid (CSF) leakage. Bathroom privileges are permitted during this period.

The question of how much information to give patients regarding adverse effects from contrast-agent administration is the subject of some debate. Particularly with respect to intravascular water-soluble contrast agents, patients may be anxious, and some authors suggest that supplying patients with information concerning possible side effects increases the likelihood of their manifestations. The best policy may be to discuss the most common and relatively benign side effects (i.e., increased body heat, metallic taste) during the period when the patient history and consent are taken.

QUESTIONS FOR PATIENT EDUCATION

select the best answer

1. Which of the following instructions apply(ies) to a patient who has undergone examination using barium sulfate?

    1. NPO
    2. Increase fluid intake
    3. Use a mild laxative
    4. Eat foods high in fiber

    (A) Choice 1 only
    (B) Choices 1 and 3
    (C) Choices 2, 3, and 4
    (D) Choice 3 only

2. All of the following are correct post-myelography instructions except:

    (A) elevate the head 35 to 40 degrees for the first 8 hours.
    (B) BRP after the first 8 hours.
    (C) NPO.
    (D) bed rest for 18 to 24 hours.

3. Which examination would employ the use of a purgative and suppository as part of the pre-examination regimen?

    (A) Myelogram
    (B) Barium enema
    (C) Bronchogram
    (D) Sialogram

4. For which examination must the patient ingest the contrast agent before arriving in the radiology department?

    (A) Small bowel series
    (B) Oral cholecystogram
    (C) Hysterosalpingogram
    (D) Sialogram

▶▶ ANSWERS TO PATIENT EDUCATION

1. The answer is (C). The patient who has undergone examination of the GI tract is typically instructed to increase fluids and fiber and to take a mild laxative to decrease the chance of barium hardening in the bowel.
2. The answer is (C). The abbreviation NPO means nothing by mouth; the patient may eat normally following myelography. BRP means bathroom privileges.
3. The answer is (B). Preparing the colon is an integral part of GI tract examinations. Most preparation regimens restrict diet and use purgatives and suppositories to cleanse the colon.
4. The answer is (B). The patient ingests the iopanoic acid approximately 14 hours before examination for oral cholecystography.

E. Administration of Contrast Media

A primary consideration for the technologist regarding administration of contrast material is that its use is based on **distribution in** and **excretion from** the body. This is markedly different from administration of medication, the purpose of which is therapeutic. Whereas therapeutic agents are administered in small quantities and at spaced intervals, contrast material is given over a short period, generally as a bolus and in relatively large quantities.

Contrast media may be administered either **orally,** as in the case of barium sulfate or meglumine diatrizoate; or **parenterally,** which means given by any route that bypasses the digestive tract (i.e., orally or rectally).

The most common parenteral routes for contrast media administration are **intravascular** (either venous or arterial), **intra-articular,** and **intrathecal. Intravenous contrast material** may be given as a **bolus,** which means all at once, or may be **infused,** a method that employs hanging the contrast material on an IV pole and allowing the contrast agent to drip in by means of gravity flow over a designated period of time.

Other parenteral routes are **topical,** applied to skin for local effect; **sublingual,** applied under the tongue; **subcutaneous,** applied under the skin, generally with a small needle; **intramuscular,** applied into the muscle; and **intradermal,** applied between the layers of skin. These methods primarily apply to medication and are generally not used in the radiology department; however, the subcutaneous route is used for the administration of local anesthetic during procedures such as myelography and arthrography.

In the radiology department, **venipuncture,** the technique that punctures a vein for the purpose of administration of contrast agent or the withdrawal of blood, has traditionally been the domain of the radiologist. Increasingly, however, technologists are assuming more of the clinical burden; therefore, it is important for technologists to be acquainted with the basic procedure. No matter the protocol is in the individual department, the technologist must remember that no medication or clinical procedure may be administered without a physician's order. The radiologist is responsible for selecting the type and amount of contrast material, as well as the route of administration.

During venipuncture, a vein is selected, most commonly the **antecubital** vein, on the anterior aspect of the proximal forearm. The vein is then palpated, and a tourniquet is applied proximally to the intended site in order to dilate the vein. The site is then cleansed with ethyl alcohol or povidone-iodine, and traction is applied to immobilize the area. The needle is held at approximately 30 degrees, and it is inserted bevel side up in the direction of the blood flow. A minute amount of resistance can be felt when the needle reaches the wall of the vein, which is sometimes described as a "pop." The needle may be cautiously advanced until blood flows back into the hub of the needle. If there is no blood flow, and the needle cannot be felt in the vein, it is best to begin again with new equipment.

Once the venipuncture is successful, the contrast agent may be connected to the needle or catheter. The technologist must ensure that all of the air has been bled out of the syringe and IV tubing, in order to prevent an inadvertent injection of air into the cardiovascular system, which is a dangerous occurrence called air **embolus** that may result in blood flow obstruction.

The successful completion of any radiographic procedure is dependent to a high degree on the readiness of the technologist. There are literally hundreds of supply items that the radiographer must be acquainted with, and working knowledge of these items in preparation for examinations is critical. The cardinal rule is: *Never bring a patient or doctor into the radiographic suite until you are ready.* In this instance, "ready" means having all pertinent supplies available, or set up, if applicable. Nothing will frustrate a doctor or a patient more than having to wait while you scurry about looking for a supply item you forgot. **Table 1-9** lists some common examinations and the supplies associated with them.

QUESTIONS FOR ADMINISTRATION OF CONTRAST MEDIA

select the best answer

1. At approximately what angle should the radiographer hold a butterfly needle when injecting the antecubital vein for an intravenous urogram (IVU) examination?
   (A) 90 degrees
   (B) 70 degrees
   (C) 45 degrees
   (D) 30 degrees

2. Which of the following examinations require(s) the technologist to have a supply of nonsterile gloves ready?

(A) UGI
(B) BE
(C) IVP
(D) All of the aforementioned

3. Which of the following examinations require(s) the use of sterile technique?

    1. Arthrogram
    2. Myelogram
    3. Double-contrast enema
    4. Double-contrast UGI

(A) Choice 2 only
(B) Choices 1 and 2
(C) Choices 3 and 4
(D) Choices 1, 2, and 3

4. Which examination would employ the use of a subcutaneous anesthetic?

(A) Hysterosalpingogram
(B) Barium enema via colostomy
(C) Video barium swallow
(D) Temporomandibular joint arthrogram

▶▶ ANSWERS FOR ADMINISTRATION OF CONTRAST MEDIA

1. The answer is (D). A butterfly needle is held at approximately 30 degrees for venipuncture.
2. The answer is (D). Universal precautions require the use of gloves whenever there is a chance of contact with body fluids, as is the case with all of these examinations.
3. The answer is (C). Intrathecal and intra-articular contrast-agent administration requires the use of sterile technique.
4. The answer is (D). Arthrography typically employs the use of lidocaine or other anesthetic to numb the skin and subcutaneous tissue before placing the needle for contrast-agent injection.

F. Complications/Reactions

The administration of contrast media may lead to complications or reactions in the patient. Of chief concern are **anaphylactic**-type reactions from intravascular water-soluble contrast agents. **Anaphylactic shock** is a severe **systemic** (pertaining to the entire body) reaction to a substance. The more quickly a patient exhibits symptoms, the more severe the reaction tends to be.

Symptoms of anaphylactic reaction may range from mild—including urticaria (hives), nausea, vomiting, and a flushed sensation—to severe—hypotension, shock, laryngeal edema, and arrhythmia. Overall reaction rates are approximately 5% to 8%; however, the majority of these are minor; life-threatening reactions occur in a range from 1 in 500 to 1 in 1,000.

The possibility of anaphylactic reaction makes it imperative for the technologist to be familiar with the

▶ TABLE 1.9. Supplies Needed for Various Examinations

Barium Enema
Enama bag
Barium
IV pole
Lubricating jelly
Towels
Nonsterile gloves

Upper Gastrointestinal (UGI) Series
Barium
Citrocarbonate (effervescent)
Cuts
Straws, emesis basin
Nonsterile gloves

Myelogram
Myelogram tray
Inflatable pillow
Hemostats
Contrast agent: Omnipaque, Isovac
Complete laboratory requisition for spinal fluid analysis
Betadyne
Razor
Sterile and nonsterile gloves
Bandages

Intravenous Urogram (IVU)
Contrast agent: Isovue, Renografin
60-cc syringe
Tourniquet
Butterfly needles (19-, 20-, 23-gauge)
Nonsterile gloves
Alcohol or Betadyne swab
Bandages

Arthrogram
Contrast agent: Isovue, Renografin
Nonsterile and sterile gloves
Arthrogram tray
Betadyne
Razor
Bandages

contents of the emergency medicine cart, usually called a crash cart. The cart contains medicines like **epinephrine, antihistamines, and IV solutions** as well as support equipment like **intubation blades, tourniquets, syringes,** and **needles.** Most carts are standardized throughout the facility, so that no matter where the emergency situation arises, it can be dealt with quickly and appropriately.

A few generalized rules that apply to injection of contrast material are:

- Never inject contrast material in an isolated setting; help should always be immediately available.
- Have the crash cart ready; check its contents on a specific schedule.
- Have a basic knowledge of the patient.
- CPR or Advanced Cardiac Life Suppoort (ACLS) certification is a must.
- Be able to identify specifically the type of reaction.
- Rapid treatment of reaction permits lower doses of drugs to reverse the reaction.

Each facility will have its own unique approach to "codes." Usually, there is a special telephone number to call, and the operator announces the code on a public address system. Some facilities are equipped with wall-mounted buttons or switches for the same purpose.

In general, nonionic contrast material produces fewer reactions; therefore, when patients who are identified as being at risk for adverse contrast-media reactions must receive such agents, nonionic media should be used.

Premedication with steroids and antihistamines reduces the incidence of anaphylactic reactions in patients who have a history of reactions, as well as frequency of repeat reactions. Premedication may occur over a period of days or immediately preceding the procedure, depending on the clinical situation.

Localized reactions may also occur from contrast-agent injection, including **extravasation,** a term meaning passage of the contrast agent into the tissues surrounding the intended vein. Elevation of the affected area is suggested, and localized moist heat may reduce pain and swelling. In the rare instances when extravasation with pain, swelling, and erythema persists beyond 18 to 24 hours, surgical treatment by a plastic surgeon is required. **Phlebitis,** which is inflammation of the vein that is often accompanied by a clot, may also occur from contrast-agent injection following venography.

Deep venous thrombosis (DVT), a condition characterized by the presence of a clot in a vein in which the vessel wall is not inflamed, is the most severe localized reaction to contrast material. The deep veins are systemic veins that accompany the arteries and are usually enclosed in a sheath that wraps both vein and artery.

Acute renal failure may occur as a direct result of contrast-media administration. Risk factors for this consequence are preexisting renal insufficiency, diabetes, dehydration, cardiovascular disease, multiple myeloma, and hypertension.

Barium aspiration may occur when a patient inadvertently inhales the contrast media. Aspiration of small amounts of barium is not clinically significant, and in fact is preferable to aspiration of meglumine diatrizoate if esophagobronchial fistula is suspected.

Although barium is an inert substance, incidences of contrast-agent reaction to barium have been reported. They are extremely rare.

Discomfort is common among women undergoing **hysterosalpingography (HSG),** but is often abated with reassurance by the technologist. Mild vaginal bleeding may also occur. There is a low incidence of pelvic infection associated with HSG, approximately 1.4%, so the technologist should inform the patient of this risk. If dilated tubes are noted at the time of examination, antibiotics are sometimes prescribed.

QUESTIONS FOR COMPLICATIONS/ REACTIONS

select the best answer

1. Which of the following is (are) considered a systemic reaction to IV contrast material?
   (A) Extravasation
   (B) Hypotension
   (C) Phlebitis
   (D) All of the aforementioned

2. Of the following contrast-media reactions, which would be considered most serious?
   (A) Deep venous thrombosis
   (B) Severe anxiety
   (C) Extravasation
   (D) Nausea

3. A patient is undergoing HSG examination and complains of severe discomfort. Which would be the most appropriate treatment?
   (A) IV sedation
   (B) Oral sedation

(C) IM sedation
(D) Reassurance

4. Following a 60-cc bolus injection of iopamidol
for an IVU examination, the radiologist leaves
the room after noting that the patient tolerated
the injection well. After obtaining the 30-
second radiograph, however, the technologist
notices that the patient is pale and diaphoretic.
The technologist's first response should be to:

(A) call a code.
(B) call the radiologist.
(C) inform the patient's nurse.
(D) observe the patient carefully.

5. The rapid onset of severe cardiovascular and
respiratory symptoms following nonionic
contrast-media injection, including cessation of
heart beat and respiration, is best described by
which term?

(A) Diaphoresis
(B) DVT
(C) Anaphylactic shock
(D) prn

▶▶ ANSWERS TO COMPLICATIONS/ REACTIONS

1. The answer is (B). **Hypotension** is considered a
systemic response to contrast material, along
with nausea, vomiting, urticaria, cardiac arrhythmia, and laryngeal edema. Extravasation and
phlebitis are localized effects.
2. The answer is (A). DVT is a serious, potentially
life-threatening situation, whereas the other
listed conditions are considered mild.
3. The answer is (D). Pain and discomfort during
HSG examination can be lessened considerably
when the technologist provides reassurance that
the sensations are expected and will soon dissipate.
4. The answer is (D). Diaphoresis is sweating, and
may be associated with contrast-agent reaction.
In the absence of other symptoms, however, the
patient should simply be carefully observed. The
situation often resolves quickly on its own.
5. The answer is (C). Anaphylactic shock is a severe
and sometimes fatal reaction to a substance.

END-OF-CHAPTER EXAMINATION

▶▶ **QUESTIONS**

Select the best answers.

1. Which examination should be performed first?
   - (A) Lumbar spine
   - (B) OCG
   - (C) BE
   - (D) IVP

2. A sphygmomanometer and stethoscope are devices used to measure which of the following?
   - (A) Respiratory rate
   - (B) Korotkoff sounds
   - (C) Pulse
   - (D) CSF pressure

3. A patient who has undergone bone marrow transplantation would most likely be placed on which of the following type of precaution?
   - (A) Fall precaution
   - (B) No-salt diet
   - (C) Contact isolation
   - (D) Neutropenic isolation

4. Which of the following procedures would be most likely to require premedication with steroids?
   - (A) Enteroclysis
   - (B) Hysterosalpingogram
   - (C) IVU
   - (D) Colostomy barium enema

5. A diaphoretic patient would exhibit which of the following?
   - (A) Hot, dry skin
   - (B) Aphasia
   - (C) Dyspnea
   - (D) Sweaty, clammy skin

6. A patient who has decubitus ulcers is most likely:
   - (A) frail, with easily torn skin.
   - (B) anxious and demanding.
   - (C) diaphoretic.
   - (D) unable to eat solid food.

7. BUN levels are an important indicator of _____. Patients with elevated BUN levels who must receive contrast material should have the _____ possible concentration of iodine injected.
   - (A) cardiac perfusion, highest
   - (B) renal function, highest
   - (C) cardiac perfusion, lowest
   - (D) renal function, lowest

8. The application of restraints to an adult patient requires:
   - (A) permission from the patient.
   - (B) permission from the patient's family.
   - (C) a physician's order.
   - (D) continuous monitoring.

9. If a patient arrives at the facility and states that his physician sent him/her for left wrist radiographs, but there is no request form, what action should the technologist take?
   - (A) Send the patient to the emergency room to be examined.
   - (B) Instruct the patient to return to his/her physician and retrieve the form.
   - (C) Verify the injury and perform the examination.
   - (D) Call the physician for confirmation.

10. Which of the following are conditions that require contact isolation?
    1. Herpes zoster
    2. TB
    3. Scabies
    4. AIDS
    - (A) Choices 1 and 3
    - (B) Choices 2 and 4
    - (C) Choice 4 only
    - (D) Choices 1, 2, and 3

11. The incidence of potentially life-threatening contrast-agent reactions when using ionic contrast media (hypotension, bronchospasm, cardiac arrest) is roughly which of the following?
    - (A) 10%
    - (B) 1%
    - (C) .1%
    - (D) .001%

(Continued)

12. The first action a technologist should take when transferring a patient from bed to wheelchair is:

    (A) position wheelchair parallel to bed.
    (B) call for help.
    (C) check the wrist ID bracelet against the requisition.
    (D) place patient in the Sims' position.

13. A patient has a pulse rate of 30, which indicates which of the following?

    (A) Pulmonary embolus
    (B) CVA
    (C) Bradycardia
    (D) Tachycardia

14. Which method of sterilization uses color-coded indicators to ensure that sterilization has been achieved?

    (A) Gas
    (B) Autoclave
    (C) Dry heat
    (D) Boiling

15. Incontinence in an unconscious patient is managed by which device?

    (A) Foley catheter
    (B) Partial rebreathing mask
    (C) Ventilator
    (D) Ventricular assist device (VAD)

16. A patient who has dyspnea is sent on a stretcher to the radiology department for PAL chest radiographic examination, but all of the exposure rooms are occupied, and so the patient must wait. The most comfortable position for the patient to wait in is which of the following?

    (A) Trendelenburg's
    (B) Fowler's
    (C) Sims'
    (D) Lateral recumbent

17. Which examination(s) would require a restricted diet 12 hours before examination?

    (A) UGI
    (B) BE
    (C) IVP
    (D) All of the aforementioned

18. For which examination is a patient typically confined to bed for 18 to 24 hours following the procedure?

    (A) ERCP
    (B) Small bowel follow-through
    (C) Cervical myelogram
    (D) T-tube cholangiogram

19. Which of the following are parenteral routes for contrast-agent administration?

    1. Oral
    2. Nasal
    3. Intravenous
    4. Intra-arterial

    (A) Choice 3 only
    (B) Choices 3 and 4
    (C) All of the aforementioned
    (D) Choices 1 and 2

20. Which is the term for redness of the skin?

    (A) Erythema
    (B) Purulent
    (C) Exfoliation
    (D) Erythrocyte

21. The concept of universal precautions is best described by which of the following?

    (A) Interaction with all patients requiring the use of personal protective equipment, such as gloves, masks, and gowns
    (B) Treatment of all body substances as infectious
    (C) Requirement of diligent hand washing before and after each patient interaction
    (D) Requirement that isolation techniques are practiced with all patients

22. A 14 × 17 cassette used to obtain a portable chest radiograph is an example of which route of infection transmission?

    (A) Direct contact
    (B) Vector
    (C) Airborne
    (D) Fomite

(Continued)

23. Which of the following is a local effect from contrast media?

    (A) Urticaria
    (B) Shortness of breath
    (C) Phlebitis
    (D) Cardiac arrest

24. The abbreviation q.s. means:

    (A) twice a day.
    (B) at night.
    (C) sufficient quantity.
    (D) after meals.

25. Viscosity has been described as the measure of friction in contrast media. The more viscous a material is, the more difficult it is to inject. A technique for reducing viscosity is:

    (A) add water to the media.
    (B) heat the contrast media.
    (C) chill the contrast media.
    (D) inject the media in conjunction with a running IV solution.

26. A patient who has cyanosis:

    1. is hypoxic.
    2. has a blue skin tint.
    3. has a cherry-red skin tint.
    4. has dry, hot skin.

    (A) All of the aforementioned
    (B) None of the aforementioned
    (C) Choices 1 and 2
    (D) Choices 3 and 4

27. The proper placement for chest tubes is:

    (A) below the level of the patient.
    (B) on a level with the patient.
    (C) at the patient's feet.
    (D) above the level of the patient.

28. The diastolic blood pressure indicates:

    (A) ventricular contraction.
    (B) atrial contraction.
    (C) ventricular relaxation.
    (D) atrial relaxation.

29. The Emergency Planning and Community Right to Know Act concerns:

    (A) biohazardous materials.
    (B) medical records.
    (C) radioactive materials.
    (D) all of the aforementioned.

30. Korotkoff sounds relate to:

    (A) bowel sounds.
    (B) lung sounds.
    (C) the tympanic membrane.
    (D) blood pressure.

▶▶ ANSWERS TO END-OF-CHAPTER EXAMINATION

1. The answer is (A). Of the listed examinations, the lumbar spine should be performed first to prevent obscuring of information by contrast media. The remaining examinations would be completed in this order: OCG, IVP, BE.

2. The answer is (B). A sphygmomanometer and stethoscope are devices used to measure blood pressure. The procedure is done by auscultation [listening to body sounds (Korotkoff sounds)].

3. The answer is (D). The purpose of neutropenic, or protective isolation, is to protect a patient who is immunocompromised. Fall precautions are generally put in place for the elderly, the mentally unstable, or patients who have vertigo or inner ear disturbances.

4. The answer is (C). Premedication with steroids and antihistamines is sometimes indicated for patients who have a known history of iodinated contrast-agent reaction. IVUs (IVPs) are done with intravenous injection of water-soluble iodinated contrast material.

5. The answer is (D). Diaphoresis is the term for sweating.

6. The answer is (A). Decubitus ulcers form when a patient lies in one position too long. They are an inflammation of the skin over a bony prominence, and occur when the affected area does not receive enough oxygen (hypoxia).

7. The answer is (D). BUN level is a renal marker. If a patient who has renal insufficiency must receive a contrast medium, the lowest level that will permit diagnostic information to be obtained should be used.

(Continued)

8. The answer is (C). Restraints require a physician's order when applied to an adult. When properly applied, they are neither harmful nor painful.

9. The answer is (D). The important action in this situation is to verify the physician's order. Although the request form is helpful and is generally required, care of the patient—who in this instance is probably in pain—is the first priority.

10. The answer is (A). Herpes zoster (shingles) and scabies are examples of conditions that would require contact isolation. Other such conditions are impetigo and conjunctivitis. Neither AIDS nor TB is transmitted via skin contact.

11. The answer is (D). Approximately 1 in 1,000 patients develops a serious reaction to ionic water-soluble contrast material. The incidence of adverse reaction using nonionic contrast media is roughly one fifth that of conventional ionic contrast-media use.

12. The answer is (C). No matter what type of transfer, the first action by the technologist is to assure the correct patient is about to be moved. Patients are often moved from room to room; they may be hard of hearing or confused. Checking the wrist band will assure the technologist that he/she is correct.

13. The answer is (C). Bradycardia is the term for slow pulse. The approximate average pulse rate for an adult is 80 bpm.

14. The answer is (B). Autoclaving, the quickest and most convenient sterilization method, uses color-coded indicators to indicate that the process is complete.

15. The answer is (A). Incontinence is the inability to control urinary or rectal function. Foley catheters are commonly used for this purpose.

16. The answer is (B). Patients who have dyspnea are generally more comfortable with the head elevated, which is Fowler's position.

17. The answer is (D). All of these examinations use a restricted diet as part of the preparation. Laxatives and suppositories are also used.

18. The answer is (C). The post-procedure regimen for myelography is usually bed rest, head elevated for the first 8 hours, and then head flat or slightly elevated following this. Bathroom privileges are also allowed after the first 8 hours.

19. The answer is (B). Parenteral routes are those routes that bypass the digestive tract.

20. The answer is (A). Erythema is redness or inflammation of the skin or mucous membranes.

21. The answer is (B). Universal precautions is a concept that requires medical personnel to treat all body fluids/substances as potentially infectious.

22. The answer is (D). A fomite is an object that has come into contact with a pathogenic organism. Common fomites in the hospital include the radiograph table, Foley catheters, and bandages.

23. The answer is (C). A local reaction is one that results from the direct effect of the contrast agent on the area. Phlebitis, which is inflammation of the vein, is one example of a local effect; extravasation is another. Systemic effects result in a change in a body system.

24. The answer is (C). The abbreviation q.s. means "in sufficient quantity."

25. The answer is (B). Heating contrast media, usually with specially designed warmers, reduces their viscosity.

26. The answer is (C). A cyanotic patient has a bluish skin tint, which is indicative of lack of oxygen in the skin tissue. This phenomenon is easily observed in the lips and gums.

27. The answer is (A). Chest tubes should be placed below the level of the patient to allow drainage. The tube itself should never be taut.

28. The answer is (C). Diastolic pressure, which is the bottom number in a pressure reading, indicates relaxation of the ventricle. An easy way to remember which number is which is to think: D represents down.

29. The answer is (A). The right-to-know legislation concerns an employee's right to knowledge of any biohazardous material that he/she may encounter in the workplace.

30. The answer is (D). Korotkoff sounds are the sounds heard during auscultation for blood pressure.

Radiation Protection

I. PATIENT PROTECTION
A. Biological Effects of Radiation

All living matter is composed of atoms that are joined into molecules by the bonding of electrons. **Ionizing radiation** displaces electrons and thus breaks the bonds holding the molecules together. It has been demonstrated that the biological effects of radiation stem from **ionization of tissue (Figure 2-1)**. Ionization is the process in which a neutrally charged atom gains or loses an electron, thereby acquiring a positive or negative charge. An **ion** is an atom or group of atoms that has acquired an electric charge from the gain or loss of an electron. A **cation** is a positively charged ion (has lost an electron), and an **anion** is a negatively charged ion (has gained an electron).

The x-ray beam itself consists of many individual bits of energy called **photons** that travel at the speed of light. X-rays are described as either **hard** or **soft** based on their penetrating ability. Hard x-rays are those of higher penetrating ability and are obtained by either selecting higher kilovoltage peak (kVp) at the time of exposure or using **filters** with an element that has a high atomic number, such as copper. Highly penetrating x-ray photons (hard) have **high frequency** and **short wavelength.** Conversely, soft x-rays are obtained by using lower voltages or filters with elements that have a low atomic number, such as aluminum; soft x-ray photons have **low frequency** and **long wavelength.**

When passing through the body, the x-ray beam is **attenuated,** which results in a lower energy beam. Attenuation consists of two processes: **absorption** of a portion of the x-ray beam through various interactions, and the emission of **secondary** and **scatter radiation.** Many photons pass through the body without any interaction whatsoever. Secondary radiation is the radiation emitted by atoms that have absorbed x-ray photons. Scatter radiation is radiation that has **changed direction** as a result of interaction with atoms.

Following the penetration of the body by x-ray photons, four types of reactions can occur: the photoelectric effect, coherent or unmodified scatter, the Compton effect, and pair production.

The **photoelectric effect (Figure 2-2)** involves relatively low-energy photons. It occurs when the incoming or **incident photon** has an energy level slightly higher than that required to remove an electron from an inner (usually K or L) shell of a given atom. When the interaction occurs, the incident photon releases all of its energy and is **truly absorbed.** The atom then releases its K shell electron and leaves a hole—the atom is then said to be in an excited state. The hole in the K shell is then immediately filled by an electron from the L shell, and the difference in energies between the two shells is given up as a characteristic ray, so called because the energy level is typical of the element concerned. The photoelectric effect occurs more frequently when the absorbing atoms are of high atomic number, that is, bone, teeth, contrast media; this **effect** plays a significant role in patient dose.

The second reaction, **coherent** or **unmodified scatter,** occurs with very low-energy incident photons that set a bound electron into motion. The motion creates an energy wave identical to that of the incident photon, but in a different direction. This interaction results in the incident photon "bouncing off" the orbital electron, without losing energy or experiencing a change in frequency or wavelength. Unmodified scatter occurs at kVp levels below that required for diagnostic radiology.

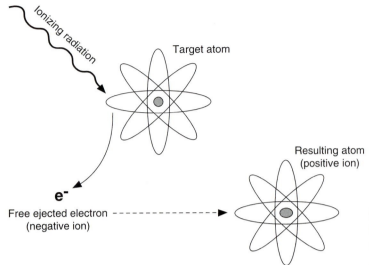

FIGURE 2-1. Ionization. Incident ionizing radiation transfers energy to the target atom, ejecting an orbital electron. The resulting free electron and positive ion are known as an ion pair.

The third reaction, the **Compton effect** (see Figure 2-2), occurs when the incident photon dislodges a loosely bound electron, and, having discharged part of its energy, the photon then proceeds in a different direction. The dislodged electron is referred to as a **Compton** or **recoil electron.** The emerging photon is called a **scattered photon.** Because the photon has released some energy on the interaction with the electron, it is of longer frequency and wavelength.

When the energy of the incident photon increases, the chance of the Compton interaction occurring decreases. However, at higher energy levels the

scattered photons also have higher energy, enough so that they pass through the body and reach the film. Scatter radiation that reaches the film contributes to **increased film fog** and **decreased detail.**

Pair production, which is the fourth type of reaction, is an interaction that takes place at energy levels of at least 1.02 megaelectron volts (MeV). It occurs when an incident photon of at least 1.02 MeV interacts with the nucleus and disappears, giving birth to a pair of electrons: one positive **(positron),** and one negative **(negatron).**

The result of these interactions is a complex

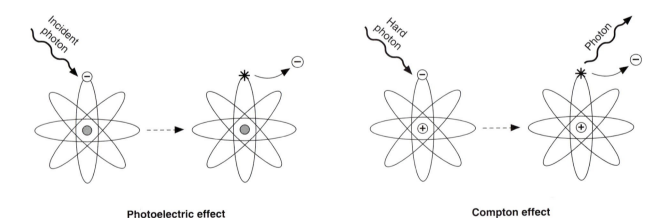

Photoelectric effect   **Compton effect**

FIGURE 2-2. Two reactions that can occur following penetration of the body by x-ray photons are of interest to the radiologic technologist: the photoelectric effect and the Compton effect. The **photoelectric effect** is an all-or-nothing energy exchange. The photon imparts all its energy to the ejected electron and vanishes. The ejected electron departs with the inherent energy of the incident photon. In the **Compton effect,** a high-energy incident photon strikes an orbital electron, resulting in partial energy transfer. The orbital electron is ejected, and the photon continues in a new "scattered" direction at a lower energy state.

shower of electrons that decrease in energy as each interaction takes place. As electrons pass through tissue, they create a track of ionized molecules. The manner in which energy is deposited in tissue along this track, measured in terms of distribution (per length of particle track), is called the **linear energy transfer (LET)** of radiation. LET is considered a qualitative measure of radiation; x-rays in the diagnostic range have a low LET.

Biological damage resulting from ionization can be either **direct** or **indirect.** A direct interaction occurs when a charged particle strikes the deoxyribonucleic acid (DNA) molecule. Evidence suggests that direct interaction with DNA is the most critical in terms of lethal cell damage; this type of interaction most often occurs with high LET radiation.

Indirect interactions result from the production of **free radicals.** Free radicals are atoms or molecules that contain unpaired electrons and are therefore highly unstable and reactive. Radiation absorption may occur in a cell water molecule, for example, and the resulting free radical may diffuse to the DNA, where it surrenders its energy, which produces a biological lesion. Two thirds of the biological effects that result from ionizing x-rays are of this indirect variety. As energy levels increase to high LET, **direct effects** become more prominent.

The biological consequence of a given dose of radiation varies according to the quality of the radiation absorbed. Thus, an absorbed dose of x-ray has quite a different biological effect from that of an identical dose of alpha particles or neutrons. Two concepts are used to characterize this difference. **Relative biological effectiveness (RBE)** is a measurement used to determine the relative toxicity (potential to create biological damage) of a given dose of one type of radiation compared with the toxicity of another type of radiation (e.g., x-ray versus alpha particles). RBE is expressed as the ratio of the amount of energy of a given type of radiation required to produce a given biological effect to the energy required to produce that same biological effect when using 200 kilo electron volts (keV) of x-ray.

The **quality factor (Q)** or **(QF)** is a similar measurement that is used primarily to determine occupational exposure dose limits. The Q is expressed as a numerical value assigned to each given type of radiation and is used in determining the following formula:

$$rad \times QF = rem$$

[where radiation absorbed dose (rad) is an expression of absorbed dose, and roentgen-equivalent-man (rem) is the unit used to express dose equivalent for radiation safety purposes].

The overall relationship between radiation dose and biological effects is referred to as the **dose-effect** or **dose-response** relationship. Radiation effects are classified into two categories: **threshold effects,** in which a specified minimum dose must be exceeded before the effect is observed, and **non-threshold effects,** for which no threshold can be observed, and therefore no dose—no matter how small—is considered safe.

Biological experiments are performed on animals to obtain dose-response data. The radiation dose to which 50% of animals respond is used as an index of effectiveness. When the death of the animal is used as the data endpoint, the 50% dose is referred to as lethal dose $(LD)_{50}$. More commonly, when 50% of animals die within 30 days, the index is called **$LD_{50}/30$ dose.**

Another means of describing the dose-response relationship is the **dose-response curve (Figure 2-3).** These curves demonstrate the quantitative relationship between dose and effect and can be linear (in a straight line) or non-linear (curved). For the purposes of diagnostic x-rays, the linear non-threshold and the linear threshold curves are most often used. The Committee on Biologic Effects of Ionizing Radiation (BEIR) has designated the **linear non-threshold** curve as the appropriate measurement tool for radiation protection standards. The linear non-threshold curve demonstrates biological responses such as cancer and genetic effects, which are sometimes called **stochastic** (meaning random) effects. In

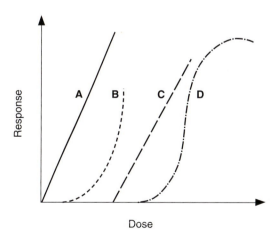

FIGURE 2-3. Dose-response curve: (A) Linear, non-threshold. (B) Non-linear, non-threshold. (C) Linear, threshold. (D) Non-linear, threshold.

theory, even extremely low doses of radiation may cause biological damage; therefore, when discussing non-threshold or stochastic effects, it is important to remember there is no safe dose or dose below which there will be no biological response. Threshold curves, on the other hand, describe interactions at which a certain dose must be given before a biological response occurs. Erythema is an example of these **non-stochastic effects.**

The biological effects of radiation can be further classified according to its manifestations. There are three main types to consider: **long-term (late) effects,** including cancer and cataracts; and life-shortening **somatic effects,** by which the human embryo, thyroid, bone marrow, and skin may be affected; and **genetic effects** (those that produce fetal anomalies).

Long-term effects, which manifest themselves long after the initial exposure has occurred, are of chief concern among technologists. History has provided us with abundant examples of possible long-term consequences, which can be attributed to either a single, large overexposure or a continuing low-level exposure. Long-term effects are generally described with linear, non-threshold dose-response curves.

In the 1940s, for example, children who had enlarged thymus glands were treated with radiation, and some patients developed **thyroid cancer** as adults. **Radiation-induced cancer** is most frequently seen in the skin; bone; thyroid; and hematopoietic systems (i.e., development of blood cells in the blood-forming organs, such as the bone marrow). Early radiation workers had an extremely high incidence of skin carcinoma as well. Many radium dial painters in the early 1920s died from anemia and bone cancer that was traced to exposure to radium. In like fashion, a high percentage of European radium mine workers suffered bronchogenic (lung) carcinoma within 15 years of beginning work in the mines. Bone marrow, thyroid, and lung cancer are all examples of somatic (i.e., pertaining to the body) effects of radiation.

Among the most probable forms of malignancy to occur from total body radiation overexposure is **leukemia.** Leukemia is a malignant cancer of the blood-forming organs. Radiation workers have a much higher incidence of leukemia than do their medical counterparts who do not use radiation in their work. Other examples of individuals who have a higher incidence of leukemia include the victims of Hiroshima and Nagasaki, patients treated with radiotherapy for ankylosing spondylitis, and children irradiated in utero.

Naturally, persons who have cancer also experience **life shortening,** but radiation also decreases the life span by **hastening the aging process.** In laboratory animals, the age-specific death rate is much lower in the irradiated group than in the controls. But because there are so many variables, it is impossible to uniquely attribute shorter life span to radiation in human subjects. Some authors have theorized that the level of radiation encountered by radiation workers is lower than necessary to significantly decrease the age-specific death rates.

Radiation-induced cataracts (**cataractogenesis**) also occur; this is an example of a biological effect measured by linear threshold dose-response curve. The threshold varies according to type of radiation used, with neutrons being most biologically efficient (causing the most damage). In laboratory animals, cataractogenesis has been determined to be a function of age, with younger eyes being more sensitive than those of older animals. Data obtained from radiotherapy patients reveal the cataractogenic threshold to be approximately 200 rad, whereas it is between 15 and 45 rad of neutrons. No cataractogenesis has been reported in workers who have been exposed to acceptable levels of radiation from occupational exposure.

Hematopoietic syndrome occurs following **acute exposure** to radiation greater than 200 rad. The disease is recognized by depression or ablation (erosion) of the **bone marrow.** In the 200-roentgen (R) range, spontaneous regrowth of the marrow may occur; exposure greater than 700 R leads to irreversible consequences. The clinical course of hematopoietic syndrome is characterized by nausea and vomiting within hours of the overexposure event; the individual feels fatigued and experiences a generalized malaise. Epilation (hair loss) occurs in the second to third week after overexposure, should the victim survive the other clinical manifestations. Other acute consequences include **gastrointestinal (GI) syndrome,** which occurs at exposure levels greater than 1000 R, and leads to death within 1 to 2 weeks; and **central nervous system syndrome,** a consequence of greater than a 2000-R total body exposure.

A low-energy, or diagnostic range, exposure of approximately 300 R results in **erythema** (redness and inflammation of the skin and mucous membranes). A greater exposure may lead to pigmentation change, blistering, necrosis, and ulceration. Among early radiation workers, **radiation dermatitis** was a relatively common consequence.

As previously mentioned, **thyroid carcinogenesis** (the process of initiating cancer) is a known result of radiation overexposure. In addition to pediatric patients who were treated for enlarged thymus, Japanese atomic bomb survivors and Marshall Islands residents exposed to radioactive fallout demonstrated increased incidence of thyroid cancer. Data from bomb survivors demonstrate that children are more susceptible than adults, females are at two to three times greater risk for the disease, thyroid nodules and goiters frequently accompany the disease, and the development of the disease is to a great degree dependent on the production of thyroid hormones. As production increases, so does carcinogenic risk.

Prenatal exposure to radiation is known to produce **fetal anomalies** (congenital malformation) and **malignant diseases.** The fetus is particularly **radiosensitive** during the first trimester of pregnancy. Skeletal and neurologic anomalies, mental retardation, and malignant disease all may occur if radiation is delivered in sufficient quantity. Fetal irradiation during the first 2 weeks of gestation may result in spontaneous abortion. High-risk examinations during this period include pelvis; kidney, ureter, and bladder (KUB); lumbar spine; intravenous pyelogram; and fluoroscopic examinations.

It is generally agreed that harmful effects stemming from irradiation during the first trimester require fetal doses exceeding 20 rad in order to be biologically effective. The technologist should be aware that although most diagnostic examinations deliver fetal doses in the range of 1 to 2 rad, he/she still bears an ethical responsibility to protect female patients of childbearing age in this regard. Therefore, patients in this category should always be questioned concerning the possibility of pregnancy and the date of their last menstrual period. Ten days following the onset of menstruation is considered the least likely time for a fertilized ovum to be present; therefore, many facilities use the **10-day rule** as a guide for scheduling female patients of childbearing age.

Sixty-eight percent of radiation exposure to the population at large stems from natural background radiation (e.g., cosmic rays, radon, and so on). The remaining total dose is largely attributable to radiation delivered during medical and dental examinations (31%); nuclear fallout, nuclear energy plants, and occupational exposure account for the remaining 1%. When taken into account with other variables such as geographic location, altitude of residency, accessibility to health care, and general health, this distribution makes it difficult to describe a dose that is genetically significant, that is, a radiation dose that will have meaningful impact (to the population as a whole) on future births.

Therefore, the concept of **genetically significant dose (GSD)** was devised. The GSD can be defined as the average annual gonadal dose to the childbearing age population, which is estimated to be 20 millirem (mrem). The GSD takes into account that although some individuals may receive no dose at all, others may be exposed to large doses, whereas still others are past reproductive years or will not produce children. The impact of a large dose on certain individuals is lessened when it is averaged with that of the entire population.

In 1906, the French scientists Bergonie and Tribondeau performed the seminal research in the field of **radiosensitivity.** The scientists determined that cells that are immature—for example, undifferentiated or stem cells—and highly mitotic cells—that is, highly proliferative cells— have increased radiosensitivity. Human cells are classified as either germ cells, which are involved with reproduction, or somatic cells. Cell division of germ cells is called **meiosis. Mitosis** (somatic cell division) can be divided into four stages: **prophase, metaphase, anaphase, and telophase. Interphase** is a resting cycle. Cells are most radiosensitive during the period when chromosomes line up along the nuclear equator, a process that occurs during metaphase. Developing tissue is also highly radiosensitive. As a general rule, technologists should recall that undeveloped tissue and cells are more radiosensitive than their developed counterparts.

Tissue in an oxygenated state is more radiosensitive than hypoxic tissue. Because of this tendency, avascular tumors (i.e., tumors with no blood flow, and therefore no oxygen content) are especially difficult to treat with radiotherapy. In some instances, hyperbaric therapy is used in conjunction with radiotherapy to increase tissue radiosensitivity.

QUESTIONS FOR BIOLOGICAL EFFECTS OF RADIATION

select the best answer

1. Which of the following is a possible consequence of a typical diagnostic exposure?
   (A) Cataracts
   (B) Gastrointestinal syndrome
   (C) Hematopoietic syndrome
   (D) None of the aforementioned

2. The 10-day rule is a guide concerning which of the following time periods?
   (A) Ten days past the first trimester
   (B) Ten days following the onset of menstruation

(C) The first 10 days of gestation
(D) Ten days following birth

3. Which of the following statements is true?

(A) Avascular tumors have increased radiosensitivity when compared with vascular tumors.
(B) Oxygenation level in treatment of tumors is irrelevant.
(C) Hypoxic tumors have decreased radiosensitivity versus vascular tumors.
(D) Hypoxic tumors cannot be treated with radiotherapy.

4. All of the following are considered late, or long-term, effects of irradiation except:

(A) leukemia.
(B) bronchogenic carcinoma.
(C) cataractogenesis.
(D) erythema.

5. Of the following dose-response curves, which is the correct curve for use with a typical diagnostic dose?

(A) Linear, non-threshold
(B) Non-linear, threshold
(C) Linear, threshold
(D) Non-linear, non-threshold

6. Which of the following statements is (are) true concerning the RBE?

(A) RBE is a qualitative measure.
(B) RBE uses 200 keV as an index of effectiveness.
(C) RBE compares one type of dose with another in order to determine relative toxicity.
(D) All of the aforementioned are true.

7. A one-time, 200-R dose directly to the hair follicles would most likely result in:

(A) moist desquamation.
(B) epilation.
(C) hirsutism.
(D) hematopoietic syndrome.

8. According to the laws of Bergonie and Tribondeau, which of the following cell types would be least radiosensitive?

(A) Muscle cells
(B) Gonadal cells
(C) Eye cells
(D) Bone marrow cells

▶▶ ANSWERS TO BIOLOGICAL EFFECTS OF RADIATION

1. The answer is (D). All of the listed biological effects require a far greater dose to occur than the typical dose delivered in a diagnostic setting.
2. The answer is (B). The period 10 days following the onset of menstruation is considered the least likely time for a fertilized ovum to be present. Some facilities use this period to schedule radiographic examinations on female patients of childbearing age.
3. The answer is (C). Oxygen levels in tissue are related to radiosensitivity. The higher the O_2 levels, the higher the radiosensitivity.
4. The answer is (D). Biological effects from radiation can be classified as acute and chronic effects. Chronic effects include various cancers and the development of cataracts, and may be caused by either a single high-level overexposure or a low-level dose delivered over time. Acute effects generally stem from a single event, and include erythema, gastrointestinal syndrome, and central nervous syndrome.
5. The answer is (A). The BEIR has determined that the correct tool for measuring biological response from a given dose of the type typically delivered in diagnostic x-ray is the linear, non-threshold curve.
6. The answer is (D). An absorbed dose of x-ray has quite a different biological effect from that of an identical dose of alpha particles or neutrons. **RBE** is a measurement used to determine the relative toxicity (potential to create biological damage) of a given dose of one type of radiation compared with that of another (e.g., x-ray versus alpha particles). RBE is expressed as the ratio of the amount of energy of a given type of radiation required to produce a given biological effect to the energy required to produce that same biological effect when using 200 keV of x-ray.
7. The answer is (B). The hair follicles of the skin are extremely radiosensitive, and a 200-R exposure would most likely result in hair loss. Epilation is a term for hair loss. Hirsutism is a term for abnormal hair growth affecting the entire body.
8. The answer is (A). Bergonie and Tribondeau determined that immature cells, that is, undifferentiated stem or precursor cells, such as those found in bone marrow, or highly mitotic cells, that is, highly proliferative cells, such as those found in the gonads or lens of the eye, are most radiosensitive. Myocytes, or muscle cells, are mature, differ-

entiated cells, and are therefore fairly radioresistant.

B. Minimizing Patient Exposure

The previous section (Section A) provides information regarding the possible health consequences from exposure to ionizing radiation. It should be clear from this information that the technologist bears an ethical responsibility to keep the patient's exposure to a minimum, while maximizing the diagnostic benefit. The following sections (1 through 9) explore various means of achieving this goal.

1. EXPOSURE FACTORS

Kilovoltage peak is the exposure factor that controls quality (penetrating ability) of the x-ray beam. As kVp increases, overall energy and frequency of the beam increase, whereas wavelength decreases. Higher kVp technique delivers a smaller absorbed dose to the patient, as higher energy photons tend to pass through the body unchanged to expose the film.

Milliamperage (mA) is the exposure factor that controls the quantity (intensity) of photons produced in a given exposure. Increasing tube current frees more electrons per second at the filament, thus increasing the exposure rate; however, mA has no effect on the average energy level of the x-ray beam. Generally speaking, then, using high kVp, low mA technique yields the lowest patient dose.

2. GENERATORS

It is important to consider patient exposure from the standpoint of how radiant energy is produced. Remember that x-rays are produced when a fast-moving stream of electrons undergoes rapid deceleration. In order to reproduce these conditions most efficiently, the x-ray circuit must be rectified in order to change incoming alternating current—which changes direction as it enters its negative cycle—to unidirectional current (pulsating direct current). The rectifier is located between the secondary coil of the high-voltage transformer and the x-ray tube. Rectifiers are solid-state diodes constructed of semiconductors such as silicon or selenium, which conduct electricity in only one direction.

With single-phase generators, the voltage constantly rises and falls from zero to maximum. The end result is an x-ray beam that varies in energy considerably over the length of exposure time. A three-phase generator, on the other hand, operates on three-phase current, which is comprised of three single-phase currents separated by one third of a cycle (120 degrees). Whereas single-phase current can be identified by a sine wave that alternatively falls to zero, three-phase current is characterized by a voltage ripple, which is also variable according to the type of rectification used to produce it. There are three types of three-phase circuits: six-pulse, six-rectifier; six-pulse, twelve-rectifier; and twelve-pulse, twelve-rectifier.

Comparison of single- and three-phase generators reveals that three-phase current produces an x-ray beam of higher average energy. Therefore, taking the increased energy into account in terms of its effect on the radiograph, it can be seen that in order to produce a radiograph of identical density, less technique is required with the three-phase generator than with the single-phase generator.

A 100-kVp, single-phase–generated x-ray beam is roughly equivalent to the beam generated by an 85-kVp device. If the technologist were to select 100 kVp on both types of equipment, the three-phase mA necessary to reproduce the same radiographic density would be 0.40% that of the single-phase generator. However, this adjustment would lessen contrast on the radiograph, so adjustment of technique to obtain identical contrast and density will produce a radiation exposure to the patient that is the same for both types of equipment.

3. SHIELDING

A primary method of minimizing patient exposure is through use of protective lead (Pb) shielding. Two areas of the body are of chief concern with respect to the rationale for shielding: (1) the gonads, in order to reduce the danger of injury to genetic material, and (2) the blood-forming bone marrow, to reduce somatic injury.

Gonadal shielding should be used whenever possible; however, there are times it is not possible, because use of shielding will obscure diagnostic information on the radiograph. Otherwise, gonadal shielding should be used if the gonads lie directly in or within a 5-cm distance from the x-ray beam, as well as when the patient has reproductive potential. At most facilities, patients under the age of 55 are considered to be within this group. Shielding male patients is relatively easy, because the testicles lie outside of the body, whereas shielding of the ovaries is restricted by uncertainty regarding their specific location.

There are four primary types of lead shielding to consider, and all must consist of at least a 0.5-mm lead equivalent in order to be effective. **Flat, contact** shields are the most common type and usually consist of lead-impregnated pieces of vinyl placed over the patient's gonads. This type of shield is most effective with the patient in a simple prone or supine position, because any obliquity makes the shield harder to secure.

Shadow shields are leaded material attached directly to the x-ray tube by means of an arm extension. The shield casts a shadow that corresponds in the illuminated field to the desired area. Shadow shields require an initial monetary investment that is higher than that for other shield types, but they tend to last longer and are more cost effective in the long range. Shadow shields may not be used for fluoroscopic procedures; however, they are advantageous in conjunction with maintaining a sterile field.

Contour shields are perhaps the most effective method of gonadal shielding. They are shaped to enclose the testicles and are held in place by disposable briefs. Contour shields can be used in any position without worry about the shielding sliding out of correct position. **Breast shields** are used when developing breast tissue is a concern. This type of patient protection is generally used in conjunction with scoliosis series and is either incorporated in the vertebral compensating filter or as a leaded vest.

Placement of lead shielding is of utmost importance, because improper placement can lead to patient re-exposure. Patients can be shielded via lead aprons, thus decreasing somatic dose, when the area of diagnostic interest is other than that of the shielded area. Common examples are shielding with half aprons during chest radiography, and shielding with aprons for extremity radiography.

Patients often inquire about the dose of radiation that is acquired during a given procedure. **Table 2-1,** which is compiled from National Council for Radiation Protection and Measurements (NCRP) reports, can be used as a general guide in your department. Of course, dose varies according to facility and patient size; the data presented in this table are considered to be accurate to ±8% to 15%.

4. BEAM RESTRICTION

Beam restriction devices limit the size of the primary beam to the area of diagnostic interest. The purpose of primary beam restriction is the reduction of low-energy photons reaching the patient and film, thus reducing patient dose and improving image quality via the reduction of secondary and scatter radiation. A reduction in scatter results in reduced film fog. Remember, secondary radiation is that radiation **emit-**

TABLE 2.1. Radiation Doses for Various Procedures			
Examination	Entrance Exposure Per Film (mrem)	Male Gonadal Dose (mrad)	Female Gonadal Dose (mrad)
Skull	330	0	0
Chest	44	0	1
UGI	710	1	170
BE	1,320	175	900
Lumbar Spine	1,920	220	720
Pelvis	610	360	210
KUB	670	100	220
Hip	560	600	125
Hand	100	0	0

ted by atoms that have absorbed x-ray photons. Scatter radiation is radiation that has **changed direction** as a result of interaction with atoms.

Collimators, which consist of a series of lead shutters mounted to the x-ray tube head, are the most widely used and most efficient beam restriction device. One set of lead shutters is placed adjacent to the tube port window to control image-degrading **off-focus** radiation. Off-focus radiation is that part of the beam that strikes other than the focal track of the anode. Another set of shutters, more familiar to the technologist, controls the length and width of the primary beam reaching the patient. These are the shutters that shape the collimated border on the film.

Cones are circular, lead-lined beam restriction devices that attach to the x-ray tube head and limit the beam to a fixed size. Some cones have extension devices that operate by means of a side-mounted screw, which when loosened allows the cone to extend. Some typical examinations that employ the use of cones are those for the paranasal sinus and spot views of L5–S1.

Some chest and head units employ simple lead **aperture diaphragms,** which are lead devices with a central opening that dictates the amount of beam restriction. Although head units may use differing sizes of aperture diaphragms that can be switched according to desired examination, chest units tend to use a one-size, fixed type of device.

5. FILTRATION

Filtration also reduces secondary and scatter radiation by eliminating low-energy photons that would other-

► **TABLE 2.2.**   NCRP Filtration Standards
<50 KVP filtration must equal 0.5 mm Al equivalent
50–70 KVP filtration must equal 1.5 mm Al equivalent
>70 KVP filtration must equal 2.5 mm Al equivalent

wise increase skin and organ dose. Removing low-energy photons has the effect of increasing average beam energy. **Inherent filtration** elements are those already present in the x-ray tube that have a filtering effect. Examples of inherent filtration elements are the x-ray tube housing and oil coolant. It should be noted that over the life of the x-ray tube, tungsten evaporates and forms deposits on the inner surface of the glass envelope. These deposits act as additional filtration, but decrease tube output. Therefore, the technologist should recall that inherent filtration increases with time. **Added filtration** elements are the collimator and mirror, as well as thin sheets of aluminum (Al) that can be added to the tube, generally through a thin slit in the side of the x-ray tube head.

Total filtration for the x-ray unit is derived from the following formula:

Total filtration = inherent filtration + added filtration

The NCRP measures filtration for standard x-ray tubes by means of **aluminum equivalent.** The required amount of filtration is dependent on the operating kVp. NCRP filtration standards are presented in **Table 2-2.**

Some mammography equipment uses molybdenum (Mo) targets. These tubes operate using Mo filtration equaling 0.0025 to 0.0030 Mo. Fractional tungsten (W) x-ray tubes, used with magnification radiography, must be 0.5-mm Al equivalent.

The **half-value layer (HVL)** of an x-ray beam is an important measurement related to filtration. HVL is defined as the thickness of a material necessary to reduce the exposure rate by one half. Thus, if a given exposure rate is 100 R/min and requires 3.5 mm of aluminum filtration to reduce the rate to 50 R/min, the HVL is equal to 3.5-mm Al.

6. PATIENT POSITIONING

Due to the nature of the x-ray beam, skin dose is always greater than that of the exit dose. Therefore, placing more radiosensitive body parts away from the primary beam is an effective means of further minimizing patient exposure. For example, dose to the lens of the eye is lessened by posteroanterior (PA) versus anteroposterior (AP) positioning, and gonadal dose can be reduced by performing abdominal radiography in the PA position whenever feasible. Likewise, breast-tissue dose is decreased by using the PA position.

7. FILMS AND SCREENS

Rare earth screens are in general four times faster than traditional calcium tungstate screens, and therefore require proportionately less radiation to produce a comparable density. Similarly, faster film speed decreases technique requirements. It should be noted that increasing film speed and screen speed results in a reduction in recorded detail; however, in most cases, a rare earth/fast-film screen system produces adequate diagnostic detail.

8. GRIDS AND AIR-GAP TECHNIQUE

Grids are lead devices, either moving (bucky) or stationary, designed to reduce scatter radiation that would otherwise reach the film and reduce image quality. Scatter reaching the film is undesirable, but does contribute to overall film density. Therefore, grid use requires a significant increase in selected technical factors. In this case, improvement in quality of the finished radiograph far outweighs the attendant increase in patient dose. Technologists must acquaint themselves with the technical considerations of grid use in order to prevent re-exposure to the patient.

The **air-gap technique** is sometimes used in place of a grid. By placing a distance in between the body part and film, exiting photons from the patient continue divergence and thus never reach the film. A lateral cervical spine performed without a grid is an example of this technique, because the shoulders of the patient place a natural distance between the patient and film. Using **increased object film distance (OFD)** for the purposes of magnification is another common use of the air-gap technique; a 20-cm air gap is roughly equivalent in image cleanup capability to the use of a 15–1 grid. Technologists should remember, however, that placing the part closer to the tube also increases dose, as governed by the inverse square law.

9. AUTOMATIC EXPOSURE CONTROL

Automatic exposure devices (AED) or automatic exposure controls (AECs) are devices used to regulate patient exposure and consistently reproduce diagnostic-quality radiographs. There are two primary types. An **ion chamber** is a device positioned beneath the tabletop or upright stand but above the bucky and radiographic film. X-rays emerge from the patient and ionize the air within the chamber. When a predetermined level relative to the body part thickness that is being exposed is reached, the exposure is terminated. A **phototimer** uses a fluorescent screen that emits light when it is irradiated to charge a photomultiplier tube. Once the charge relative to the body part thickness is reached, the exposure terminates. A **backup timer** is used in conjunction with both types of devices to prevent overexposure to the patient and x-ray tube in case of AEC malfunction. If the exposure time exceeds that of the backup time, the exposure is terminated.

QUESTIONS FOR MINIMIZING PATIENT EXPOSURE

select the best answer

1. All other factors being equal, which of the listed technical settings will yield the lowest patient dose?
   (A) 5 milliampere-seconds (mAs), 70 kVp
   (B) 10 mAs, 60 kVp
   (C) 20 mAs, 51 kVp
   (D) 2.5 mAs, 80 kVp

2. A type of shielding that attaches to the x-ray tube is:
   (A) contour.
   (B) flat.
   (C) shadow.
   (D) breast.

3. The purpose of primary beam restriction is to:
   (A) improve image quality.
   (B) increase overall energy level of the x-ray beam.
   (C) reduce exposure time.
   (D) none of the aforementioned.

4. According to NCRP guidelines, at least how much filtration is required of an exposure room used primarily for examinations of the GI tract?
   (A) 2.5 mm Al
   (B) 0.0025 mm Al
   (C) 1.5 mm Mo
   (D) 0.5 mm Al

5. Gonadal shielding can be used effectively on male patients for which of the following examinations?
   1. KUB
   2. Hip
   3. Forearm

   (A) Choice 1 only
   (B) Choice 3 only
   (C) Choices 2 and 3
   (D) Choices 1, 2, and 3

6. Which of the following are examples of inherent filtration elements?
   (A) Collimator
   (B) Oil coolant
   (C) Aluminum inserts
   (D) Mirror

7. How do rare earth screens minimize patient exposure?
   (A) Rare earth screens have wider exposure latitude.
   (B) Rare earth screens produce better detail.
   (C) Rare earth screens produce more light.
   (D) Rare earth screens need higher kVp in order to function.

8. Which of the following exposure rooms would commonly employ an aperture diaphragm?
   1. Dedicated chest room
   2. Specials room
   3. Franklin head unit

   (A) Choice 2 only
   (B) Choices 1 and 3
   (C) Choice 3 only
   (D) Choices 1, 2, and 3

▶▶ ANSWERS TO MINIMIZING PATIENT EXPOSURE

1. The answer is (D). Although these exposure factors are rough equivalents, in general high-kVp, low-mAs exposures yield the lowest patient dose.
2. The answer is (C). A shadow shield is a leaded device that is a attached to the x-ray tube head by means of a flexible arm. A shadow in the illuminated x-ray field indicates the shielded area on the patient.
3. The answer is (B). Increasing the energy level of the beam has the effect of reducing absorbed dose to the patient by reducing the number of low-energy photons that have only sufficient energy to penetrate the skin and be absorbed.

4. The answer is (A). GI examinations are generally performed using barium sulfate, a highly dense material that necessitates exposures be made using at least 100 kVp in order to penetrate the material adequately. Therefore, according to NCRP guidelines, the filtration requirements for such a room must exceed a 2.5-mm Al equivalent.

5. The answer is (D). Although care must be taken not to obscure diagnostic information with respect to the KUB and hip films, shielding of male patients is easily accomplished, and the finished radiograph should demonstrate evidence of gonadal shielding.

6. The answer is (B). Inherent filtration is that filtration intrinsic in the x-ray tube. Examples are oil coolant and the x-ray tube housing.

7. The answer is (C). By producing more light to expose the radiographic film, rare earth screens reduce the amount of radiation required to produce a given density on radiographic film.

8. The answer is (B). Aperture diaphragms are commonly associated with chest rooms and head units.

II. PERSONNEL PROTECTION
A. Sources of Radiation Exposure
1. EXPOSURE TO PRIMARY BEAM

The objective of a radiologic personnel protection program is to maintain the occupational exposure rate as far as possible below the maximum permissible dose. Obviously, exposure to the **primary beam** represents the greatest danger to technologists. Therefore, when it is necessary to hold or restrain a patient for the purpose of maintaining the required position, occupationally exposed personnel should never be used.

Instead, the technologist should attempt to use a mechanical restraining device which, when properly used, supplies the needed support. In the event it is necessary to hold the patient, a male or nonpregnant female adult should be employed. Careful attention by the technologist should be given to the placement of these individuals; they should be positioned as far as possible from the useful beam, and never directly in its path.

2. SECONDARY RADIATION

Secondary and scatter radiation, particularly high-energy Compton scatter emerging from the patient, represents the greatest occupational exposure hazard to the technologist. Although the patient is the greatest source of scatter, other objects to consider are the radiograph table, the bucky slot cover, and the control booth wall or protective barrier. The intensity of scatter radiation 1 meter from the patient is 0.10% that of the primary beam.

3. LEAKAGE RADIATION

Radiation emanating from the tube housing in a differing direction from the useful beam is considered **leakage radiation.** NCRP guidelines state that leakage radiation should not exceed 100 milliroentgen (mR) per hour at a distance of 1 meter from the x-ray tube.

select the best answer

1. An elderly patient arrives via stretcher at the radiography department and is unable to stand for chest radiographic examination. Attempts to provide the patient with support equipment have failed. Realizing that you require someone to hold the patient to complete the examination, you should:

   (A) call another technologist to assist.
   (B) perform a supine examination.
   (C) call a nurse to assist.
   (D) ask an adult family member to assist.

2. The greatest threat of occupational exposure arises from:

   (A) Compton scatter.
   (B) primary beam.
   (C) Thompson scatter.
   (D) photoelectric effect.

3. According to NCRP guidelines, leakage radiation should not exceed:

   (A) 100 R/hr at 1 m.
   (B) 1000 mR/min at 10 m.
   (C) 100 mR/hr at 1 m.
   (D) 100 mR/hr at 10 m.

▶▶ **ANSWERS TO SOURCES OF RADIATION EXPOSURE**

1. The answer is (D). Technologists should never modify a requested examination without a physi-

cian's order. In such a situation, every attempt should be made to employ the assistance of non–occupationally exposed personnel, such as an adult family member.

2. The answer is (A). For the technologist, the greatest risk of occupational radiation exposure comes from Compton scatter, particularly that associated with high kVp–produced fluoroscopy. Recall that Compton scatter is the result of an incident photon first removing a loosely bound electron and then proceeding at a lower energy level in a different direction. The photoelectric effect results in the complete absorption of the incident photon. Thompson scatter, another name for coherent or unmodified scatter, is the result of an incident photon interacting with an electron bound with identical energy, with production of an electromagnetic wave of identical energy but in a different direction.

3. The answer is (C). NCRP guidelines state that radiation emanating from the tube housing and proceeding in a direction other than the primary beam should not exceed 100 mR/hr at a distance of 1 meter.

B. Basic Methods of Protection

The fundamental principles of occupational radiation protection are based on three key ideas: time, distance, and shielding.

1. TIME

Decreasing the amount of time spent exposed to ionizing radiation minimizes occupational exposure. To some degree, the technologist can facilitate a reduction in fluoroscopy exposure by better organizing the exposure room and having increased awareness of the radiologist's needs. The more smoothly an examination proceeds, the less time is spent with the fluoroscope turned on. Similarly, a conscientious technologist will take every measure possible to increase his/her store of knowledge concerning the examinations performed, thus reducing the necessity of repeat exposures. In some instances, as in use of the C-arm in the operating room, or in the GI laboratory during endoscopic retrograde cholangiopancreatography procedures, the technologist may be required to perform the actual fluoroscopy. In these cases, intermittent exposure rather than continuous exposure techniques for fluoroscopy are best. More modern units have a "last image hold" feature that automatically saves the last image taken, thus reducing the need for uninterrupted fluoroscopy.

2. DISTANCE

The **inverse square law** states that the intensity of the x-ray beam is inversely proportional to the square of the distance between the x-ray source and the area of interest. Therefore, doubling the amount of distance results in a fourfold decrease in exposure intensity. This principle is especially important to recall when performing portable radiography, a clinical situation in which distance is the primary means of exposure reduction.

3. SHIELDING

Placement of lead barriers between the technologist and the radiation source also reduces occupational exposure. **Primary barriers** such as the lead walls and door of the exposure suite have high attenuation rates and are effective protection from the useful beam. **Secondary barriers** are designed to provide additional protection from leakage (from the tube housing) and scatter radiation (primarily from the patient). Examples of secondary barriers are the walls of the exposure room that are more than 7 feet in height, lead aprons and gloves, and the control booth. Recall that the primary beam should never be directed at the control booth.

QUESTIONS FOR BASIC METHODS OF PROTECTION

select the best answer

1. If the known dose for a given exposure is 50 mrem at a distance of 40 inches, what will the exposure be at 80 inches?
   (A) 100 mrem
   (B) 200 mrem
   (C) 25 mrem
   (D) 12.5 mrem

2. Which of the following is a secondary radiation barrier?
   (A) Lead-lined door
   (B) Collimation
   (C) Lead apron
   (D) Filtration

3. If a known exposure produces a 10-mrem exposure at 1 second, what exposure would result from a 0.75-second exposure, using otherwise identical technical factors?
   (A) 7.5 mrem
   (B) 75 mrem
   (C) 40 mrem
   (D) 5 mrem

▶▶ ANSWERS TO BASIC METHODS OF PROTECTION

1. The answer is (D). According to the inverse square law, $I_o/I_n = D_n^2 / D_o^2$; therefore, to solve, $50/x = 80^2/40^2$; $6400x = 80,000$; $x = 12.5$.
2. The answer is (C). Other examples of secondary barriers include walls of the exposure suite that are more than 7 feet in height, lead gloves, glasses, thyroid protection, and the control booth.
3. The answer is (A). The relationship between time and exposure rate is directly proportional. Therefore, a 0.25 reduction in time would result in a 0.25 reduction in dose.

C. NCRP Recommendations for Protective Devices

In 1928, the NCRP (see end of section for NCRP correspondence information) was founded as the Advisory Committee on X-ray and Radium Protection and was later reorganized as the National Committee on Radiation Protection. A congressional charter was granted in 1964 to the National Council on Radiation Protection and Measurements, which allowed 75 scientists to serve 6-year terms as members. The NCRP is a nonprofit corporation chartered by Congress to:

- Collect, analyze, develop, and disseminate for the public interest information and recommendations about (1) protection against radiation and (2) radiation measurements, quantities, and units, particularly those concerned with radiation protection
- Provide a means by which organizations concerned with the scientific and related aspects of radiation protection and radiation quantities, units, and measurements can cooperate for effective use of their combined resources, as well as to stimulate the work of such organizations
- Develop basic concepts about radiation quantities, units, and measurements; the application of these concepts; and radiation protection
- Cooperate with the International Commission on Radiological Protection, the International Commission on Radiation Units and Measurements, and other national and international organizations—government and private—that are concerned with radiation quantities, units, measurements, and radiation protection

Primary barriers, or barriers that protect the technologist from the primary beam, must have greater attenuation capacity than that of secondary barriers. NCRP guidelines state that primary barriers must consist of a lead lining 1/16 of an inch thick and must extend to a height of 7 feet, whereas secondary barriers, those barriers that protect against leakage and secondary radiation, require the thickness of the lead lining to be 1/32 of an inch.

Required thickness of primary and secondary barriers is further governed by **distance** from the x-ray source. Decreasing the distance from source to barrier increases the required thickness. **Occupancy factor** refers to the population of the space adjacent to the x-ray source: greater occupancy requires greater protection. **Use factor** is a term that refers to the amount of time a particular location is exposed to the useful beam. Increased use requires increased thickness. **Workload** refers to cumulative examinations performed per week. Greater workload requires greater thickness of shielding.

Guidelines further stipulate that (1) technologists must be physically present in the control booth when making the exposure, and (2) the exposure switch and cord should be configured in such a way that the control booth operation is the only way of making the exposure. Leaded glass, a feature in control booths that permits observation of the patient, must be a 1.5-mm Pb equivalent.

Protective apparel requirements are governed by **NCRP Report Number 102.** The report states that lead gloves must be a 0.25-Pb equivalent, whereas lead aprons must consist of a 0.50-Pb equivalent. Technologists should recall that leaded apparel is a secondary barrier and does not provide protection from the useful beam.

Protective apparel should be stored on appropriate racks so as to prevent cracking of the rubberized lead material; this apparel should be imaged yearly as part of the radiology department's radiation protection program.

The NCRP can be reached by mail at: 7910 Woodmont Avenue, Suite 800, Bethesda, MD 20814-3095; telephone: (301) 657-2652; E-mail: ncrp@ncrp.com

QUESTIONS FOR NCRP RECOMMENDATIONS FOR PROTECTIVE DEVICES

select the best answer

1. Lead aprons must have Pb equivalents of:
   (A) > 0.50 mm.
   (B) ~ 0.50 mm.

(C) = 0.50 mm.
(D) < 0.50 mm.

2. Protective apparel such as lead aprons and gloves should be _____ at least once every_____.
   (A) worn, week
   (B) imaged, month
   (C) worn, day
   (D) imaged, year

3. Which of the following are factors in determining primary-barrier Pb requirements?
   1. Distance from source to barrier
   2. Average age of exposed population
   3. Reproductive potential of exposed population
   4. Number of examinations performed per week

   (A) Choices 1 and 3
   (B) Choices 1 and 4
   (C) Choice 3 only
   (D) Choice 4 only

▶▶ **ANSWERS TO NCRP RECOMMENDATIONS FOR PROTECTIVE DEVICES**

1. The answer is (C). Lead aprons must consist of material equal to 0.50-mm Pb equivalent. Lead gloves must be a 0.25-Pb equivalent.
2. The answer is (D). As part of the departmental radiation safety program, secondary barriers such as leaded apparel should be imaged with either plain film radiography or fluoroscopy at least once a year.
3. The answer is (B). The factors that influence required thickness of a given barrier are distance, workload, occupancy factor, and use factor. Age and reproductive potential, although important considerations from the standpoint of biological effects, are not related to determining barrier thickness requirements.

D. Special Considerations

1. MOBILE UNITS

Occupational radiation dose is greatest in two areas: portable radiography and fluoroscopy. In order to prevent overexposure when performing these modalities, the technologist must be mindful of radiation protection fundamentals, that is, time, shielding, and distance. Each portable unit should have protective lead equipment—including aprons, gloves, and glasses—

assigned to it, and the technologist should attain maximum distance from the x-ray tube during the exposure. NCRP guidelines state that the exposure cord must permit the technologist to stand at least 6 feet from the x-ray source. Some mobile units feature cordless designs that permit remote exposures. Mobile fluoroscopic units (C-arm units) must permit a 12-inch source-to-skin distance (SSD) as well.

2. FLUOROSCOPY

Another protective device designed to curb occupational exposure is the **protective drape** or **curtain.** The curtain is constructed of at least a 0.25-mm Pb equivalent and is attached to the fluoroscope tower in order to reduce scatter emanating from the patient. The curtain is positioned between the patient and the technologist and physician when the fluoroscope tower is pulled across the examination table.

The **bucky slot/cover** must also be of a 0.25-Pb equivalent to attenuate scattered radiation, which is emitted approximately at the level of the gonads with under-table fluoroscopic tubes. A **cumulative timing device** must be present to give persons present in the radiographic suite a signal (either an audible, visible, or combination signal) when a given amount of time, usually 5 minutes, has elapsed.

NCRP guidelines (CFR-21) provide further specifications regarding fluoroscopy, mobile x-ray, and mobile fluoroscopy. Tabletop intensity of the beam must be less than 10 R/min (or 2.1 R/min/mA), and should preferably be less than 5 R/min. Fluoroscopic milliamperage must not exceed 5 mA, although this is not a factor with image-intensified fluoroscopy, which generally uses relatively high kVp technique and settings between 1 and 3 mA. Modern fluoroscopic units use automatic exposure controls, so technique varies widely according to the part being imaged, with thicker body parts such as the abdomen requiring more exposure than body parts of lesser density, such as the chest.

The **image intensifier** is classified as a primary barrier and therefore must have at least a 2.0-mm Pb equivalent. The monitor must demonstrate evidence of beam collimation on the viewed image. Total filtration of the fluoroscopy unit must be equal to or greater than a 2.5-mm Al equivalent.

QUESTIONS FOR SPECIAL CONSIDERATIONS

select the best answer

1. What is the maximum amount of time that can elapse before the fluoroscopic cumulative timer must be reset?

(A) 5 minutes
(B) 10 minutes
(C) 15 minutes
(D) 20 minutes

2. An exposure is made using the following technical factors: 50 mAs, 70 kVp, 40″ SID. In order to reduce patient dose and maintain the same approximate density, which of the following combinations of exposure factors should be used?

(A) 50 mAs, 80 kVp, 40″ SID
(B) 25 mAs, 80 kVp, 40″ SID
(C) 60 mAs, 60 kVp, 48″ SID
(D) 50 mAs, 70 kVp, 72″ SID

3. According to NCRP guidelines, at least how far should a technologist stand from the exposure source during a portable abdomen examination?

(A) 2 feet
(B) 4 feet
(C) 6 feet
(D) 8 feet

4. What SSD must be maintained during a mobile fluoroscopy–guided surgical repair of an intertrochanteric fracture?

(A) 1 foot
(B) 2 feet
(C) 6 inches
(D) 3 feet

▶▶ ANSWERS TO SPECIAL CONSIDERATIONS

1. The answer is (A). The cumulative timer is a protective device. It reminds the technologist and radiologist of the actual amount of radiation used for the procedure.

2. The answer is (B). Increasing kVp with a corresponding appropriate reduction in mAs will reduce patient dose while maintaining density, albeit with a slightly longer scale contrast using these factors. Simply changing distance will reduce patient dose but results in an underexposed radiograph. Similarly, increasing kVp as the sole adjustment will increase average beam intensity, thus reducing patient dose, but in the absence of mAs reduction, this technique will produce film that is too dark.

3. The answer is (C). NCRP guidelines state that the exposure cord on mobile x-ray units must permit technologists to stand at least 6 feet away from the tube during the exposure. Distance is the primary means of radiation protection during portable radiography.

4. The answer is (A). One of the most common uses for the C-arm unit is during image-guided surgical repairs. NCRP guidelines indicate that a 12″ SSD must be maintained during mobile fluoroscopic procedures.

III. RADIATION EXPOSURE AND MONITORING
A. Basic Properties of Radiation

An x-ray is a **highly penetrating, electrically neutral** energy form that is part of the **electromagnetic spectrum and travels at the speed of light** (3×10^8 m/sec). Unlike light, an x-ray **cannot be focused** by means of a lens but can be restricted by the use of lead shutters, as is the case with collimators in the x-ray unit. The x-ray is **not affected by magnetic or electrical fields.** The x-ray beam is comprised of discrete bits of energy called **photons (or quanta)** that have **heterogeneous (made up of dissimilar elements) energy levels** and behave both as **particles and waves.** The useful range of energy in diagnostic radiology is approximately 25 to 140 kVp.

The x-ray **releases minute amounts of heat** when traveling through matter and **ionizes tissue,** causing chemical and biological changes. Radiation causes fluorescence in certain crystals; this property is used with fluoroscopy and intensifying screens. Similarly, the x-ray affects photographic film, producing a latent image that can be processed chemically. A typical x-ray beam produces secondary and scatter radiation when interacting with matter.

QUESTIONS FOR BASIC PROPERTIES OF RADIATION

select the best answer

1. The characteristic of x-rays that permits image-intensified fluoroscopy is called:
(A) screen lag.
(B) heterogeneous energy level.
(C) fluorescence.
(D) excitation.

2. _____ is the property of x-rays that induces chemical and biological changes in living matter.

(A) Somatic effect
(B) Genetic effect
(C) Ionization
(D) Heat

3. Which of the following types of tissue would be most likely to absorb the highest dose of radiation?
   (A) Blood
   (B) Bone
   (C) Heart
   (D) Liver

4. Which of the following types of radiation are considered electromagnetic in nature?
   1. X-ray
   2. Alpha
   3. Beta
   4. Gamma

   (A) Choice 1 only
   (B) Choices 2 and 3
   (C) Choice 4 only
   (D) Choices 1 and 4

▶▶**ANSWERS TO BASIC PROPERTIES OF RADIATION**

1. The answer is (C). X-rays induce fluorescence in certain crystals such as cesium iodide and zinc cadmium sulfate, which are similar in nature to intensifying screens. The primary difference between the fluoroscopic image and an image produced with intensifying screens is that the fluoroscopic image persists only during excitation of the screen by x-ray. It is this property that permits real-time visualization of anatomy and physiology during fluoroscopy.
2. The answer is (C). X-rays interact with biological tissue, causing ionization, the process in which a neutral atom gains or loses an electron. Ionization produces a wide array of biological effects, including cell death and mutation.
3. The answer is (B). Of the tissue listed, bone is the type possessing the greatest attenuation coefficient; therefore, it would absorb the greatest dose. Blood-filled organs such as the heart and liver would be the next greatest absorbers of radiation; blood absorbs the least amount of radiation.
4. The answer is (D). Alpha and beta are particulate radiation forms; alpha consists of two protons and two neutrons, and beta is identical to an electron. Both gamma rays and x-rays are part of the electromagnetic spectrum, behaving in a similar

manner to other forms of the spectrum, such as visible light, radiowaves, and infrared light.

B. Units of Measurement

1. RADIATION ADSORBED DOSE (GRAY)

The term rad is an acronym for **radiation absorbed dose.** Recall that as radiation interacts with living tissue, it deposits energy. Rad is the amount of deposited energy per gram of irradiated matter, specifically, 1 rad = energy absorption of 100 erg per gram. The rad can be applied to any type of radiation, whether electromagnetic or particulate. In the International System (SI), the rad is replaced by the **gray (Gy),** with 1 Gy = 1 joule/kg; thus, 1 Gy = 100 rad, or 1 centigray = 1 rad.

2. REM (SIEVERT)

The term **rem** is an acronym for **roentgen equivalent man** and is the proper unit to express occupational exposure or **dose equivalent (DE).** Remember that different types of radiation produce differing biological effects; therefore, a quality factor (QF) assigned to each type of radiation is used to predict biological outcomes. By definition, DE is measured in rem and is the product of absorbed dose and the quality factor of the type of radiation involved. Therefore:

$$DE = absorbed\ dose \times QF$$

or

$$rem = rad \times QF$$

With respect to x-rays, gamma rays, and beta particles, the QF is assigned a value of 1.
Therefore:

$$DE = rad \times 1$$

or

1 rad = 1 rem for x-rays, gamma rays, and beta particles

The SI unit for rem is the **sievert (Sv).** 1 Sv = 100 rem, as 100 rad = 1 Gy.

3. ROENTGEN (COULOMB PER KILOGRAM)

Roentgen is a measure of the quantity of ionization that occurs in air as measured by ionization chambers and is expressed as R/min or R/hr. You may recall that leakage radiation is measured in such terms. The roentgen is only used to measure energies up to 3 MeV. The SI unit for the roentgen is known as the

exposure unit and is expressed in coulomb per kilogram (C/kg).

To find exposure rate:

exposure rate (R/min) = exposure in R per time in minutes

Total exposure is determined by:

$$exposure\ (R) = exposure\ rate \times time$$

QUESTIONS FOR UNITS OF MEASUREMENT

select the best answer

1. Which of the following units is measured with an ionization chamber?
   (A) LET
   (B) DE
   (C) C/kg
   (D) rad

2. Which of the following measurements requires multiplication by the QF in order to attain it?
   (A) rem
   (B) rad
   (C) R
   (D) Gy

3. Which of the following is the equivalent of 100 ergs per gram?
   (A) QF
   (B) Gy
   (C) Sv
   (D) C/kg

▶▶ ANSWERS TO UNITS OF MEASUREMENT

1. The answer is (C). The SI unit for roentgen—the unit that expresses ionization in air measured with an ionization chamber—is the exposure unit, which is expressed as C/kg.
2. The answer is (A). Rem, or sievert, is the correct unit to express occupational dose. It is derived from the product of the absorbed dose (rad) and the QF. For x-ray, gamma, and beta particles, the QF is 1; thus, 1 rem = 1 rad.
3. The answer is (B). Rad, the measurement for absorbed dose, is the amount of deposited energy per gram of irradiated matter, specifically, 1 rad energy absorption of 100 erg per gram. The Gy is the SI unit for the rad.

C. Dosimeters (Types and Uses)

Monitoring whole body exposure is a means of evaluating radiation safety practices in the workplace; the NCRP recommends monthly monitoring for occupationally exposed individuals who are likely to receive one fourth of the total dose equivalent.

The **film badge** is the most common means of tracking occupational radiation dose. It consists of a special dosimetry film, much like dental film, in a plastic container. The container is comprised of a window and a series of aluminum and copper filters, which serve to indicate the energy level at which the individual has been exposed. Radiation passing through a copper filter is of higher energy than that which passes through the window of the badge; and in the same manner, radiation passing through an aluminum filter is of still higher energy. The film is backed with lead foil to absorb scatter radiation from behind the badge.

Generally speaking, film badges are supplied by commercial laboratories and are collected and processed once a month. After processing, dosimetric comparisons are made against control film exposed at known values, and the results are reported to the radiology department. The badge should generally be worn on the hip or chest, but during fluoroscopy it should be worn over the lead apron at the neck. Pregnant female personnel should wear an additional badge underneath the apron during both fluoroscopy and mobile procedures in order to monitor fetal exposure.

1. THERMOLUMINESCENT DOSIMETER

The thermoluminescent dosimeter (TLD) is a more sensitive device than the film badge and operates on the principle that crystalline materials such as lithium fluoride (LiF) store energy when exposed to ionizing radiation. When the TLD is measured, the LiF crystals are heated, a process that returns the electrons to their normal state and releases the stored energy in the form of light. The light is then measured by a photomultiplier tube, which in turn gives a measure of the radiation exposure. The TLD is widely regarded as superior to the more familiar film badge and may one day replace it. Its advantages include the following:

Cost—detectors are inexpensive

Durability—detectors are sealed in Teflon

Response to radiation is proportional up to 400 R and independent of radiation energy from 50 kV to 20 MeV

Accuracy is ± 5% versus ± 50% with film badges

Response of crystalline material is similar to that of human tissue

2. POCKET DOSIMETER

Pocket dosimeters are the most sensitive type of occupational monitors available. They do not provide a permanent legal record of exposure; however, they are useful when an individual is likely to receive a high exposure over a short period of time. The instrument resembles a fountain pen and contains a thimble-sized ionization chamber at one end. This type of instrument can either be read by means of an electrometer or is self reading.

QUESTIONS FOR DOSIMETERS (TYPES AND USES)

select the best answer

1. Which of the following will provide an immediate reading for a one-time, high-level exposure?

   (A) TLD
   (B) Film badge
   (C) Lithium fluoride crystal
   (D) Pocket dosimeter

2. Which of the following is not a characteristic of a TLD?

   (A) Uses laser film
   (B) Possesses crystals that store energy
   (C) Converts energy to light when heated
   (D) Yields readings accurate to ± 5%

3. Which of the following instruments yields the must accurate measure of occupational radiation exposure?

   (A) Geiger counter
   (B) Cutie pie
   (C) TLD
   (D) Pocket dosimeter

4. Which of the following is (are) considered a disadvantage of a film badge?

   (A) Cost
   (B) Inaccuracy
   (C) Durability
   (D) All of the aforementioned

▶▶ ANSWERS TO DOSIMETERS (TYPES AND USES)

1. The answer is (D). The pocket dosimeter is a kind of personalized ionization chamber used when a high dose of radiation is likely. Some models permit immediate readings of exposure, generally expressed in mrem. The TLD and film badge are used for monthly assessment of radiation exposure. LiF crystals are the material used for TLDs.

2. The answer is (A). The TLD operates on the principle that LiF crystals store energy and give off light measured by a photomultiplier tube when heated under controlled conditions. It is much more accurate than the film badge, which has a margin of error of ± 50%.

3. The answer is (D). The Geiger counter and cutie pie are radiation survey instruments. The TLD is more accurate than the film badge, but the pocket dosimeter is more accurate still.

4. The answer is (D). Although the film badge is certainly the most common means of measuring monthly occupational exposure, it possesses many disadvantages when compared to other available means, including higher cost, wide margin of error, and lack of durability.

D. NCRP Recommendations for Personnel Monitoring

It should be clear from your review of the radiation protection material that an upper exposure limit should be established concerning occupationally exposed individuals. Such a limit is outlined in NCRP Report No. 116, *Limitation of Exposure to Ionizing Radiation,* published in 1993, which defines the occupational dose equivalent. Pertinent maximum exposure levels are presented in **Table 2-3.**

Ultimately, however, responsibility for mainte-

▶ **TABLE 2.3.** Ionizing Radiation Exposure Limits

For Yearly Occupational Dose: 50 mSv/Yr
For Cumulative Occupational Dose: 10 mSv/Yr × Age in years
15 mSv/Yr: lens of the eye
500 mSv: skin, hands and feet

For General Public:
1 mSv: continuous exposure
5 mSv: infrequent exposure
50 mSv: lens of the eye, skin, hands and feet

For developing embryo: 0.5 mSv/month

NCRP Report 116: Limitation of Exposure to Ionizing Radiation, 1993.

nance of the radiation dose record falls upon the technologist. If you change place of employment, it is up to you to assure that your record follows you from place to place, so that accurate cumulative records are maintained.

1. ALARA

Obviously, even with closely monitored radiation exposure and established guidelines, it is to the technologist's benefit to practice effective radiation safety measures at all times. Awareness of sound radiation safety principles will lead to occupational exposure rates far below the maximum permissible dose (MPD).

A radiology department that practices such an awareness is said to have a program based on the **ALARA** concept, an acronym that stands for maintaining exposure rates at a level that is **as low as reasonably achievable.**

2. CUMULATIVE DOSE RECORDS

Maintenance and evaluation of a cumulative dose record in a radiology department are the responsibility of the radiation safety officer. To reiterate, most departments use commercial laboratories to obtain monthly film badge readings; these laboratories issue a monthly report.

END-OF-CHAPTER EXAMINATION

▶▶ **QUESTIONS**

Select the best answer.

1. What is the MPD for a 46-year-old technologist?

   (A) 46 mR
   (B) 0.46 R
   (C) 4.6 R
   (D) 140 R

2. All of the following are factors that influence absorbed dose in the patient except:

   (A) kVp.
   (B) attenuation coefficient.
   (C) focal spot size.
   (D) filtration.

3. According to NCRP regulations, fluoroscopic mA must not exceed:

   (A) 50 mA.
   (B) 500 mA.
   (C) 5 mA.
   (D) 100 mA.

4. Which of the following is not a long-term biological effect of radiation exposure?

   (A) Gastrointestinal syndrome
   (B) Cataracts
   (C) Cancer
   (D) Life-span shortening

5. A patient with profound mental retardation arrives in the radiology department for flat and upright abdomen examination. Attempts to attain cooperation for the examination fail; it is apparent that the patient must be held if the examination is to be successful. Of the following, the best individual to hold the patient is:

   (A) another technologist.
   (B) the patient's mother.
   (C) an orderly.
   (D) a nurse.

6. Which of the following is not a fundamental property of the x-ray?

   (A) Exists as both a wave and a particle of energy
   (B) Consists of discrete bits of energy traveling at the speed of light
   (C) Can be focused only by a collimator
   (D) Produces secondary and scatter radiation

7. Which of the following is the SI unit of measurement for exposure in air?

   (A) Gy
   (B) Sv
   (C) C/kg
   (D) Roentgen

8. The intensity of scatter radiation 1 meter from the patient is:

   (A) 50% greater than the useful beam.
   (B) 10% less than the useful beam.
   (C) 50% less than the useful beam.
   (D) 90% less than the useful beam.

9. Referring to the drawing below, which dose-response curve would be used to illustrate a long-term effect from radiation exposure?

   (A) Linear, non-threshold
   (B) Non-linear, non-threshold
   (C) Linear, threshold
   (D) Non-linear, threshold

10. A 13-year-old girl comes to the radiology department for scoliosis evaluation. In order to produce the highest degree of radiation protection for developing breast tissue, which of the following positions should be employed?

    (A) Anteroposterior
    (B) Posteroanterior
    (C) Left anterior oblique
    (D) Right anterior oblique

(Continued)

11. Why can an air-gap technique be used in place of a grid in some instances?

    (A) Inverse square law
    (B) 50/15 rule
    (C) Heterogeneous beam
    (D) Beam divergence

12. The primary purpose of filtration is to:

    (A) increase detail.
    (B) decrease patient skin dose.
    (C) reduce technologist dose.
    (D) reduce film fog.

13. Of the following technical factors, which, if any, serve(s) to simultaneously affect overall quality and quantity of the x-ray beam?

    1. kVp
    2. OFD
    3. HVL

    (A) All of the aforementioned
    (B) None of the aforementioned
    (C) Choice 3 only
    (D) Choices 1 and 3

14. Which of the following is an example of a primary barrier?

    (A) Lead apron
    (B) Lead gloves
    (C) Exposure room door
    (D) Control booth

15. If a given exposure rate at 40 inches SSD is 80 R/min, what is the rate at 72 inches?

    (A) 24.69 R/min
    (B) 56 R/min
    (C) 280 R/min
    (D) 16 R/min

16. Avascular tumors treated with radiotherapy are sometimes also treated with hyperbaric therapy because:

    (A) oxygen helps repair radiation burns.
    (B) tumors are more sensitive in oxygenated conditions.
    (C) tumors are less sensitive in oxygenated conditions.
    (D) hyperbaric therapy aids patient comfort level.

17. The difference between gamma rays and x-rays is:

    (A) size.
    (B) source.
    (C) penetrating ability.
    (D) charge.

18. The maximum annual exposure for the general population is _____ R/year, which is _____ that permissible for occupationally exposed individuals.

    (A) 5 millisievert (mSv)/yr; 0.1%
    (B) 50 mSv/yr; 0.1%
    (C) 500 mSv/yr; 0.1%
    (D) 0.5 mSv/yr; 0.1%

19. Which of the following statements is true?

    (A) As LET decreases, RBE increases.
    (B) As LET increases, RBE decreases.
    (C) As LET decreases, RBE decreases.
    (D) LET and RBE are unrelated.

20. The BEIR has determined the linear, non-threshold curve to be the appropriate curve to measure occupational exposure to ionizing radiation. Which of the following biological effects would be measured by a linear, threshold curve?

    (A) Leukemia
    (B) Thyroid cancer
    (C) Bone cancer
    (D) Cataracts

21. Of the following technical factors, which is most important in reducing patient dose?

    (A) Collimation
    (B) Appropriate FFD
    (C) Focal spot size
    (D) Correct positioning

22. The exposure switch and cord on a mobile x-ray unit must permit the operator to stand at least _____ from the x-ray source?

    (A) 2 feet
    (B) 4 feet
    (C) 6 feet
    (D) 8 feet

(Continued)

23. Where can leakage radiation be found in the R/F exposure room?

    (A) Tube housing
    (B) Radioactive isotope lead container
    (C) Control booth
    (D) Ion chamber

24. The cumulative timer on the fluoroscopy unit is a protective device to remind the physician and technologist of the amount of exposure acquired in a given procedure. How often must the cumulative timer be reset?

    (A) Every 2 minutes
    (B) Every 3 minutes
    (C) Every 5 minutes
    (D) Every 10 minutes

25. Of all of the types of radiation monitoring devices, the film badge is the most familiar. How does it measure radiation exposure?

    (A) Heated crystals that emit light
    (B) By a series of metallic filters and film
    (C) Measurement of ions in a chamber
    (D) Measurement of free electrons by quenching gases and high voltage

26. What is the HVL of an exposure of 140 R/min?

    (A) 2.5 mm Al; 70 R/min
    (B) 0.5 mm Al; 14 R/min
    (C) 1.5 mm Al; 140 R/min
    (D) 3.0 mm Al; 7 R/min

27. Which of the following is determined by the product of absorbed dose and the QF?

    (A) Gray
    (B) LET
    (C) RBE
    (D) Sievert

28. Which of the following modalities is likely to produce the highest occupational dose?

    (A) Diagnostic radiography
    (B) Mammography
    (C) Helical computed tomography scan
    (D) Magnification radiography

29. If a given fluoroscopic procedure took 1 hour to perform, and the exposure rate was 48 mrem/hr, how much dose would be received if the procedure time was cut in half?

    (A) 12 mrem/hr
    (B) 24 rem/hr
    (C) 24 mrem/hr
    (D) 6 mrem/hr

30. According to NCRP guidelines, a radiation protection quality-control program should include at least yearly inspection of which of the following?

    1. Collimator accuracy
    2. Linearity
    3. Reproducibility

    (A) None of the aforementioned
    (B) All of the aforementioned
    (C) Choice 2 only
    (D) Choices 1 and 3 only

▶▶ **ANSWERS TO END-OF-CHAPTER EXAMINATION**

1. The answer is (A). MPD or DE is obtained by using the formula: DE = 1R × age in years.> Substituting known values, we find: 1 × 46 = 46 R.

2. The answer is (C). kVp is the primary factor in determination of average beam intensity. Increased intensity means less absorbed dose because many high-energy photons pass through the patient unabsorbed. Likewise, filtration increases beam intensity by filtering low-energy photons. Attenuation coefficient of the part being examined is also important; the higher the density, the more absorption occurs. Focal spot has no influence on absorbed dose.

3. The answer is (C). Although regulations limit fluoroscopic mA to 5, with image-intensified fluoroscopy, the mA generally ranges from 1 to 3, depending on the body part being examined.

4. The answer is (A). Gastrointestinal syndrome is the result of acute whole body radiation exposure in the supralethal range, that is, 600 to 1000 R. Symptoms include loss of appetite, nausea, vomiting, intractable diarrhea, and a dramatic drop in white blood cell count.

5. The answer is (B). Radiology personnel should never be used to hold patients. If no family member or friend is available, other medical personnel can be used. Except for the patient, no person should be placed directly in the path of the useful beam.

(Continued)

6. The answer is (C). Collimators on the x-ray unit are merely a means of restricting the x-ray beam; x-ray cannot be focused. Quantum theory states that x-ray exits as a shower of photons traveling at the speed of light, devoid of electrical charge.

7. The answer is (C). The SI unit for exposure in air is coulombs per kilogram—replacing the colder roentgen—and designated by C/kg. The rad, unit for radiation absorbed dose, has been replaced by the Gy; and the rem, unit for roentgen-equivalent-man, has been replaced by the Sv.

8. The answer is (D). The wording of this question is important. Secondary and scatter radiation, particularly high-energy Compton scatter emerging from the patient, represents the greatest occupational exposure hazard to the technologist. Although the patient is the greatest source of scatter, other objects to consider are the radiograph table, bucky slot cover, and the control booth wall or protective barrier. The intensity of scatter radiation 1 meter from the patient is 0.10% (90% less) that of the primary beam.

9. The answer is (A). The linear non-threshold curve demonstrates long-term (or stochastic) effects, such as cancer and leukemia. These are all-or-nothing, or random biological effects, that is, effects that cannot be marked by degrees of severity. With a non-threshold curve, there is no safe dose below which it can be predicted that no biological response will occur. The BEIR has designated the linear non-threshold curve as the appropriate curve for use with radiation protection standards.

10. The answer is (B). Radiation dose is always greater at the entrance point when compared with its exit. Therefore, placing developing breast tissue nearest the film in the PA position will afford the greatest degree of radiation protection in this patient

11. The answer is (D). The air-gap technique, whereby a distance between the patient and film is used, can be substituted for a grid in some instances, because scattered photons emerging from the patient continue their divergent path and never reach the film. This technique is used with lateral cervical spine examinations. When used in conjunction with chest radiography, the SID must be increased in order to reduce magnification and maintain detail, which requires a corresponding increase in technique, usually in mAs.

12. The answer is (B). Metallic filtration in the x-ray unit, usually aluminum, serves to increase overall average beam energy by eliminating long-wave, low-energy photons, thus reducing patient skin dose.

13. The answer is (D). Although kVp is primarily a qualitative factor, it also affects the number of photons produced at the target. HVL is the amount of material necessary to decrease the intensity of the x-ray beam by half, thereby affecting beam quality and quantity. Increasing OFD, as in the air-gap technique, has an effect similar to that of a grid; so increasing OFD affects film density but does not affect overall beam energy or quantity.

14. The answer is (C). Primary barriers such as the lead walls and door of the exposure suite have high attenuation rates and are effective protection from the useful beam. Secondary barriers are designed to provide additional protection from leakage (from the tube housing) and scatter radiation (primarily from the patient). Examples of secondary barriers are the walls of the exposure room that are more than 7 feet in height, lead aprons and gloves, and the control booth.

15. The answer is (A). Use the inverse square law to solve. $\text{Intensity}_{old}/\text{Intensity}_{new} = \text{distance}_{new}^2/\text{distance}_{old}^2$. Substituting values; $80/x = 5184/1600$; $5184x = 128,000$; $x = 24.69$ R/min.

16. The answer is (B). Biological tissue is more reactive to radiation in an oxygenated state. Therefore, avascular tumors, having little or no oxygen supply, may respond to radiotherapy more satisfactorily in the presence of high-pressure oxygen treatment.

17. The answer is (B). The x-ray and gamma ray photon are identical, except for their origin. Gamma rays are emitted by a radioactive atom, whereas the x-ray is the product of a high-speed electron's sudden deceleration and interaction with target material.

18. The answer is (A). According to NCRP guidelines, annual occupational dose should not exceed 5 R/yr (50 mSv/yr). The MPD of the general population is one tenth that of the occupational population.

(Continued)

19. The answer is (C). LET, linear energy transfer, is a measure of transferred energy rate (per unit length of path) to biological tissue, which is affected by radiation type and attenuation coefficient. RBE, relative biological effectiveness, is a measure of biological response to ionization from a given exposure. Therefore, as LET decreases, so does RBE.

20. The answer is (D). Cataracts are a biological consequence that can be reliably predicted from an exposure in the range of 200 R. Therefore, a threshold exists that, when exceeded, can be expected to produce cataracts. Various forms of cancer are measured by linear, non-threshold curves.

21. The answer is (A). Beam restriction via collimation is the most important listed factor in minimizing patient dose. Correct positioning is important in terms of producing a diagnostic film and reducing retakes, particularly when using AED. Correct FFD selection is important for the same reason. Focal spot size must be appropriate for the examination and is a factor when considering heat unit (HU) production and detail. Overall, however, restricting the beam to the area of interest reduces the volume of irradiated tissue, lessens scatter, and improves radiographic contrast by reducing fog.

22. The answer is (C). The three cardinal principles for reducing occupational exposure are time, shielding, and distance. NCRP regulations state that an x-ray portable unit must allow the operator to stand at least 6 feet from the exposure source. Many units are equipped with remote switches that permit even further distance.

23. The answer is (A). Leakage radiation is defined as radiation emitted from the tube housing in directions other than that of the primary beam. NCRP regulations state that static leakage radiation should not exceed 100 mR/hr 1 meter from the x-ray tube. R/F is an abbreviation for radiography/fluoroscopy.

24. The answer is (C). As a personnel protection procedure, the cumulative timer on the fluoroscopy unit must be reset every 5 minutes.

25. The answer is (B). The film badge consists of a series of copper and aluminum filters and film. Radiation that passes behind the Al filter is more energetic than that passing through the open window of the badge. Likewise, radiation passing through the copper filter is of higher energy than that which passes through the aluminum. Film badges are collected once a month and measure doses as small as 10 mSv. A report is generated from the measurements and sent to the referring radiology department.

26. The answer is (A). Half-value layer is the amount of material necessary to reduce the exposure rate by half. If 2.5 mm Al reduces a 140 R/min exposure to 70 R/min, then the HVL equals 2.5 mm Al.

27. The answer is (D). Sievert, or rem (roentgen-equivalent-man), is determined by multiplication of the absorbed dose (rad, or gray) and the QF, a qualitative designation assigned to different types of radiation.

28. The answer is (A). Mammography uses extremely low kV exposure factors that produce very little scatter, and CT scan uses a highly collimated beam that is associated with low occupational dose. Magnification radiography is produced with special equipment that employs very small focal spots and increased OFD. The highest doses are associated with diagnostic radiography, particularly with fluoroscopy and portable x-ray procedures.

29. The answer is (C). Time and exposure rate have a proportional relationship. Cutting the time by half also reduces the exposure rate by half.

30. The answer is (B). Reproducibility is a term meaning that a given exposure will repeatedly produce the same results on film. Linearity refers to differing combinations of mA and time that equal the same mAs and produce consistent film density. Light localized collimation must be accurate to within 2% of the displayed field.

CHAPTER 3

Equipment Operation and Maintenance

I. RADIOGRAPHIC EQUIPMENT
A. Components of the Basic Radiographic Unit

1. OPERATING CONSOLE

The **operating console** or **control panel** of the x-ray unit is an apparatus operated by the radiographer for the purpose of making an exposure. From the console, the technologist selects desired technical factors, such as kilovoltage peak (kVp), milliampere-seconds (mA-s), automatic exposure, and so forth; mode of operation, as in fluoroscopic, radiographic, or tomographic modes; as well as any accessory devices such as table or wall bucky that should operate during the exposure.

Also present on the panel are meters, which are usually digital readouts on more modern equipment, and traditional analog meters on older units. These devices indicate various facets of equipment operation. The console may include milliammeter, filament ammeter, mA-s meter, and kilovoltmeter.

Some units also have a line voltage compensator, which allows the operator to adjust for variance in incoming line voltage in older models, and an internal device that detects and automatically adjusts line voltage on newer models. Remember, a small fluctuation in the incoming voltage to the primary side of the transformer means a large fluctuation on the secondary side. There are numerous adaptations of the basic configuration, but almost all units are comprised of some variant of these basic features.

2. X-RAY TUBE

A typical x-ray tube used for medical x-ray diagnosis is **a thermionic diode,** comprised of a negatively charged **tungsten filament cathode;** a positively charged **tungsten anode;** a **glass tube or envelope,** which operates in a vacuum; and **two circuits,** one that heats the cathode filament, and one that drives the space charge electrons to the anode.

3. CATHODE

The cathode **filament** serves as the electron source for the tube. The filament is a small coil (approximately 2 cm) of tungsten wire, mounted on two sturdy wires that both support and carry current to it. Low-voltage [approximately 10 volts (V) and 3–5 amps (A)] filament current is supplied, which produces electrons by **thermionic emission.**

Electrons remain around the filament in a negatively charged cloud called a **space charge** until sufficient kilovoltage is applied to the anode, which creates a potential difference across the x-ray tube, and produces a stream of electrons flowing to the anode. Increasing tube current [milliamperage (mA)] will result in filament temperatures to >2200°C, due to the high resistance of tungsten, and increases the number of electrons produced. A **focusing cup** or **cathode block** surrounds the filaments and aids in directing electrons toward the anode. **X-ray** tube output is therefore directly proportional to x-ray tube current, with typical ranges of 25 to 1000 mA for radiography and 3 to 5 mA for fluoroscopy.

Modern x-ray tubes generally feature dual filaments of differing size mounted side by side, which results in two **focal spot** sizes. Such tubes are referred to as **double-focus** tubes. Only one filament is activated during each exposure, and this filament is selected at the control panel when the operator chooses the mA station.

Over time, the cathode filament thins as a result of prolonged heat exposure. The resulting loss of cross-sectional area produces increased resistance, and subsequent greater filament temperature. Greater filament temperature will naturally produce greater tube current and a greater number of source electrons. Because filament circuitry is designed to produce constant current, filament current of older x-ray tubes must be adjusted downward to obtain proper electron emission.

4. ANODE

The x-ray tube **anode** is the 2″ to 5″ target electrode in which swiftly moving electrons are suddenly decelerated, which produces heat and x-rays. There are two types of anodes: rotating and stationary. **Stationary anodes** can be found in some mobile x-ray units and are constructed of a tungsten target, which is used because of its high melting point (3370°C) and high atomic number (Z = 74), embedded in a copper block (**Figure 3-1**).

5. ROTATING ANODES

A **rotating anode** increases target area and heat loading capacity. In addition to the tungsten target material, rhenium (Z = 75) and rhodium (Z = 45) are incorporated in the target to reduce heat-induced pitting and cracking. Rhenium metal is very hard; with the exception of tungsten, it is the least fusible of all common metals. Rhenium melts at approximately 3180°C (approximately 5756°F), and has a specific gravity of 20.53. The atomic weight of rhenium is 186.207.

Along with rhenium, rhodium is one of the transition elements of the periodic table. Rhodium is very durable, insoluble in ordinary acids, and very difficult to fuse. Aqueous solutions of many of its salts are rose colored, from which its name is derived. **Figure 3-2** shows the periodic table representations of rhenium and rhodium.

A typical anode speed is roughly 3500 rpm, with high-speed anodes rotating at speeds up to 10,000 rpm. The **induction motor** of the anode consists of two primary parts: the **stator** and the **rotor.** The stator is a series of electromagnets positioned outside of the glass envelope that are supplied with current to induce an electromagnetic field. The rotor is affected by pull exerted by these fields and rotates the anode.

The target area of the anode is called the **focal spot.** Typical focal spot sizes vary according to use; the smaller the focal spot, the greater the detail, and the more heat is produced. Intense heat loading from protracted use of small focal spots may produce melting at the target; therefore, small focal spots are generally only used for radiography of smaller body parts.

The **actual focal spot** is the target area bombarded by electrons, which is determined by filament size and dimensions of the **focusing cup,** whereas the **effective focal spot** is the dimension of the x-ray source as viewed from the image. The optimum

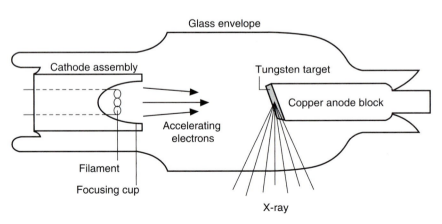

Figure 3-1. A simplified x-ray tube with stationary anode. The tungsten target is embedded in a copper block that conducts heat away from the target and to the oil coolant surrounding the glass envelope.

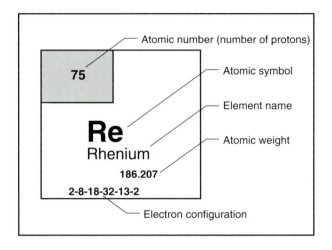

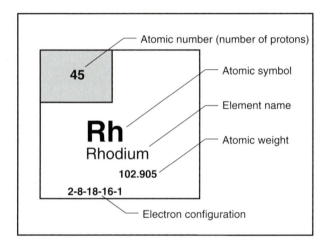

Figure 3-2. Periodic table representations of rhenium and rhodium.

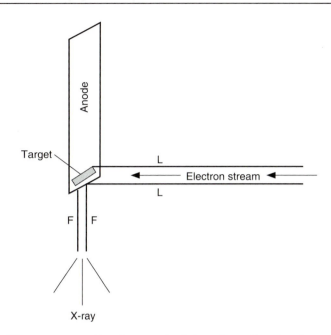

Figure 3-3. Line focus principle, where F = focal spot size, and L = an incoming stream of accelerated electrons. F is smaller than L due to the target angle.

effective focal spot is one that produces the greatest detail, while permitting adequate heat loading. **Figure 3-3** demonstrates the **line focus principle,** which minimizes the apparent size of the focal spot by orienting the anode at a small angle with respect to the direction of the x-ray beam.

It is crucial to remember that although decreasing target angle increases the actual focal spot, thereby increasing heat loading capacity, it also increases the **anode heel effect,** thereby decreasing the amount of film coverage. As a rule, remember that a small target angle and large focal spot provide the greatest heat loading capacity.

The **anode heel effect,** also known as **anode cutoff,** is a phenomenon relating to beam divergence and the attendant non-uniform distribution of

energy in the beam. Look at **Figure 3-4.** Note that the exposure rate is maximal in the central portion of the beam. Exposure rate is much less on the anode side of the beam.

The heel effect can be put to practical use, however, by placing thicker body parts toward the cathode end of the beam and thinner parts toward the anode. This practice results in more uniform radiographic

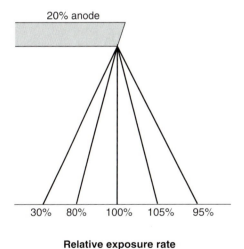

Figure 3-4. Intensity of exposure rate due to anode heel effect.

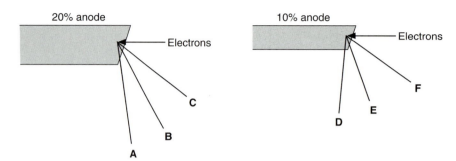

Figure 3-5. Photon "a" must pass through a greater thickness of anode than that which photon "b" or "c" passes through. This portion of he anode iscalled the "heel." Note the effect becomes more pronounced with a steeper target angle.

density on film and is most pronounced with body parts that have widely divergent densities, such as the thoracic spine. **Figure 3-5** offers an explanation for the physical basis of the heel effect.

There are a number of devices that measure focal spot accuracy. **The pinhole camera** is a metallic device with a small hole in its center. A tabletop exposure is made, and the hole acts to collimate the beam. The area that demonstrates density on film is then measured; this number represents focal spot size. The pinhole camera requires lengthy exposure times; care must be taken to avoid damaging the target.

The **star pattern resolution object** is a grid that is radiographed, demonstrating a focused area on film. The star pattern also demonstrates resolution—the smallest area between two objects—of the focal spot. The focused area is measured; the width and length are representative of the focal spot size.

6. ENVELOPE

The working parts of an x-ray tube are enclosed in a heat-resistant **glass tube or envelope** containing a nearly perfect **vacuum.** Some tubes are heated during manufacturing to expel air and other gases in a process known as **degassing.** The vacuum provides an unobstructed path for the electron stream. If the vacuum deteriorates, the electrons begin to encounter resistance from impeding air molecules, and x-ray production diminishes. The presence of air may also cause oxidation of the cathode filament.

7. TUBE HOUSING

The envelope itself is enclosed in the **tube housing.** The housing contains an oil bath that insulates and cools the tube and also acts as a shield against leakage

radiation. X-rays exit through a thin **window** in the tube housing.

8. WARM-UP PROCEDURES

The heat imparted by a sufficiently energetic single large exposure to a cold x-ray tube causes sudden expansion of the anode, which may crack it. Therefore, most tube manufacturers recommend suitable **tube warm-up procedures** to prevent anode damage. The procedures generally consist of a series of exposures carried out at progressively higher milliamperes (mA) and kilovolts (kV); these exposures take only a few minutes to perform. Technologists should consult the manufacturer's user manual for more specific information.

9. TUBE RATING CHARTS

The high cost of x-ray tubes demands that both technologists and radiology administrators guard against the life span of the tube. Overheating the filament, anode, or tube housing shortens tube life.

Applying excessive current (mA) to the filament may cause burnout by raising its temperature beyond the rated limit. Similarly, using the "boost and hold" properties of the x-ray switch, whereby filament temperature is increased to a standby level and then suddenly increased again to the desired mA when the exposure is made, shortens tube life. Although the "standby mode" is useful relative to radiography for infants and uncooperative patients because it permits the exposure to be made at the instant when the patient is held in place, technologists should recall that excessive use compromises tube viability.

Undue filament heating causes a reduction in its diameter. A decrease of only 10% will result in tube failure. Further, as the filament deposits vaporized tungsten on the tube glass wall, x-ray production is decreased, and the insert itself may become punctured by electrical spark-over.

Localized melting or cracking of the anode occurs when the temperature exceeds a limiting value. The thermal stress that is the cause of the cracking is set up in the anode due to differences in temperature between the focal track and the inside of the disk.

Although most modern radiographic units have built-in safety devices that prevent tube overloading, technologists must be able to use manufacturer-supplied **tube rating charts,** which are easy-to-use graphical representations of safe exposure factors for each individual unit. Tube loading capacity varies from unit to unit, based on focal spot size, mode of operation, generator capacity, type of rectification, and so forth; therefore, tube rating charts are supplied with each x-ray tube. The chart that is mounted in the control booth for reference must represent the tube that is actually installed in the room. This is of particular importance following x-ray tube replace-

ment, because a replacement tube's heat loading capacity may vary significantly from the original tube.

On the chart, the vertical or y-axis represents kVp, the horizontal or x-axis represents the maximum exposure time in seconds, and the diagonally traversing lines represent various mA stations. The chart is simple to use. Suppose you were going to make an exposure using 300 mA and 80 kVp. To determine maximum allowable exposure time, draw a line beginning at the point on the y-axis representing 80 kVp across to the intersection point at 300 mA. Next, draw a line vertically downward to the x-axis, which represents maximum allowable exposure. On the tube represented by **Figure 3-6**, the maximum exposure the tube will tolerate using these factors is 3 seconds.

Multiple exposures cause heat to accumulate in the anode. Again, exceeding the anode heat rating may cause anode failure. The heat storage capacity for a given anode is measured in **heat units (HU),** which are determined by the following formula:

$$HU = kV \times mA \times sec$$
$$(single\text{-}phase)$$

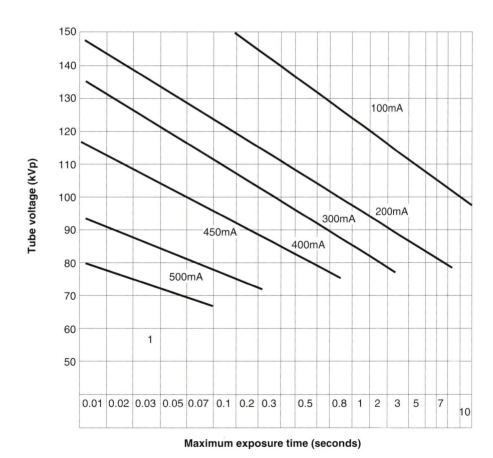

Figure 3-6. Tube rating chart: typical 3-phase, 12-pulse, 1-mm focal spot.

$$HU = kV \times mA \times sec \times 1.35$$
(three-phase, six-pulse)

$$HU = kV \times mA \times sec \times 1.41$$
(three-phase, twelve-pulse)

Use of this formula points out the increased effectiveness of high kilovoltage technique relative to tube life. For example, suppose an exposure is made on a single-phase unit at 300 mA, 1 sec, 60 kV. Using the HU formula, these factors yield:

$$HU = 300 \, mA \times 60 \, kV \times 1 \, sec = 18,000 \, HU$$

However, using the 50/15 rule, by which radiographic density is maintained by reducing mAs by half and increasing kV by 15%, we find:

$$HU = 150 \, mA \times 69 \, kV \times 1 \, sec = 10,350 \, HU$$

Over time, similar reduction in HU production may significantly extend tube life.

The heat storage capacity of anodes varies, ranging from 70,000 to 400,000 HU. The rate at which a given anode cools is measured by an **anode cooling chart.** With this chart, the y-axis on the left represents heat measured in HU stored in the anode. The x-axis at the bottom indicates the amount of cooling time necessary to permit further heat loading. The chart in **Figure 3-7** shows a tube which is rated at 200,000 HU. After 2 minutes, the tube is cooled to approximately 110,000 HU, permitting additional exposures of approximately 90,000 HU.

The ability of the tube housing to store and dissipate heat is measured with a **tube housing cooling chart,** which is used in the same manner as an anode cooling chart. Rapid sequence exposures used in angiography and cineradiography demand that special cooling charts be used. These charts give the maximum allowable HU produced in *a single exposure* on the left hand y-axis, and the *total number of exposures* on the bottom x-axis. The various curves demonstrate number of *exposures per second.*

10. AUTOMATIC EXPOSURE CONTROL

An **automatic exposure control or device** (AEC or AED) is a sophisticated timer used to produce uniform radiographic results. The radiographer selects the AEC at the control panel, instead of manually selecting mAs and kV. The device functions in conjunction with the x-ray bucky, and therefore may not be used for tabletop radiography.

There are two types of AEC—the **ionization chamber** and the **photomultiplier tube**—both of which are equipped with **sensors,** or **cells,** which are radiation detectors that signal the exposure switch, instructing it to terminate the exposure once a known correct value has been attained. The ionization chamber is found beneath the x-ray tabletop above the bucky and x-ray cassette. When the AEC is used, the patient is positioned centrally over the sensor, and an exposure is made. Once a predetermined amount of ionization has occurred, as measured by a connected **electrometer,** the exposure is terminated.

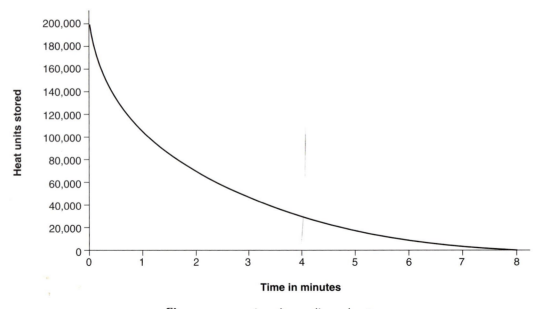

Figure 3-7. Anode cooling chart.

The **photomultiplier tube,** or **phototimer,** is also located under the table, but behind the x-ray cassette. The phototimer is comprised of a fluorescent screen that produces light when activated by x-rays. The fluorescent light in turn charges a photomultiplier tube that is also connected to an electrometer, which signals the x-ray switch to terminate the exposure once the correct charge is reached. Some phototimers are designed for use with special cassettes that have very little foil backing. A **backup timer** is used as a protective device to stop the exposure in case of AEC malfunction.

11. EXPOSURE CONTROLS

There are three primary x-ray circuits. The **high voltage, or secondary circuit,** includes the x-ray tube itself, the high-voltage transformer, and the rectification system. The **filament circuit** controls filament current, and hence is responsible for supplying the correct amount of current to the filament for the desired mA. The remainder of x-ray devices are found in the **low-voltage, or primary x-ray circuit.** These are primarily devices found on the x-ray console.

The technologist is chiefly concerned with the kVp, mA, and time exposure controls. When kVp is selected, the operator is engaging the autotransformer, which is a variable transformer operating on alternating current on the low-voltage x-ray circuit. The kVp selector on the control panel corresponds with a movable contact that selects the appropriate number of coils on the autotransformer. Milliamperage selection is a function of the filament circuit. Increasing the filament current increases the space charge around the cathode, and hence increases the number of electrons and the mA.

Most modern x-ray equipment uses an electronic timer to regulate the length of the exposure. This type of timer is based on a capacitor-resistor circuit and is capable of exposures as short as a millisecond [ms (.001 sec)]. The timer is also located on the low-voltage side of the x-ray circuit. Another type of timer, called an mAs timer, may still be found on older units and some portable equipment. The mA-s timer terminates the exposure once the designated mA-s is reached.

12. BEAM RESTRICTION DEVICES

Beam restriction devices, such as the x-ray tube **collimator,** and accessory devices, such as **diaphragms** and **flared and cylinder cones,** restrict the primary beam to desired dimensions; these devices are attached to the tube housing.

Collimators consist of a series of lead shutters mounted to the tube head and are the most widely used and most efficient beam restriction device. One set of lead shutters is placed adjacent to the tube port window to control image-degrading **off-focus** radiation. Off-focus radiation is that part of the beam that strikes other than the focal track of the anode. Another set of shutters, more familiar to the technologist, controls the length and width of the primary beam reaching the patient. These are the shutters that shape the collimated border on the film.

Cones are circular, lead-lined beam restriction devices that attach to the x-ray tube head and limit the beam to a fixed size. Some cones have extension devices that operate by means of a side-mounted screw, which when loosened allows the cone to extend. Some typical examinations that employ the use of cones are the paranasal sinus view and spot views of L5–S1.

Some chest and head units employ simple lead **aperture diaphragms,** which are lead devices with a central opening that dictates the amount of beam restriction. Although head units may use differing sizes of aperture diaphragms that can be switched according to desired examination, chest units tend to use a one-size, fixed type of device.

QUESTIONS FOR COMPONENTS OF THE BASIC RADIOGRAPHIC UNIT

select the best answer

1. Which of the following combinations will permit the greatest heat-loading capacity?
   (A) 1-mm actual focal spot, 10-degree target angle
   (B) 0.5-mm actual focal spot, 10-degree target angle
   (C) 1-mm actual focal spot, 20-degree target angle
   (D) 0.5-mm actual focal spot, 20-degree target angle

2. The device that selects kVp is a:
   (A) rheostat.
   (B) capacitor.
   (C) autotransformer.
   (D) resistor.

3. A double-focus x-ray tube has two:
   (A) filters.
   (B) windows.
   (C) filaments.
   (D) rectifiers.

4. An alternative means of expressing 500 mA and 80 kVp is:

   (A) 5 A; 800 V.
   (B) 0.5 A; 80,000 V.
   (C) 50 A; 80,000 V.
   (D) 0.5 A; 8000 V.

5. The star pattern test is used to measure:

   (A) focal spot resolution.
   (B) half-wave rectification.
   (C) incoming line voltage.
   (D) tube cooling properties.

6. How many heat units are produced on a three-phase, six-pulse machine using the following factors: 300 mA, 80 kVp, 0.5 sec?

   (A) 24,000 HU
   (B) 12,000 HU
   (C) 48,000 HU
   (D) 16,200 HU

7. Which of the following represents a typical filament current?

   (A) 300 A
   (B) 3 A
   (C) 30 A
   (D) 0.3 A

8. All of the following relate to the x-ray cathode except:

   (A) space charge.
   (B) thermionic emission.
   (C) filament current.
   (D) focal track.

9. Refer to the anode cooling chart in Figure 3-7. Suppose that you are midway through a lengthy series of films on a large patient; the machine notifies you of a technique overload. Assuming that you have reached the capacity for this machine, how long would you have to wait before continuing with a series of films that would generate 140,000 HU?

   (A) Less than 1 minute
   (B) Two minutes
   (C) Three minutes
   (D) Four minutes

10. An AEC will adjust exposure time for all of the following except:

    (A) pathologic process in the patient.
    (B) high-kilovoltage technique.
    (C) screen speed.
    (D) exceptionally large patients.

11. Which of the following are beam restriction devices?

    (A) Grids, cones, collimator
    (B) Collimator, cone, diaphragm
    (D) Grid, AEC, collimator
    (E) Cone, AEC, radiolucent sponge

▶▶ ANSWERS TO COMPONENTS OF BASIC RADIOGRAPHIC UNIT

1. The answer is (A). The smallest target angle and largest actual focal spot will permit the greatest heat-loading capacity. Decreasing target angle (making it steeper) increases the effective focal spot. However, recall that steeper target angles also increase the anode heel effect, which makes focal film distance (FFD) and film size an issue.

2. The answer is (C). The autotransformer is a variable transformer that operates on alternating current on the low-voltage x-ray circuit. The kVp selector on the control panel corresponds with a movable contact that selects the appropriate number of coils on the autotransformer.

3. The answer is (C). A double-focus x-ray tube has two filaments and two focal spots. When the small focal spot is selected at the control panel, the small filament is heated, and electrons are driven across to a smaller portion of the anode focal track. Conversely, when the operator selects a large focal spot, the large filament is heated, and electrons are driven to a large portion of the focal track.

4. The answer is (B). The key to this problem is understanding that the prefix "milli" refers to thousandths and "kilo" refers to thousands. Multiplying known values in this problem yields the following:

   500 × 0.001 = 0.5 A and 80 × 1000 = 80,000 V

5. The answer is (A). The **star pattern resolution object** is a grid that is radiographed and then demonstrates a focused area on film. The star pattern also demonstrates resolution—the smallest area between two objects—of the focal spot. The focused area is measured; the width and length are representative of the focal spot size.

6. The answer is (D). Use the formula HU = mA × sec × kVp × 1.35 to solve for three-phase, six-pulse machines.

7. The answer is (B). The **filament circuit** controls filament current, and hence is responsible for supplying the correct amount of current to the

filament for the desired mA. A typical filament current is 3 to 5 A.

8. The answer is (D). Focal track is the area on the anode where electrons are directed. Space charge, thermionic emission, and filament current all relate to the production of negatively charged electrons around the cathode.

9. The answer is (D). The machine is rated at 200,000 HU. If the remainder of the films you need to take will generate 140,000 HU, you must wait at least 4 minutes until the anode cools to 60,000.

10. The answer is (C). When the AEC is initially calibrated, its components are tuned so that appropriate exposures are made for a given screen speed. Introducing a faster speed screen to an automatic exposure system will result in an overexposed radiograph, whereas a slower speed will produce a film that is underexposed.

11. The answer is (B). Examples of beam restriction devices are: collimator, which is a fixed device comprised of two sets of lead shutters incorporated in the tube head; cones, which may be cylindrical or flared, and are attached to the tube head; and diaphragms, flat lead structures with varying sizes of openings, also attached to the x-ray tube.

B. X-ray Generator, Transformers, and Rectification System

1. BASIC PRINCIPLES

Recall the discussion of basic x-ray production. X-ray and heat are produced when rapidly moving electrons are suddenly decelerated upon encountering a tungsten anode. An extremely high, positively charged kilovoltage must be applied to the anode side of the x-ray tube in order to attract negatively charged electrons at the cathode.

The device that makes production of kilovoltage possible is the **transformer,** also known as the **x-ray generator.** An electric generator, or **dynamo,** is a device that converts mechanical energy into electrical energy by electromagnetic induction.

The transformer uses **alternating current** to change voltage from low to high, in the case of a **step-up transformer,** or from high voltage to low, in the case of a **step-down transformer.** An alternating current in the primary coil sets up a magnetic field that expands and contracts in and around the coil, varying in direction and strength in the same manner as the alternating current.

The transformer transfers electrical energy from one circuit to another without the use of mechanical parts or electrical contact using the principle of **electromagnetic induction.** The principle of electromagnetic induction is that the **electromotive force** (emf) induced in any coil is directly proportional to the number of turns in the coil that link with a given magnetic flux. Thus, if a given coil on the primary side of a step-up transformer has one turn, and an adjacent or secondary coil has two turns, the emf on the secondary side of the step-up transformer is twice that of the primary side. Conversely, if the secondary side of a step-down transformer has one turn and the primary side has two turns, the induced emf is half that of the primary side.

Transformer characteristics may be summarized using the following formula:

$$Vs/Vp = Ns/Np$$

where **Vs** is the voltage in the secondary coil; **Vp** is the voltage in the primary coil; **Ns** is the number of turns in the secondary coil; and **Np** is the number of turns in the primary coil.

According to the law of conservation of energy, however, outgoing power on the secondary side cannot exceed that of the incoming side. Therefore, it is important to recall what happens to *current* with an induced emf. Apply what you know about transformers to the following formula: power equals voltage multiplied by amperage, or **P = I × V.** With the induced emf a transformer produces, it can be concluded that:

$$IsVs = IpVp$$

where **Is** = the current in the secondary coil; **Ip** = current in the primary coil; **Vs** = the voltage in the secondary coil; and **Vp** = the voltage in the primary coil.

Use the following practical example: Suppose a given step-up transformer has a **turns ratio,** that is, the number of turns on the primary side compared with the secondary side, of 1:600. Further suppose that this transformer is supplied with 60 A and 220 V. What is the kVp and mA output?

Filling in the known values into the previously mentioned equations yields:

$$\frac{x}{220} = \frac{600}{1}$$

$$x = (600)(220) = 132,000 \ V$$
$$x = 132 \ kVp$$

and

$$\frac{600}{1} = \frac{60}{x}$$

$$600x = 60$$
$$x = 0.1 \ amp, \ or \ 100 \ mA$$

To summarize, a step-up transformer increases voltage and decreases amperage, whereas a step-down transformer decreases voltage and increases amperage. Another name for the step-down transformer in the x-ray circuit is the filament transformer. Its function is to regulate the voltage and current supplied to the filament circuit.

There are four main types of transformers to consider. The **air core transformer** consists of two insulated coils lying side by side with no physical connection; this transformer uses the principle of **mutual induction,** wherein one coil with a continuously moving magnetic field (AC) induces a current in a second coil. The **open core transformer** consists of an iron core inserted into an insulated coil of wire. Open core transformers are subject to power loss at the ends of the cores, which is a condition known as **leakage flux.**

A **closed core transformer** is comprised of heavily insulated, continuous coils around a laminated (i.e., made up of thin layers) square or circular core. The closed core provides a contiguous path for magnetic flux, which minimizes leakage flux. Alternating current in the primary side creates a magnetic flux in the iron core; because the flux links with both coils, it induces the same voltage **per turn** in both coils. The closed core transformer is more efficient than the open core transformer, and is therefore most commonly used for x-ray generators.

Shell transformers are the most sophisticated type of transformer and are used for commercial purposes. A laminated silicon core is used, and both primary and secondary sides are heavily insulated from each other and wound around the central core.

2. POWER LOSSES IN TRANSFORMERS

The efficiency of a transformer may be described as the ratio of power input to power output. Depending on the type, transformers exhibit up to approximately a 5% power loss from input to output, with the lost energy surrendered as heat. **Copper losses** are the loss of electric power due to **resistance** of the coil, and may be minimized by using wire of adequate diameter.

The magnetic flux in the transformer core induces **eddy currents** (swirling currents), which in turn produce heat. Electrical energy given up as heat results in power loss. Eddy current power loss can be diminished by using laminated silicon steel plates, which are insulated from each other, and reduce the size of the eddy currents.

Recall that the magnetic flux in the core of a transformer is created using alternating current. The continually changing direction of the current causes a concurrent rearrangement of the magnetic domains in the core. The repeated change of direction of magnetic flux produces heat and attendant power loss, known as **hysteresis losses.** Hysteresis loss is minimized by using a material with good permeability, such as the laminated silicon steel core.

3. AUTOTRANSFORMER

Because the relationship between the primary and secondary side of the transformer is a fixed one, that is, for a given input, there will be a given output depending upon the number of windings on the secondary side, standard transformers do not meet the requirements of modern x-ray equipment, which require a dynamic range of kilovoltage production. To obtain an adequate variety of kilovoltages, therefore, a device known as an **autotransformer** is connected between the source of the AC and the primary side of the transformer. The autotransformer consists of a solitary coil wound around an iron core. The coil acts in both a primary and secondary fashion, and operates on the principle of **self-induction.** Insulation is omitted at uniform intervals along the core, and the bare points are connected or tapped to a movable contact, which is in actuality the kVp selector on the x-ray control panel.

The autotransformer law is as follows:

$$\frac{Autotransformer \ secondary \ voltage}{autotransformer \ primary \ voltage}$$

$$= \frac{number \ of \ tapped \ turns}{number \ of \ primary \ turns}$$

Consider the following practical example: Assume that a given autotransformer is supplied with 240-V power and has tapped 3 turns on a coil with 10 primary turns. What is the autotransformer secondary voltage? To solve, fill in known values, using the autotransformer formula:

$$\frac{Autotransformer \ secondary \ voltage}{240} = \frac{3}{10}$$

Consider the following: a given autotransformer has 3000 windings. If it is supplied with 220 V, and 400 windings are tapped, what is sent to the primary of the step-up transformer? Use the transformer law to solve.

$$\frac{x \ (voltage \ sent \ to \ primary)}{220} = \frac{400}{3000}$$

$$3000x = 88000$$

$$x = 29.3 \ volts \ sent \ to \ the \ primary$$

4. RECTIFIERS

Optimum conditions for x-ray tube operation require a current that travels in one direction only. As you have seen, important components such as the transformer and the autotransformer require alternating current, which continually varies in amplitude and alternately varies in charge. Therefore, x-ray current must be **rectified** or altered to unidirectional current before it reaches the x-ray tube.

In simple terms, a **rectifier** modifies alternating current (AC) so that it becomes direct current (DC).

An x-ray circuit rectifier is located between the secondary side of the step-up transformer and the x-ray tube itself. **Full-wave rectification** occurs when the negative amplitude of the alternating current is changed to a positive alternation by using at least four **diodes** that produce two pulses per cycle. **Half-wave rectification** occurs by elimination of the negative alternation of AC. Rectifiers are constructed of materials such as silicon or germanium, which are semiconductors. Semiconductors conduct electricity in a unidirectional fashion.

5. PHASE AND PULSE

Kilovoltage peak is the maximum voltage that crosses the x-ray tube during one cycle. **Figure 3-8A** describes a **single-phase current.** Although the negative alternation has been eliminated by rectification, amplitude of the energy level constantly rises and falls. Single-phase current possesses 100% **voltage ripple,** because expressed as a percentage, the overall energy level varies 100% over the course of one cycle.

Obviously, constant change in amplitude results in an x-ray beam of lower energy. To address this difficulty, **three-phase generators,** which obtain power from three lines of current, each 120 degrees out of phase (superimposed) from the other are used. **Three-phase, six-pulse** generators typically produce voltage ripples of approximately 13%, whereas **three-phase, twelve-pulse** generators operate with an approximate 4% ripple. **Figure 3-8 B** and **C** demonstrate three-phase currents.

Newer, high-frequency generators produce an energy level consistent with that of three-phase, twelve-pulse generators.

select the best answer

1. The principle that allows the primary side of the high-voltage (step-up) transformer to generate voltage in the secondary side is called:
   - (A) self-induction.
   - (B) mutual induction.
   - (C) Newton's law.
   - (D) hysteresis loss.

2. Which type of rectification eliminates the negative alternation of alternating current?
   - (A) Half-wave
   - (B) Full-wave
   - (C) Three-phase
   - (D) Inverse

3. Which device maintains electron flow from cathode to anode?
   - (A) Stator
   - (B) Rotor
   - (C) High-frequency generator
   - (D) Diode rectifier

4. Which of the following is the *most important* advantage of the three-phase generator over the single-phase generator?
   - (A) Permits higher mA selections
   - (B) Permits higher kVp selections
   - (C) Increases average photon energy
   - (D) Permits smaller focal spots

5. Which of the following components is responsible for regulation of kVp?
   - (A) High-tension transformer
   - (B) Step-up transformer
   - (C) Autotransformer
   - (D) Capacitor

6. Where in the x-ray circuit is the step-down transformer located?
   - (A) Anode
   - (B) Filament circuit
   - (C) High-voltage side
   - (D) Rectification system

7. Which type of waveform is associated with an approximate 13% voltage ripple?
   - (A) Three-phase, twelve-pulse
   - (B) Three-phase, six-pulse

A

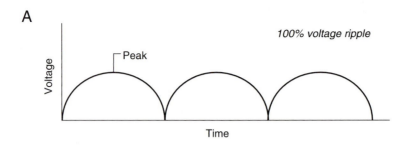

Single phase / full wave rectification

B

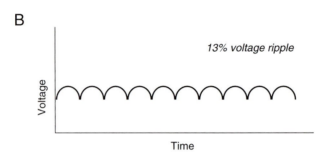

Three phase six pulse

C

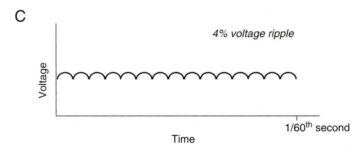

Three phase twelve pulse

Figure 3-8. (A) Single-phase, full-wave rectification. (B) Three-phase, six-pulse current. (C)Three-phase, twelve-pulse current.

(C) Single-phase
(D) Half-wave rectified

▶▶ ANSWERS TO X-RAY GENERATORS, TRANSFORMERS, AND RECTIFICATION SYSTEM

1. The answer is (B). Mutual induction occurs when an alternating current in the primary coil of the transformer links with the secondary coil, inducing in it an alternating, or opposing, current by electromagnetic induction. Because the AC in the secondary coil also induces an opposing current in the primary coil, the process is known as mutual induction.

2. The answer is (A). Half-wave rectification is achieved by elimination of the negative alternation of alternating current; this may be achieved either by self-rectification, whereby the x-ray

tube only allows electron flow during the positive half of the alternation, or via the use of diodes, which change the polarity of the transformer during the negative alternation, eliminating current flow.

3. The answer is (D). A rectifier modifies AC to pulsating DC, unidirectional current. If true AC were applied to the x-ray tube, the filament would be destroyed as polarity changed and electrons rushed back in the other direction. A diode operates by reversing the polarity of the transformer secondary, rendering it nonconductive.

4. The answer is (A). Although the three-phase waveform does produce higher energy photons, thus slightly increasing beam energy, its primary advantage over single-phase current is that of the nearly constant potential and almost constant x-ray production. These factors result in a higher *quantity* of x-ray per exposure time, and thus allow for higher mA stations. High mA stations are extremely important in special procedures radiography, where multiple rapid exposures are necessary.

5. The answer is (C). The autotransformer consists of a solitary coil wound around an iron core. The coil acts as both primary and secondary, and operates on the principle of **self-induction.** Insulation is omitted at uniform intervals along the core, and the bare points are connected or tapped to a movable contact, which is in actuality the kVp selector on the x-ray control panel.

6. The answer is (B). Another name for the step-down transformer in the x-ray circuit is the filament transformer. Its function is to regulate the voltage and current supplied to the filament circuit.

7. The answer is (B). Single-phase current has a 100% voltage ripple; that is, it rises and falls continuously from zero to maximum. Three-phase currents are generated from three lines, each 120 degrees from the other, with three-phase, six-pulse current possessing a 13% voltage ripple, and three-phase, twelve-pulse current possessing a 4% ripple.

C. Fluoroscopic Unit

1. IMAGE INTENSIFIER

Fluoroscopy is a radiographic method that permits direct observation of a desired body part or system on a fluorescent screen. The **fluoroscope** uses a standard x-ray tube in conjunction with the fluorescent

screen; however, the tube operates at current averaging 1 to 3 mA.

Early versions of the fluoroscope were crude by today's standards and required the fluoroscopist to *dark adapt* his or her eyes to a darkened examining room in order to adequately visualize the part being examined.

Brightening of the fluoroscopic image was achieved with the advent of the **image intensifier,** a device that coverts an x-ray image to a light image of greater intensity. With the image intensifier, x-ray photons pass through the patient, striking the **input screen,** a 5- to 12-inch in diameter slightly convex device comprised of **cesium iodide (CsI).**

Emerging fluorescent light strikes a photocathode, which frees electrons of varying densities and duplicates the light image. The electrons are then accelerated via an applied high voltage of approximately 25 to 35 kVp and are focused with a negatively charged **electrostatic focusing lens** toward the **output screen.** The output screen, which is comprised of even smaller crystals of cesium iodide, reconverts electrons into a light pattern that is typically 4000 to 7000 times brighter than a conventional fluoroscopy screen. The whole of these components are sealed within a vacuum glass envelope.

The amplification of light photons exiting the output phosphor is known as **brightness gain** and is dependent on two main properties of the image intensifier. First, the output screen is approximately 1/80th the size of the input screen. Because light photons are forced into a much smaller area, brightness is amplified correspondingly (approximately $80\times$) through a process known as **minification gain.** Minification gain may be expressed numerically as the ratio of diameters of both input and output screens squared:

$$\left(\frac{input\ screen\ diameter}{output\ screen\ diameter}\right)^2$$

Second, acceleration of electrons toward the output phosphor yields a multiplication of light photons at the output screen, a phenomenon known as **flux gain.** The numerical expression of flux gain is the ratio of photons at the output screen to the photons at the input screen.

Taking these factors into consideration:

brightness gain = flux gain × minification gain.

Contrast, brightness, and resolution are reduced as much as 25% at the edge of an intensified image primarily because there is lower exposure rate at the periphery. The less than perfect process of electron focusing at the photocathode also contributes to this characteristic of image intensification called **vignetting.**

The poor focusing of electrons at the periphery of the output screen is also responsible for the **pincushion effect,** which is loss of recorded detail through distortion of lines at the edge of an image.

Lag is the continued luminescence of the phosphor after x-ray stimulation has stopped. CsI screens have lag times of approximately 1 ms, which is of little concern.

The image **field of view** is an important image quality factor. A larger field of view results in more minification of the image, a focal point closer to the output screen, and less magnification of the perceived image. Cumulatively, these factors produce a brighter image, with less exposure required.

2. VIEWING SYSTEMS

Older model image intensifiers transferred the fluoroscopic image via its optical system to **a mirror viewing apparatus.** Image resolution was good with mirror systems, but was clumsy to use in actual practice and only permitted viewing by a single person. Modern fluoroscopic systems use a closed-circuit television system for viewing. An **objective lens** transfers the image from the output phosphor to a **beam splitter,** which divides the image between two devices, such as the television screen and the spot film device.

Television systems are classified as **vidicon** or **plumbicon** camera systems. Vidicon systems possess high-image lag, which reduces noise, but results in overlap of images. Plumbicon systems have less lag, but more noise.

3. IMAGE RECORDING SYSTEMS

Permanent records of the fluoroscopic procedures may be obtained in a number of ways. Film recording systems obtain image data directly from the image intensifier, because television cameras exhibit an inherent loss of image detail.

Photospot film records the image onto 70-mm, 90-mm, or 105-mm roll-type film, or onto 100-mm (9 × 9) cut film. With roll film, there is no need to change cassettes, and the device permits fairly rapid-sequence exposures of up to 12 frames per second. Although roll film has the disadvantage of small film size, there is a substantial film cost savings over cut film, and it requires less patient exposure because of the film size being exposed.

Cinefluorography is a series of rapidly ob-

tained photospot images taken on 35-mm film, which produces images that are 18 by 24 mm. Cinefluorography has its widest use in cardiac imaging and involves a system using a **grid-controlled x-ray tube** that synchronizes the x-ray pulse and the cine shutter. Image frequency with most cine devices is in multiples or fractions of 30 frames per second: 15, 30, 60, or 90 frames-per-second rates may be used, with 30 per second being most common.

The most common types of film associated with cine are **panchromatic,** which is sensitive to all light, and **orthochromatic,** which is sensitive to all but red light. Both types of film are available in either 16-mm or 35-mm varieties; 35-mm film provides greater detail, but also greater patient dose. With either type, patient dose associated with cinefluorography is greater than with conventional image-intensified fluoroscopy, because the output screen must be bright enough to expose the cine film. Roughly 85% to 95% of the output screen's light is used to expose film, with the remainder being used for the television monitor.

Fluoroscopic procedures may also be recorded on videotape, which permits immediate viewing of the examination. Videotape also provides the advantage of slow-speed playback and single-frame viewing and sound, but has less resolution than does film.

4. AUTOMATIC BRIGHTNESS CONTROL

When a range of body part densities are to be studied with a single examination, a component known as the **automatic brightness control** compensates for varied attenuation of the beam by adjusting mA and kVp according to patient body part thickness in order to maintain a consistent image.

5. DIGITAL FLUOROSCOPY

Digital fluoroscopy is an imaging system that uses an **analog-to-digital converter** to sample a video signal from the camera and convert it to a binary number stored on a computer. The image may be enhanced before viewing, and permanent films may be obtained by a laser camera. In general, spatial resolution of digital images is less satisfactory than that of conventional film; however, this disadvantage is somewhat offset by the image processing that digital imaging permits.

QUESTIONS FOR FLUOROSCOPIC UNIT

select the best answer

1. The function of the beam splitter in a conventional fluoroscopic imaging system is to:

(A) divide the x-ray beam between the input and output phosphor.

(B) divide the image between the photocathode and output phosphor.

(C) split the image data between the television monitor and photospot film camera.

(D) split the electrons between the input phosphor and photocathode.

2. A given image intensification system has an input phosphor measuring 12 inches and an output phosphor measuring 1 inch. If the flux gain is 50, what is the brightness gain?

(A) 6500

(B) 7000

(C) 7200

(D) 10,000

3. Which component of the image intensifier changes fluorescent light into electrons?

(A) Photocathode

(B) Electrostatic focusing lens

(C) Input phosphor

(D) Output phosphor

4. Flux gain can be described as:

(A) multiplication of electrons at the photocathode.

(B) multiplication of light photons at the output screen.

(C) inherent increase of signal-to-noise ratio with image intensification.

(D) ratio of kilovoltage from primary to secondary in a step-up transformer.

5. All of the following are methods of permanently recording the fluoroscopic image except:

(A) 105-mm camera.

(B) cinefluorography.

(C) mirror optics system.

(D) videotape.

▶▶ ANSWERS TO FLUOROSCOPIC UNIT

1. The answer is (C). The beam-splitting mirror permits continued monitoring of the patient on the television monitor while a permanent record of the examination on film is obtained. From 85% to 95% of the available light is used to expose the film, with the remainder of light used for the monitor.

2. The answer is (C). To solve, recall the formulas:

$$\left(\frac{input\ screen\ diameter}{output\ screen\ diameter}\right)^2$$

and

$$brightness\ gain = flux\ gain \times minification\ gain.$$

$$\left(\frac{12}{1}\right)^2 = 144$$

$$144 \times 50 = 7200$$

3. The answer is (A). The path is as follows: X-ray photons reach the input phosphor made of cesium iodide. For each absorbed x-ray photon, approximately 5000 light photons are emitted. The fluorescent light strikes a photocathode, releasing electrons. These electrons are accelerated by means of a negatively charged focusing lens, and forced through the neck of the tube where they are further accelerated by a potential difference of 25 to 35 kVp to the output phosphor.

4. The answer is (B). Flux gain is the increased number of light photons released from the output phosphor compared with that of the input phosphor. The product of flux gain and minification gain, which is the increase in brightness due to image size reduction, equals brightness gain, which is a numeric expression of image intensifier brightness.

5. The answer is (C). Mirror optics systems were used in older fluoroscopic units, but these systems only permitted viewing, not recording, of the image. Permanent records of real-time events examined with fluoroscopy may be obtained in a number of ways. Spot film (9 × 9) cassettes have long been used, but are gradually being replaced by 105-mm spot film cameras that allow multiframe exposures at lower patient dose. Cinefluorography is a method that is useful for recording rapid biologic events, such as esophageal motility during esophagram examinations. The fluoroscopic image may be transferred to videotape, which permits instantaneous viewing without image processing.

D. Types of Units

Generally speaking, x-ray units are classified according to their purpose and energy output. For example, a certain unit will be described as a mammography machine, a head unit, or perhaps a 150-kV chest unit. The operating characteristics of a given unit are important for the technologist to recognize. The mammography unit, for example, is constructed for use with extremely low kilovoltage in the range of 25 to 40 kVp. You certainly would not want to take a patient scheduled for a standard PA and lateral line chest examination into the mammography room.

1. STATIONARY

The majority of equipment you will encounter in a radiology department is **stationary**—that is, it is fixed in place and is not intended to be moved. Some examples of fixed equipment include radiographic and fluoroscopic (R+F) rooms, tomographic rooms, cystography rooms, special procedure rooms, computed tomography (CT) scanners, magnetic resonance imaging (MRI) scanners, and nuclear medicine rooms.

2. MOBILE

Mobile, or **portable, x-ray units** are used when, for varying reasons, the patient is unable to travel to the radiology department. Some commonplace uses for portable radiography equipment include daily chest or abdominal examinations for intensive care unit (ICU) patients; these units are sometimes referred to as "morning portables." Because it is common practice for virtually all ICU patients to receive this type of examination, they are usually carried out by the technologist all at once, and usually early in the morning, before physicians begin their morning rounds.

Other uses for mobile radiography are: standard radiographs or fluoroscopy performed in the operating suite, fluoroscopy performed for central line placement, and radiographic services for trauma or unstable patients who are in the emergency room. Both nuclear medicine and ultrasound can be performed with mobile units.

For technical reasons, most portable examinations are of lesser radiographic quality than comparable examinations performed in the radiology department. Therefore, it is preferable to carry out most examinations with fixed equipment if the patient's condition permits these procedures.

3. DEDICATED OR SPECIALIZED

As previously mentioned, some types of equipment, the mammography unit, for example, are designed for one specific intent. This type of equipment is sometimes referred to as **dedicated** equipment. Chest units, head units, cystography units, and to-

mography units are all examples of specialized or dedicated equipment.

QUESTIONS FOR TYPES OF UNITS

select the best answer

1. A Franklin head unit is an example of which type of radiographic machinery?

   (A) Fixed
   (B) Dedicated
   (C) Mobile
   (D) Fluoroscopy

2. A patient arrives via ambulance at the emergency room, on a backboard and in a cervical collar, following a motor vehicle accident. The most likely examination to be ordered first is:

   (A) portable chest.
   (B) lateral skull.
   (C) rib series.
   (D) portable cross-table lateral cervical spine.

▶▶ **ANSWERS TO TYPES OF UNITS**

1. The answer is (B). The Franklin unit is a well-known variety of radiography equipment designed to produce high-quality radiographs of the skull and facial bones. In it, the patient is seated upright at a bucky, and the tube arm swings in a wide arc around the patient, which allows a wide variety of views to be obtained in a relatively easy fashion. Today, however, head units are not used as often, because CT and MRI are now the preferred modalities for examining the head.

2. The answer is (D). In the absence of other life-threatening emergencies, the emergency room physician's first priority is to rule out a fracture of the cervical spine. Generally, a portable cross-table lateral view of the cervical spine will be obtained with the patient still on the backboard, and the cervical collar in place. If the film appears grossly normal, the collar will generally be removed, and an entire cervical spine series will be obtained. Some physicians prefer to obtain anteroposterior and odontoid views with the patient still immobilized; however, these films are of limited quality due to the immobilized position of the patient.

II. EVALUATION OF RADIOGRAPHIC EQUIPMENT AND ACCESSORIES
A. Equipment Calibration

In order to maintain radiographic equipment in proper working order, radiology departments establish a schedule for preventive maintenance and **quality control (QC).** QC is a documented, systematic plan for maintaining standards. Components of the radiology department evaluated by a QC program include the automatic processor, x-ray tube, and x-ray generator. Such a program is supervised by a designated QC technologist and includes input from staff technologists, radiologists, service engineers, and a radiation physicist.

1. KILOVOLTAGE PEAK

Kilovoltage accuracy is crucial to radiographic contrast and is generally evaluated with digital kVp meters in the diagnostic range of approximately 40 to 150 kVp. Digital equipment has replaced the **Wisconsin test cassette,** which was formerly used for this purpose. When tested, selected kVp must not differ more than 5 kVp from the actual kVp produced. Mammography units must be accurate to within 1 kVp.

2. MILLIAMPERAGE

Competence of the mA station is a key factor in the determination of radiographic density and patient dose. An **aluminum step wedge, or penetrometer,** is used for this evaluation. Performing this test involves making a series of exposures at a constant kVp. Consistent mAs values are used, with the time being adjusted downward as mA is adjusted upward. X-ray output is measured in terms of milliroentgen (mR) per mA-s and must be accurate to within ± 10% for consecutive mA stations.

A digital ion chamber, or dosimeter, is used to assess mA **linearity.** Linearity is a term that refers to *exposure consistency* using differing mA and time values to produce the same mAs. Do not confuse linearity with **reproducibility,** which refers to *exposure output during repeated exposures using the same settings.*

3. TIME

Like mA, accuracy of the radiographic timer is a determinant for patient dose and radiographic density. The **digital dosimeter** is simpler and more accurate

mA station	mR/mAs
(A) 200	42
(B) 300	47
(C) 400	44
(D) 500	41

than the **spinning top test,** which was formerly used, and is now the instrument of choice for this evaluation. Exposure time must be accurate to within 5%.

QUESTIONS FOR EQUIPMENT CALIBRATION

select the best answer

1. Refer to the table below. Assume that the correct output at the 100-mA station is 40 mR/mA-s. Which of the of the following mA stations requires calibration of linearity?

2. Which of the following instruments may be used to test the accuracy of the x-ray unit timer?
    1. Spinning top
    2. Digital dosimeter
    3. Wisconsin cassette
   (A) All of the aforementioned
   (B) None of the aforementioned
   (C) Choices 1 and 3
   (D) Choices 1 and 2

3. Suppose that an exposure made using 500 mA, 0.02 sec, and 70 kVp yields an exposure output of 250 mR. What is the mR/mAs?
   (A) 50
   (B) 25
   (C) 12.5
   (D) 75

4. Calibration of kVp is a key determinant in which of the following factors on the exposed x-ray film?
   (A) Contrast
   (B) Exposure latitude
   (C) Density
   (D) Screen lag

▶▶ ANSWERS TO EQUIPMENT CALIBRATION

1. The answer is (B). Linearity is a term that refers to *exposure consistency* using differing mA and time

values to produce the same mAs; linearity must be accurate to within 10% of the consecutive mA, that is, to within 10% of either the mA station above or below the mA station being tested.

If the correct value for 100 mA is 40 mR/mA-s, then the 200-mA station must be accurate to within 10% of that value. In other words, it must have values between 36 and 44 mR/mA-s. Therefore, linearity is within acceptable limits between 100- and 200-mA stations. However, the 300-mA station has an mR/mA-s value of 47, meaning that the station above it (400 mA) and the station below it (300 mA) must have values between the range of 42.8 and 51.7, or ± 10% of its value. Because the 200-mA station has a value of 42, linearity does not exist between the 200- and 300-mA stations.

2. The answer is (D). The spinning top test is somewhat outmoded, but may be used to test accuracy of single-phase equipment. The test uses a metallic disk with a small hole in its outer edge. Suppose a 0.1-sec exposure is made while the top spins. Because single-phase, full-wave rectified equipment should produce 120 impulses per second, the exposed film should record 12 dots if the timer is accurate. Today, however, many in the field consider the digital dosimeter to be the instrument of choice for this procedure.

3. The answer is (B). The mR/mAs is the expression used for calibration of mA stations and is determined by dividing exposure output in mR by the mAs. In this instance,

250 mR ÷ 500 mA (0.02 sec) = 25 mR/mA-s

4. The answer is (A). Kilovoltage primarily affects the quality of photons in x-ray production. As such, its main effect on the exposed radiograph is that of contrast. Exposure latitude is a film characteristic. Screen lag refers to the amount of continued phosphorescence after the exposure is terminated that a given intensifying screen exhibits. Milliamperage is the primary factor in determining quantity of photons; therefore, it primarily affects radiographic density.

B. Beam Restriction

Beam restriction devices limit the size of the x-ray beam to a desired area, and are therefore a factor in patient dose. Various devices, such as cones and diaphragms, may be attached to the x-ray tube for this purpose. Cones and diaphragms are very durable and do not require special testing beyond a simple visual inspection to ensure their accuracy.

Of concern with respect to quality control testing is the variable aperture collimator. The collimator consists of a pair of lead shutters that work in tandem to limit the x-ray beam both in the transverse and longitudinal planes. The uppermost pair of shutters is closest to the tube port and serves to reduce off-focus radiation, a factor in geometric blurring of the image. The second set of shutters is positioned at a lower point and function to size the x-ray beam.

Modern collimators include a mirror placed in the path of the beam and a light bulb that shines in the mirror. The combination of mirror and light bulb project size, location, and center of the irradiated field.

The mirror is positioned at a 45-degree angle with respect to the bulb so that it reflects the light on the patient. In order for the light shining on the patient to be an accurate indication of the x-ray field size, a properly positioned mirror and focal spot are exactly the same distance from the center of the mirror. Most technologists rely on the collimator light to ensure that the patient is positioned correctly in alignment with the central ray.

National Council for Radiation Protection and Measurements (NCRP) Report No. 102 requires that a positive variable beam limiting device (a collimator) work in conjunction with the bucky tray to ensure that the light field does not exceed ± 2% FFD. Most equipment today includes a function that automatically performs collimation to film or receptor size, but it may be de-selected, because there are many cases in which the technologist wants the beam to be less than the film size used. In any case, it is vital for the technologist to ensure that the field of radiation *never exceeds that of the actual film size being used.*

Evaluation of mirror alignment should be conducted semiannually.

QUESTIONS FOR BEAM RESTRICTION

select the best answer

1. According to guidelines established in NCRP Report No. 102, when using a 40-inch SID, how far can the illuminated field extend beyond the dimensions of the cassette?
   (A) 4 inches
   (B) 0.4 inch
   (C) 8 inches
   (D) 0.8 inch

2. The primary purpose of the pair of lead collimator shutters closest to the x-ray source is to:
   (A) size and shape the x-ray field.

(B) minimize off-focus radiation.
(C) act as a backup.
(D) reduce scatter from the tube housing.

3. The most reliable means of assuring that the x-ray tube is centered to the potter-bucky tray is to:
   (A) visually inspect the alignment before positioning the patient.
   (B) use the collimator centering light to ensure tube–part–grid alignment.
   (C) use the automatic centering device.
   (D) adjust the tube if films exhibit grid cutoff.

4. In order for the size, location, and center of an illuminated field to be accurately representative of the actual irradiated field, which two components must be exactly the same distance from the center of the mirror inside the tube head?
   (A) Anode and cathode
   (B) Anode and focal spot
   (C) Focal spot and light bulb
   (D) Anode and light bulb

▶▶ **ANSWERS TO BEAM RESTRICTION**

1. The answer is (D). NCRP guidelines provide that positive beam limitation devices (PBLs) must be accurate to within ± 2% of the SID. Therefore, using a 40-inch SID, an illuminated area of 0.8 inch extending beyond the film dimensions would be acceptable.
2. The answer is (B). Off-focus radiation is produced when electrons interact with material other than the focal track of the mode; this type of radiation may be responsible for indistinct densities on the film that do not add diagnostic information. The primary purpose of the pair of lead shutters closest to the anode is to reduce off-focus radiation.
3. The answer is (C). Almost all modern x-ray units are equipped with automatic centering devices, which are sometimes referred to as the tube détente. Centering devices consist of magnetic locks that engage when the tube is properly placed relative to the transverse plane of the table. Visual inspection is not as reliable, and the collimator light cannot be used, because many tabletops move from side to side, making it difficult to determine the center accurately. Incorrect tube centering relative to the potter-bucky tray results in grid cutoff.
4. The answer is (C). The collimator assembly con-

sists of a pair of lead shutters, a mirror, and a light bulb. The light beam is deflected by the mirror, which is at a 45-degree angle relative to the light beam. In order for the illuminated field on the patient to project accurately, the focal spot and light bulb must be exactly the same distance from the center of the mirror.

C. Recognition of Malfunctions

Maintenance of continuous quality in the radiology department is a joint effort among biomedical repair personnel, staff technologists, the QC technologist, department administrators, and office/hospital administrators. A weak link in any part of the QC chain can cause frustrating slowdowns and less than optimal performance from both technologists and equipment.

Suppose, for example, a given administrator takes a bottom-line approach to the department service contract and hires a less costly company to perform service work. Although such decisions are commonplace in today's cost-cutting environment, experience teaches that you get what you pay for. The yearly fee for such a service may be less, but discounts received on the front end are inevitably negated by increased cost of downtime and poor film quality, which necessitates repeat exposures and higher supply costs. This is one circumstance that highlights the importance of a team approach to operations.

Concerning operation of mechanical components like x-ray units and processors, however, the staff technologist is the most likely person to encounter a potential problem first, so it is crucial that technologists not only recognize machinery malfunctions when they occur, but also properly identify the necessary steps for restoring normal operations.

The sheer number of possibilities concerning recognizing and repairing malfunctions in the radiology department precludes detailed description here. However, as you will soon learn in your own workplace, there are basically two sets of conditions: those that require a service call and those that can be rectified by radiology personnel. Technologists must learn how to quickly locate service personnel and describe the situation, but when technologists themselves can take restorative actions, they should do so.

QUESTIONS FOR RECOGNITION OF MALFUNCTIONS

select the best answer

1. A lateral lumbar spine film is obtained using a normally reliable AEC device. The film appears

underexposed when processed. Possible causes for the film being too light include all of the following except:

(A) processor temperature too low.
(B) AEC out of calibration.
(C) improper positioning.
(D) improper FFD.

2. Suppose during the course of an examination the x-ray tube begins emitting a high-pitched sound, and you detect a burning smell. The appropriate action to take would be to:

1. shut down the equipment.
2. remove the patient in a quick, calm fashion.
3. notify the fire department.

(A) All of the aforementioned
(B) Choice 1 only
(C) Choices 1 and 2
(D) Choices 2 and 3

▶▶ **ANSWERS TO RECOGNITION OF MALFUNCTION**

1. The answer is (D). Automatic exposure devices will compensate for inaccurate distance; however, as FFD decreases, magnification increases. If the patient is not properly positioned over the AEC cell, the preselected amount of energy will reach the AEC detector, and the exposure will terminate too quickly, which results in an underexposed radiograph. Similarly, inadequate developer temperature will result in light films. Both proper positioning and maintenance of correct developer temperature are examples of steps that the technologist can take to ensure quality. The automatic exposure device is generally calibrated by service personnel. If the AEC was the cause of the underexposed radiograph, the proper action for the technologist would be to initiate a service call.

2. The answer is (C). A high-pitched sound and a burning smell are indications of major mechanical malfunctions, such as a tube arcing, malfunctioning rotor, or generator failure. The patient's safety is always the first priority, so shutting down the equipment and removing the patient from the area would represent appropriate measures in this instance. By law, exposure rooms must be equipped with a main breaker switch that will shut down all equipment simultaneously. In the absence of other evidence, however, notify-

ing the fire department at this stage of such an incident would be premature. Instead, inform qualified service personnel of your observations, and allow them access to the room to investigate the source of operation disruption.

D. Screens and Cassettes

In order to allow highly light-sensitive x-ray film to be used outside of the darkroom, it is encased in light-proof **cassettes.** The front of the cassette consists of low attenuating material such as carbon fiber, which readily allows the passage of x-ray photons. The back is comprised of lead, which absorbs exiting x-ray photons and reduces image-degrading backscatter. The back of the cassette contains locking latches, which when released allow access to the inside of the cassette for film removal and replacement. Design of the latches varies by manufacturer.

Maintenance of cassettes is simple but important. Cassettes should be stacked upright according to size and speed. Piling them on top of each other or haphazardly stuffing them in the passbox places them at risk for damage.

Part of the ongoing departmental QC effort should include visual inspection of cassettes for damage and cleanliness. The inside should be cleaned regularly to remove dust and lint, and damaged cassettes should be sent for repair.

Intensifying screens, which are layers of phosphor that emit light when exposed to x-rays, are mounted inside the cassette and serve to amplify the action of x-ray photons on x-ray film. Developed by Thomas Edison in 1896, early versions of the screens were composed of **calcium tungstate** ($CaWOL_4$). Calcium tungstate produces primarily blue light.

The early 1970s saw the advent of green light–emitting **rare earth screens,** which are composed of phosphors that have higher absorption efficiency than calcium tungstate. Rare earth screens require less exposure to produce densities comparable to their calcium tungstate counterparts.

High-speed screens are thicker and faster but have decreased spatial resolution when compared with thinner **slow, or detail, screens.** Generally speaking, high-speed screens are used in conjunction with larger body parts such as the abdomen and chest, whereas use of detail screens is confined to radiography of the extremities.

Intensifying screens can be the source of image artifact. Artifact can be defined as an image-degrading density on film that is not part of the demonstrated anatomy. Sources of intensifying screen-related artifacts include hair, dirt, scratches, and talcum powder, all of which may accumulate from everyday use. Bearing this in mind, technologists should recall that keeping hands clean and dry is an important consideration when working in the darkroom, and that cleaning intensifying screens with a commercially prepared nonstatic solution is part of a thorough QC program.

When the film and screen are not properly in contact, areas of blur may occur on the developed radiograph. Therefore, another significant source of artifact is poor **screen contact.** Screen contact is tested with a **wire mesh device.** To perform the test, a cassette is placed on the x-ray tabletop, and the wire mesh device rests on top of the cassette. A typical extremity-type exposure is then made, and the developed film is examined. Blurred areas on the film demonstrate areas of poor screen contact. These screens should be either discarded or sent for repair.

A similar test is performed for grid cassettes. A low exposure, which is enough to demonstrate the grid lines, is made, and the processed film is examined. Areas of uneven density indicate malaligned lead strips, and these should be repaired, if possible.

QUESTIONS FOR SCREENS AND CASSETTES

select the best answer

1. The QC test used to evaluate poor screen contact is a:

   (A) spinning top.
   (B) wire mesh.
   (C) resolution test pattern.
   (D) Wisconsin test.

2. All of the following could be the cause of intensifying screen artifact except:

   (A) phosphor thickness.
   (B) static.
   (C) oil.
   (D) talcum powder.

3. What measures can be taken to ensure reliability of grid alignment in a grid cassette?

   (A) Visual inspection
   (B) Weekly cleaning
   (C) Production of a radiograph of the grid
   (D) Wire mesh test

►► ANSWERS TO SCREENS AND CASSETTES

1. The answer is (B). The wire mesh test is used to evaluate poor screen contact. The resolution test pattern is used to test resolution in lines per inch, whereas the spinning top test is used to evaluate rectification. The Wisconsin test cassette is an outmoded means of evaluating correct kVp.

2. The answer is (A). Phosphor thickness is relative to intensifying screen speed, with increasing thickness being proportional to increased speed. Oil from hands or talcum powder residue from gloves leaves image-degrading artifact, as does static that results from the friction created when film interacts with the screen. Screens should be cleaned with commercially prepared antistatic solutions to reduce the incidence of static artifact.

3. The answer is (C). The lead strips within a grid cassette can become malaligned from ordinary use. The most reliable means of testing the lead strips is to make a low-energy exposure of the grid cassette, and then examine the processed film for areas of uneven density.

E. Shielding Accessories

Radiology departments are equipped with protective devices such as lead aprons, lead gloves, thyroid shields, and lead-imbedded glasses. All of these devices may become less effective if they are not properly maintained via an ongoing QC effort.

Lead aprons may become cracked if thrown haphazardly on the floor or carelessly folded. Technologists should use the racks provided for such items. Lead aprons should be fluoroscoped annually to ensure that no cracks in the lead material have developed, which would decrease effectiveness.

If soiled, protective devices can be cleaned with a damp cloth and warm, soapy water. If protective devices become contaminated with biohazardous material, use appropriate materials such as 1:10 water and bleach solution to cleanse the soiled item.

QUESTIONS FOR SHIELDING ACCESSORIES

select the best answer

1. Which of the following items is associated with use during a barium enema examination?

   (A) Lead apron
   (B) Lead gloves
   (C) Lead glasses
   (D) All of the aforementioned

2. An effective quality control program includes fluoroscopic examination of leaded protective accessories at least:

(A) Weekly
(B) Daily
(C) Monthly
(D) Yearly

▶▶ANSWERS TO SHIELDING ACCESSORIES

1. The answer is (D). Lead aprons, glasses, and gloves all may be used during a typical BE examination. Both the physician and technologist wear aprons, and some prefer using protective eyewear as well. The radiologist will don lead gloves if a compression device is used to manipulate the bowel during fluoroscopy.
2. The answer is (D). Protective lead apparel should be checked with fluoroscopic examination yearly to ensure the integrity of the leaded material.

END-OF-CHAPTER EXAMINATION

▶▶ QUESTIONS

Select the best answer.

1. A device that automatically compensates for variation in patient tissue density in order to produce radiographs with consistent density is called a:
   (A) backup timer.
   (B) ion chamber.
   (C) rectifier.
   (D) transformer.

2. The purpose of rectification in the x-ray circuit is to produce:
   (A) half-wave DC.
   (B) full-wave AC.
   (C) nonpulsating AC.
   (D) pulsating DC.

3. Which of the following components in a QC program is checked by visual means?
   (A) Illumination system
   (B) Intensifying screen artifacts
   (C) Intensifying screen contact
   (D) Lead aprons

4. Which image intensification device changes light photons into an electronic image?
   (A) Input phosphor
   (B) Output phosphor
   (C) Photocathode
   (D) Focusing lens

5. Of the following radiographic components, all are examples of dedicated units except:
   (A) Franklin head unit.
   (B) cystography unit.
   (C) radiography/fluoroscopy unit.
   (D) tomographic unit.

6. Which of the following formulas would be used to find current on the secondary side of a step-up transformer?

   (A) $\dfrac{V_S}{V_P} = \dfrac{N_S}{N_P}$

   (B) $\dfrac{V_S}{V_P} = \dfrac{N_P}{N_S}$

   (C) $\dfrac{V_P}{V_S} = \dfrac{N_S}{N_P}$

   (D) $\dfrac{N_S}{N_P} = \dfrac{I_P}{I_S}$

7. Most x-ray anodes are comprised of a tungsten-rhenium alloy. Which of the following characteristics of tungsten increases x-ray production?
   (A) Durability
   (B) High atomic number
   (C) High thermal conductivity
   (D) High melting point

8. Which component of the fluoroscopic unit serves to make adjustments for tissue density variations?
   (A) Automatic brightness control
   (B) Photocathode
   (C) Focusing cup
   (D) Output phosphor

9. If a digital dosimeter is not available, what simpler, less expensive device can be used to evaluate mA linearity?
   (A) Wisconsin test tool
   (B) Geiger counter
   (C) Cutie pie
   (D) Penetrometer

(Continued)

10. The star pattern resolution device is used in conjunction with what component of the x-ray tube?

    (A) Filament
    (B) Focusing cup
    (C) Focal spot
    (D) Anode

11. Which of the following formulas is used to determine HU output of a three-phase, twelve-pulse radiographic unit?

    (A) HU = mA $\times$ s $\times$ kVp
    (B) HU = mA $\times$ s $\times$ kVp $\times$ 1.35
    (C) HU = mA $\times$ s $\times$ kVp $\times$ 1.41
    (D) $\dfrac{I_1}{I_2} = \dfrac{D_2^2}{D_1^2}$

12. Using a 72-inch FFD, how far can the illuminated light field exceed the boundaries of a 14-inch $\times$ 17-inch cassette?

    (A) 1.44 inch
    (B) 0.7 inch
    (C) 0.77 inch
    (D) 0.14 inch

13. A 300-lb man comes to the radiology department for evaluation of the lumbar spine. In order to perform a phototimed examination, which of the following components could be adjusted upward from their default settings in order to prevent an inadequate exposure?

    (A) Backup timer
    (B) kVp
    (C) mA
    (D) All of the aforementioned

14. Which of the following components determines focal spot size?

    (A) Rectifier
    (B) Autotransformer
    (C) Target material
    (D) Filament size

15. A film that exhibits localized areas of blurring is most likely representative of:

    (A) artifacts.
    (B) fogged film.
    (C) poor screen–film contact.
    (D) yellowing of screen phosphor.

16. All of the following are essential components of a high-quality dedicated mammography room except:

    (A) high-frequency generator.
    (B) dedicated processor.
    (C) high radiographic contrast.
    (D) compression devices.

17. Of the following, which type of radiation is the major constituent emitted from the target?

    (A) Compton scatter
    (B) Bremsstrahlung radiation
    (C) Coherent scatter
    (D) Annihilation reaction

18. During an exposure, you note that the mA meter registers only one half the selected mA. Additionally, the resulting radiograph demonstrates only one half its expected density. The most likely cause of malfunction is:

    (A) rectifier failure.
    (B) mA station out of calibration.
    (C) Fluctuating line voltage.
    (D) Step-up transformer failure.

19. How much time is required for an exposure equaling 70 mAs when using the 200-mA small focal spot station?

    (A) 0.50 sec
    (B) 1 sec
    (C) 0.35 sec
    (D) 0.55 sec

20. Which of the following is not an acceptable part of the regimen for proper care of lead aprons?

    (A) Fluoroscoped yearly to evaluate integrity of leaded material
    (B) Laundered weekly to eliminate residual biohazardous material
    (C) Disinfected with spray material after biohazardous contamination
    (D) Hung from designated racks after use

21. Which type of x-ray unit permits dynamic imaging?

    (A) Fluoroscope
    (B) Tomographic unit
    (C) Mobile unit
    (D) Dedicated chest room

(Continued)

22. Compared with grids constructed of plastic interspace material, grids that use aluminum as the interspace material:

    (A) provide greater contrast and less patient dose.
    (B) provide less contrast and less patient dose.
    (C) provide greater contrast and greater patient dose.
    (D) provide greater scatter cleanup with less patient dose.

23. Which of the following is a true statement regarding a variable aperture collimator?

    (A) Consists of four shutters operating independently
    (B) Eliminates need for compensating filters
    (C) Consists of two pairs of shutters and a light localizing system
    (D) Can produce a variety of collimated field shapes, including circular, rectangular, and square

24. If an AEC is used to radiograph a lateral thoracic spine, and the resulting radiograph demonstrates inadequate density, what is the most likely cause?

    (A) Plus density was selected
    (B) Excessive backup time was selected
    (C) Center cell was selected
    (D) Center cell was posterior to the thoracic spine

25. What device is used to test accuracy of the x-ray timer?

    (A) Aluminum step wedge
    (B) Spinning top
    (C) Star pattern
    (D) Densitometer

26. How many half-value layers (HVL) are required to reduce a beam intensity from 560 mR to 35 mR?

    (A) 2
    (B) 3
    (C) 4
    (D) 5

27. What component of the x-ray circuit is engaged in order to reduce the selected kilovoltage?

    (A) Autotransformer
    (B) Step-up transformer
    (C) Step-down transformer
    (D) High-frequency generator

28. Of the following, which are beam restriction devices?

    (A) Compensating filters, focused grids, collimators
    (B) Collimators, flare cones, diaphragms
    (C) Aluminum filters, slit diaphragms, focused grids
    (D) Inherent filtration, mirror-guided light device, non-focused grid

29. Older intensifying screens often change in appearance from bright white to yellow. What is the radiographic result of this change?

    (A) Increase in speed
    (B) Decrease in detail
    (C) Increase in detail
    (D) Decrease in speed

30. Which of the following are methods of recording the fluoroscopic image?

    (A) 105-mm film
    (B) Optical laser disk
    (C) Magnetic tape
    (D) All of the aforementioned

▶▶ ANSWERS

1. The answer is (B). Along with the phototimer, the ion chamber is a type of automatic exposure device that automatically compensates for tissue variants in order to reproduce constant radiographic density. The device terminates the exposure once a predetermined amount of ionization has been reached.

2. The answer is (D). The rectification system is responsible for maintaining the unidirectional flow of electrons from cathode to anode. The action of the rectifier actually creates two pulsating AC pulses, but because they are in the same direction, they are referred to as pulsating DC. Three-phase current more closely resembles true DC current, although a ripple or voltage drop is still present. Voltage drops are as follows: single-phase, 100%; three-phase, six-pulse, 13.5%; and three-phase, twelve-pulse, 3.5%.

(Continued)

3. The answer is (B). Intensifying screens contaminated with dust, hair, oil, and other substances leave visual artifacts on the exposed radiograph. Screens must be visually inspected, and then cleaned with antistatic solution to keep them as artifact-free as possible. Lead aprons should be fluoroscoped once a year to detect loss of integrity; wire mesh is used to examine screen contact; and a light meter should be used in conjunction with testing of illumination systems (view boxes).

4. The answer is (C). Light photons striking the photocathode are converted to an electron image and then focused by the electrostatic lens to the output phosphor.

5. The answer is (C). Standard radiography/fluoroscopy rooms are used for a variety of examinations and are therefore considered examples of fixed equipment. Dedicated rooms, such as the type listed, or mammography rooms, are used for a singular, distinct purpose.

6. The answer is (D). *I* is the variable associated with current in equations. Letter A represents the equation used for the transformer law; letters B and C are invalid. Letter D is the variant of transformer law used to determine current on the secondary side of a step-up transformer.

7. The answer is (B). The high atomic number of tungsten serves to increase x-ray production. Tungsten's high melting point of 341°C resists pitting and cracking, and high thermal conductivity facilitates rapid heat dissipation.

8. The answer is (A). In terms of function, the automatic brightness control acts like a phototimer, adjusting technique up and down as tissue density varies, and maintaining constant brightness and contrast on the output monitor. There are additional brightness and contrast controls on the monitor itself.

9. The answer is (D). An aluminum step wedge or penetrometer may be used to evaluate mA station accuracy. With the step wedge, a series of exposures at constant kVp and constant mAs values at differing mA stations are made. If mA stations are linear, the step wedge images should be identical.

10. The answer is (C). The star pattern resolution device measures focal spot accuracy as a function of geometric blur. An exposure is made of the device that sits on top of a screen cassette, and the individual distinct elements are visually examined for areas of blur.

11. The answer is (C). Letters A and B represent the formulas for finding heat units for single-phase and three-phase, six-pulse machines, respectively; letter D is the formula for the inverse square law.

12. The answer is (A). By NCRP regulation, light field to radiation field alignment must be within ± 2% of the SID. Substituting values, therefore, 72 inches × 0.02 = 1.44 inches.

13. The answer is (D). Automatic exposure default settings are generally predetermined for either small, medium, or large body size. If a patient's size exceeds that of the default settings, an increase in technical adjustments must be made, or backup time will be inadequate. Technologists may increase time, kVp, or mA as desired in order to accomplish this.

14. The answer is (D). Most modern x-ray equipment is dual focused, which means that there are two filament sizes to choose from. When the smaller filament is selected, the smaller focal spot is selected, and less area on the disk is bombarded by electrons.

15. The answer is (C). Poor screen film contact is manifested when localized areas of blurring occur on the processed radiograph. In order to evaluate the condition of screens for contact, a wire mesh test is used.

16. The answer is (A). The technical factors used in conjunction with mammography are relatively low, with typical exposures made in the range of 25 to 40 kVp; therefore, a high-frequency generator would not be required. A dedicated processor, that is, one used only for mammography, is key in maintaining the discerning levels of processor QC now associated with mammography by law. Compression devices help the mammographer even out the difference in density between the thicker chest wall and thinner nipple area. Additionally, compression aids in reducing scatter and object film distance (OFD).

(Continued)

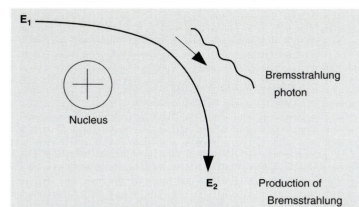

E_1

Bremsstrahlung
photon

Nucleus

E_2 Production of
Bremsstrahlung

Figure 3-A.   Bremsstrahlung radiation.

17. The answer is (B). As an electron approaches the positive field of a tungsten atom, the negatively charged electron is deviated from its path, according to the law that governs opposite attraction. In deviating, the electron decelerates, and the lost kinetic energy is given up as "braking" or Bremsstrahlung radiation, which represents 80% to 85% of the useful beam. Compton and coherent scatter are interactions between electrons and tissue. Annihilation reaction occurs at energy levels higher than that associated with diagnostic radiation.

18. The answer is (A). When the listed conditions are present, the most likely culprit is rectifier failure. Such equipment is said to be "half-waving." Half-waving occurs when inverse voltage is not used. Single-phase rectifiers are tested with a spinning top test, and three-phase equipment is tested with the synchronous type of spinning top or with an oscilloscope.

19. The answer is (C). To solve, use the formula: mA $\times$ S = mAs:

$$200x = 70$$
$$x = 70/200$$
$$x = 0.35$$

20. The answer is (B). Lead aprons are normally cleaned with a damp cloth or sprayed with a disinfectant material and wiped down. Protective leaded apparel is not designed for laundering, however; this would subject the aprons to excessive moisture.

21. The answer is (A). The term dynamic refers to a part in motion. One of the most important aspects of the fluoroscopic unit is its ability to examine anatomy in motion, such as is performed with barium swallow examinations. Another way of thinking about this concept is that fluoroscopy permits examination of physiology, which is the study of living organism functions.

22. The answer is (C). When compared with grids constructed with plastic interspace material, grids that use aluminum have greater cleanup ability, and therefore provide greater radiographic contrast. Unfortunately, greater patient dose is required as compared with grids that use plastic.

23. The answer is (C). The variable aperture collimator consists of a longitudinal and transverse pair of lead shutters that can shape the x-ray field in square or rectangular shapes. Compensating filters are used in conjunction with radiography of body parts that possess a wide range of densities, such as body parts radiographed for scoliosis series; these filters are not part of the collimator system.

24. The answer is (D). When using AEC devices, proper positioning is critical. If the cell of the AEC was posterior to the spine during the exposure, the preselected quantity of ionization would take place too quickly, because the spine is not positioned over the cell. If positioned correctly, the thoracic spine would attenuate the correct amount of useful beam, which would result in proper density displayed on the radiograph.

25. The answer is (B). Along with testing rectifier failure, the spinning top test is used to check accuracy of the x-ray timer. Using single-phase, full-wave rectification, which produces 120 pulses per second, an exposure of 0.10 sec should produce 12 dots on a processed radiograph. The visualization of fewer or more dots is indicative of timer inaccuracy. Remember, the spinning top is used only with single-phase equipment. Three-phase equipment must be tested using an oscilloscope or synchronous spinning top.

26. The answer is (C). Half-value layer is defined as the amount of aluminum filtration required to reduce beam intensity by half. Therefore, 560/2 = 280; 280/2 = 140; 140/2 = 70; 70/2 = 35. Each division is equal to 1 HVL.

(Continued)

27. The answer is (A). In the x-ray circuit, the autotransformer is used to select kVp. Placed between the AC source and the primary side of the transformer, its function is to allow varying voltage input to the primary side of the transformer. The autotransformer has multiple turns, or "taps," which are selected when kVp is changed.

28. The answer is (B). The x-ray unit has three primary types of beam restriction: collimators; cones, both flared and cylindrical; and diaphragms. The mirror is a component of the collimator, but is not the means of restriction. Filtration serves to increase the average beam intensity by filtering of soft photons. Grids eliminate scatter radiation created by the patient before it reaches the film.

29. The answer is (D). As screens become discolored over time, light emission is reduced, and thus speed decreases.

30. The answer is (D). Cameras that use 105-mm film have largely replaced those units that use conventional spot films; the former have become the preferred recording medium. Although they possess the disadvantage of a smaller image on film, with 105 mm, less patient dose is required, and the camera is less work-intensive. More modern departments now use magnetic tape or optical disk as the recording medium, which can store many examination results on a single tape or disk.

CHAPTER 4

Image Production and Evaluation

I. SELECTION OF TECHNICAL FACTORS
A. Density

MILLIAMPERE-SECONDS (mAs)

The term **radiographic technique** describes the combination of settings on the x-ray unit control panel that produce a certain effect on radiographic film. There are two groups of exposure factors: **exposure technique factors** and **image quality factors.**

Exposure technique factors determine the characteristics of exposure to both film and patient, and include kilovoltage peak (kVp), milliampere-seconds, and distance. Image quality factors provide an orderly structure by which to produce and compare radiographs, and include distortion, density, contrast, and detail.

Radiographic **density** may be defined as the overall degree of blackening on the x-ray film. An aluminum stepwedge (discussed in Chapter 3) can be used to measure the amount of density present on a radiograph. The stepwedge numerically demonstrates the amount of transmitted light through a film. An optical density of 3 or 4 is numerically equivalent to completely black, whereas a measurement of 0.2 represents a clear film.

Radiographs that demonstrate inappropriate density must be repeated. A film that is "dark" has a high optical density. The film is overexposed; too much radiation reached the film. Conversely, a "light" radiograph has a low optical density, and is underexposed; too little radiation was used.

Although technologists think of density in terms of overall blackness, the radiologist may refer to density as a pathologic or anatomic change that absorbs x-rays. For example, a neoplasm (tumor) in the lung absorbs more radiation than does the surrounding tissue; therefore, that area on the radiograph would be described by the radiologist as less dense. Similarly, an area of decreased physical density, such as the demineralized portion of a hip in a patient who has osteoporosis, will produce an area of increased density on film.

The primary controlling factor of radiographic density is mAs. Remember, mAs is the product of milliamperage (mA) and time (S), and is a *quantitative* measure of x-ray photon production. Density increases directly as mAs increases. Therefore, if a change of density is required on a radiograph, then mAs is the correct exposure factor to modify. *A 30% to 40% change in mAs is required to produce a significant change in density on the processed radiograph.* This rule is especially important to recall in the workplace. When repeat films for density are necessary, the most common error made is inadequate upward or downward adjustment.

For example, a commonly suggested way to compensate for a light radiograph is to adjust up or down one time station. Not only is this suggestion impractical for reasons of nonspecificity (the percentage of change would depend on the range of time involved), but as you have seen from your own experience, one step in time will rarely produce a 30% increase in mAs.

A 30% increase in mAs will produce an increase in density just perceptible to the human eye. A substantial visible change would require at least a 50% increase in mAs, and a film that is grossly underexposed would require doubling of the mAs, or 100% increase in technique. Because the relationship between mAs and density is proportional, you can recall an easy rule of thumb: double the mAs = double the density.

The mA required for a given density is inversely proportional to exposure time, with all other factors constant. The mathematical relationship may be expressed by using the following formula:

$$\frac{Original\ mA}{New\ mA} = \frac{New\ Time}{Original\ Time} \quad (1)$$

Examine for yourself the ramifications of this formula by carrying out a few simple test problems. For example, if you were called upon to radiograph a child's abdomen, and the technique chart called for an exposure using 200 mA and 0.6 sec, how could you most effectively decrease exposure time in order to reduce motion artifact, assuming a maximum of 600 mA was available on the machine?

$$\frac{200\ mA}{600\ mA} = \frac{X}{0.6}$$
$$600X = 120 \quad (2)$$
$$X = 0.2\ sec$$

Using the maximum mA in this example reduces the exposure time by one third, while maintaining a constant density. This sample problem is an example of the **reciprocity law,** which states: *Any combination of mA and time that produces an identical mAs will produce an identical density on film.* The reciprocity law will attain more significance as we continue to discuss radiographic technique variables. You will see that there are many times when adjusting either mA or exposure time upward or downward can be used to advantage to produce a more desirable radiograph. **Table 4-1** lists mAs values, which form a useful reference for the workplace.

The effect of kilovoltage on radiographic density is indirect. Although an increase in kVp results in increased density on the radiograph, it does so because more electrons of shorter wavelength and higher energy are produced at the target. Because more electrons are produced, kVp is regarded as a secondary quantitative factor in photon production. Remember, though, kVp is first and foremost a qualitative factor.

Unlike mAs, the relationship between kVp and density is not directly proportional. Doubling the kVp will not double the density on the processed radiograph. The chief effect of kVp is qualitative, that is, it controls the penetrating abilities of the primary beam.

There is, however, a rule of thumb to recall concerning kVp and density. A 15% increase in kVp will have the same effect as doubling the mAs on the radiograph. Conversely, decreasing kilovoltage by 15%

is equivalent to halving mAs. This is sometimes called the 50–15 rule, or the 15% rule. This guideline will become more important in the discussion on contrast.

A caveat to the rule of mAs governing density is: the kilovoltage used in conjunction with the selected mAs must be sufficient to penetrate the part being examined. No amount of mAs can compensate for inadequate kVp.

DISTANCE

The relationship between radiographic density and FFD (focal film distance) is governed by the **inverse square law,** which states: The intensity of the x-ray beam varies inversely with the square of the distance; where I = beam intensity, and D = FFD. In practice, however, changing FFD as a means of varying density is rarely done. Most FFDs are used by convention. For example, posterior–anterior and lateral (PAL) chest radiographs are performed at 72 degrees FFD, and bucky abdominal examinations are performed at 40 degrees. These distances are used in practice primarily because grid manufacturers design grids to be used at a given distance, and because FFD impacts radiographic magnification. But because every examination is not carried out in the standard manner, particularly with respect to trauma or surgical radiography, the radiographer must understand the impact of variable distance on density. Consider again the inverse square law. The equation for *exposure rate* can be stated:

$$\frac{I_1}{I_2} = \frac{D_2^2}{D_1^2} \quad (3)$$

Use this formula to determine exposure rate, as in this sample exercise:

A radiograph is made at 40 inches, which results in an exposure rate of 100 milliroentgen (mR) per minute. What is the new rate at 72 inches?

$$\frac{100}{X} = \frac{72_2^2}{40_1^2} \quad (4)$$

Substituting,

$$5184X = 160,000$$
$$X = 30.86\ mR/min$$

Note then that the primary concept is *exposure rate decreases as distance increases:* an inverse relationship. In practice, however, the inverse square law must be restated in order to find new mAs values when the FFD is changed. The formula is then stated:

$$\frac{I_1}{I_2} = \frac{D_1^2}{D_2^2} \quad (5)$$

▶ **TABLE 4-1.** mAs Values

Time (Decimal)	Time (Fraction)	25 mA	50 mA	100 mA	200 mA	300 mA	400 mA	500 mA	600 mA
0.00830	$\frac{1}{120}$	0.2075	0.4	0.83	1.66	2.49	3.32	4.15	4.98
0.01000	$\frac{1}{100}$	0.25	0.5	1	2	3	4	5	6
0.01600	$\frac{1}{62}$	0.4	0.8	1.6	3.2	4.8	6.4	8	9.6
0.02000	$\frac{1}{50}$	0.5	1.0	2	4	6	8	10	12
0.02500	$\frac{1}{40}$	0.625	1.3	2.5	5	7.5	10	12.5	15
0.03500	$\frac{2}{57}$	0.875	1.8	3.5	7	10.5	14	17.5	21
0.05000	$\frac{1}{20}$	1.25	2.5	5	10	15	20	25	30
0.06700	$\frac{1}{15}$	1.675	3.4	6.7	13.4	20.1	26.8	33.5	40.2
0.08300	$\frac{1}{12}$	2.075	4.2	8.3	16.6	24.9	33.2	41.5	49.8
0.01000	$\frac{1}{10}$	2.5	5.0	10	20	30	40	50	60
0.12500	$\frac{1}{8}$	3.125	6.3	12.5	25	37.5	50	62.5	75
0.13300	$\frac{2}{15}$	3.325	6.7	13.3	26.6	39.9	53.2	66.5	79.8
0.15000	$\frac{3}{20}$	3.75	7.5	15	30	45	60	75	90
0.16700	$\frac{1}{6}$	4.175	8.4	16.7	33.4	50.1	66.8	83.5	100.2
0.20000	$\frac{1}{5}$	5	10.0	20	40	60	80	100	120
0.25000	$\frac{1}{4}$	6.25	12.5	25	50	75	100	125	150
0.30000	$\frac{3}{10}$	7.5	15.0	30	60	90	120	150	180
0.40000	$\frac{2}{5}$	10	20.0	40	80	120	160	200	240
0.50000	$\frac{1}{2}$	12.5	25.0	50	100	150	200	250	300
0.66000	$\frac{33}{50}$	16.5	33.0	66	132	198	264	330	396
0.75000	$\frac{3}{4}$	18.75	37.5	75	150	225	300	375	450

This formula represents a direct relationship and is sometimes referred to as the **distance maintenance formula.**

Try this practical exercise. If an upright bucky cervical spine examination were to be carried out using 25 mAs at 40 inches, how many mAs would be required using 72 inches?

$$\frac{25}{x} = \frac{40^2}{72^2} \qquad (6)$$
$$1600X = 129,600$$
$$X = 81 \text{ mAs}$$

As distance is increased, mAs must be increased in order to maintain consistent density. Will you have time to make these computations in the workplace? Practically speaking, no. Instead, think in general terms. If the FFD is doubled, then four times the mAs is required to maintain density. Conversely, if FFD is halved, then one quarter the mAs is required to maintain the same density.

FILM SCREEN COMBINATIONS

The characteristics of both film and intensifying screens are important factors that affect radiographic density. Both are described in terms of **speed,** which can be defined as the ability of either film or intensifying screen to respond to x-ray exposure.

There are varied classifications of intensifying screens; in general, they may be described as either slow (detail), par (medium), or fast screens. The faster the screen, the less radiation is required to produce a given density. Rare earth screens, composed of such phosphors as gadolinium, lanthanum, and yttrium, are faster than the traditional calcium tungstate screens.

The same distinction may be made concerning film speed. The faster the film speed, the less radiation required to produce a given density.

Some manufacturers assign a numeric value to film or screens or the combination of both. This value is based on the mAs value required to produce a given exposure. For example, using a 100-speed system (film and screen), an exposure of 60 mAs at 80 kVp is required to produce an acceptable film. A 200-speed system would require only 30 mAs to produce the same density, a 300-speed system needs 15 mAs, and so on.

GRIDS

Grids are x-ray accessory devices constructed of alternating strips of lead foil and radiolucent filler material. Their purpose is to absorb secondary and scatter radiation (the Compton effect) produced by the patient before the x-ray photons reach the film. The lead strips are aligned in the same direction as the primary beam, and the interspace material permits passage of the "cleaned up" beam. Grids may be either stationary or moving.

Use of a grid is recommended when body parts that are 10 to 13 cm or larger are examined; techniques required to penetrate body parts of this thickness produce enough scatter radiation to significantly detract from image quality. Chest radiography represents a significant exception to this rule. Because the chest is composed primarily of air, less scatter radiation is produced than with other body parts of similar thickness. Therefore, chest radiography may be performed using a nongrid technique.

Note that many radiologists prefer high kilovoltage grid technique over that of screen radiography, and many facilities use grid chests in their standard protocol.

Scatter radiation is responsible for as much as 50% of radiographic density. Using a grid reduces the actual number of photons reaching the film or image receptor, therefore reducing radiographic density. In order to maintain density when using a grid, a significant increase in mAs is required. The specifics of grid compensation technique will be discussed later in this chapter.

FILTRATION

Recall that the purpose of filtration is to reduce low-energy wavelengths emerging from the tube, thus increasing the overall average beam intensity. Filtration may be inherent (tube housing, coolant) or added (aluminum strips). However, any material that attenuates the primary beam reduces radiographic density.

The reduction in density caused by standard inherent and added filtration is not visibly appreciable. There are, however, specialized compensating filters such as wedge and trough filters whose purpose is to reduce density on a specific area of the radiograph. A common example of this filter type is the compensating filter used in conjunction with scoliosis radiography, where density at the proximal end of the radiograph is much less than at the distal end. Using the filter produces a radiograph with consistent density on the entire film.

A common wedge filter is used for foot radiography, where the proximal tarsal end of the body part is much thicker than the thinner toe end. Trough filters, which are thick at the ends and thin in the middle,

are used to visualize the thicker, mediastinal portion of the chest without overexposure of the lung parenchyma.

BEAM RESTRICTION

Beam restriction devices such as collimators, cones, and aperture diaphragms reduce the volume of irradiated tissue, causing reduction in density on the finished radiograph. A tightly collimated radiograph will require a compensatory increase in mAs. There is no specific guideline concerning this compensation; experience is the best teacher. In general, the increase is small.

Of course, the reverse is also true. As field size increases, more scatter radiation is produced, which increases film density. Beam size should never exceed film or receptor borders. A visibly collimated border should appear on all films whenever feasible.

ANATOMIC AND PATHOLOGIC FACTORS

Selection of density-related technical factors is dependent on tissue thickness and composition. Pathologic conditions may alter distribution of density in a given part, and technical adjustments must be made in order to maintain consistent density.

For example, elderly women are statistically likely to have osteoporosis, a demineralizing condition of the bone. In this case, technique must be adjusted downward from standard exposure factors; otherwise, the finished radiograph will be overexposed—demineralized bone attenuates less radiation than does normal bone. Another very common clinical situation is that of the intensive care patient who has pneumonia or another space-occupying infiltrate. Because these patients generally have daily portable chest films ordered, it is imperative that the radiographer realize and make technical adjustment for the clinical condition of these patients. The presence of high-density fluid in the thorax requires an upward adjustment in technique in order to produce a diagnostic film. Patients who have advanced disease may require quite a dramatic increase.

Similarly, makeup of tissue is altered by normal biologic factors, such as age, sex, body type, and level of activity. A young, healthy athletic male will possess much denser tissue and require much higher levels of exposure than an elderly woman, even though they may be similar in terms of tissue thickness.

TABLE 4-2. Density Factor Relationships

Factor Increased	Effect on Density
mAs	Increase
kVp	Increase
FFD	Decrease
Part thickness	Decrease
Pathologic condition	Variable, according to condition
Developer time	Increase
Density setting on AEC	Increase
Beam restriction	Decrease
Grid ratio	Decrease

mAs = milliampere-seconds; kUp = kilovolt peak; FFD = focal film distance; AEC = automatic exposure control.

DENSITY FACTOR RELATIONSHIPS

The effects of various factors on film density are presented in **Table 4-2.**

ANODE HEEL EFFECT

The variance in density along the longitudinal axis of the tube is known as the anode heel effect. Photons traveling toward the cathode end of the tube encounter less target material; therefore, the density produced at the cathode end of the tube is greater than that of the anode end **(Figure 4-1)**.

The heel effect may be used to advantage during

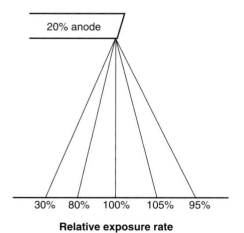

FIGURE 4-1. The anode heel effect. Note that exposure intensity is greatest at the cathode end.

radiography of long body parts with wide tissue variance, most prominently, the femur and thoracic spine. The heel effect is most pronounced using a short target film distance (TFD), steep target angle (small focal spot), and large film area.

QUESTIONS FOR DENSITY

select the best answer

1. Which of the following conditions requires a downward adjustment from routine exposure factors in order to maintain proper density on the finished radiograph?
   1. Emphysema
   2. Congestive heart failure
   3. Osteoporosis
   (A) All of the aforementioned
   (B) None of the aforementioned
   (C) Choices 2 and 3
   (D) Choices 1 and 3

2. Consider the following set of exposure factors: (a) 400 mA, 0.25 seconds; (b) 200 mA, 0.50 seconds; (c) 100 mA, 1 sec. With all other factors remaining constant, all three combinations will produce identical radiographic density, illustrating the principle of:
   (A) inverse square law.
   (B) reciprocity.
   (C) resolution.
   (D) geometric unsharpness.

3. The inverse square law states that if a given set of exposure factors is used at 36 inches TFD, then the radiographer must _____ in order to maintain density at 72 inches?
   (A) Double the mAs
   (B) Halve the mAs
   (C) Use 4 × the mAs
   (D) Increase the kVp 15%

4. Which of the following combinations of elements is used in the construction of a typical grid?
   (A) Lead strips and aluminum interspace
   (B) Aluminum strips and lead interspace
   (C) Plastic strips and aluminum interspace material
   (D) Aluminum strips and plastic interspace material

5. Which of the following factors make the anode heel effect less noticeable?

   1. Short FFD
   2. Large film area exposed
   3. Small focal spot

   (A) Choice 2 only
   (B) Choices 1 and 2
   (C) Choice 3 only
   (D) Choice 1 only

6. An extremely thin woman comes to the radiology department for PAL chest examination. When positioning her, you collimate the light field several inches on either side of a 14 × 17 cassette. The proper technique for compensation would be:

   (A) increase the kVp.
   (B) decrease the kVp.
   (C) increase the mAs.
   (D) decrease the mAs.

7. A trough filter is used in conjunction with which type of radiography?

   (A) Scoliosis survey
   (B) PA chest with emphasis on mediastinum
   (C) Mammography
   (D) Long bone survey

8. As intensifying screen speed increases, density:

   (A) increases.
   (B) decreases.
   (C) is unchanged.
   (D) becomes unpredictable.

▶▶▶ **ANSWERS TO DENSITY**

1. The answer is (D). Congestive heart failure (CHF) is a condition characterized by abnormal accumulation of fluid in the chest. The presence of CHF necessitates increasing technique to ensure adequate penetration. Emphysema is abnormal alveolar distention with air, and osteoporosis is demineralization of bone tissue. Both are conditions that require downward adjustment in technique in order to maintain optimum density.

2. The answer is (B). The product of mA and time (s) is mAs. Either variable may be changed, and density will be maintained as long as the product of the two variables is the same. This principle is known as the reciprocity law. In the problem, the three listed examples are differing combinations equaling 100 mAs, and all three will produce identical density on film. Strictly speaking, the reciprocity law applies only to direct exposure radiography, because exposures using intensifying

screens may demonstrate a comparative loss of density when exposure times are exceedingly long. In actual practice, however, this tendency is compensated for with the characteristics of film emulsion, so the radiographer may regard all mAs combinations as reliable.

3. The answer is (C). An x-ray beam diminishes in intensity as it moves farther from the source. Using the distance maintenance restatement of the inverse square law, the radiographer finds that when distance is doubled, then mAs must be increased by a factor of 4 in order to maintain density. For example, if 10 mAs were used as the original technique in this example, then the solution could be found by:

$$\frac{10^2}{X} = \frac{36^2}{72^2} \qquad (7)$$

$$1296X = 51,840$$
$$X = 40 \text{ mAs}$$

4. The answer is (A). A grid is constructed of alternate lead strips and radiolucent interspace material. The lead strips attenuate scatter radiation before it reaches the film, and the radiolucent interspace material is plastic or aluminum. Some older grids used cardboard as the interspace material; however, it was discovered that cardboard was adversely affected by humidity.

5. The answer is (D). The x-ray beam is most uniform nearest the central portion of the beam; therefore, the anode heel effect is least discernible when a large FFD, small field size, and large focal spot are used.

6. The answer is (C). Decreasing the volume of irradiated tissue reduces production of scatter radiation. Consequently, less density is produced on film. The proper compensation to increase density is an increase in mAs.

7. The answer is (B). The trough filter is a type of compensating filter that is thin in the central portion and thicker on the ends. It is used for chest radiography to penetrate the mediastinum without overpenetrating the lung and pulmonary markings.

8. The answer is (A). Screen speed is a measure of light emission from screen phosphors. The faster the screen, the more light is produced and the higher will be the density on the finished radiograph.

B. Contrast

Contrast may be broadly defined as the variation in density present on the radiograph. There are three important interrelated types of contrast for the radiologic technologist to consider. First, **radiologic contrast** refers to the difference in density between adjacent structures on the radiograph. **Scale of contrast** refers to the range of optical densities from lightest to darkest present on the radiograph. This contrast type may either be **short scale,** with dramatic differences from black to white, or **long scale,** with a gradually changing array of densities on the film.

Short-scale contrast is associated with high mAs and low kVp technique, whereas long-scale contrast is associated with high kVp and low mAs technique. The longer the scale of contrast, the wider the range of densities that may be radiographically evident. The ability of film to respond to exposure by reproducing a wide range of density is called **exposure latitude.**

Second, the measure of x-ray intensity transmitted through one part of anatomy on a given radiograph compared with that of a more attenuating or less attenuating adjacent structure on the radiograph is known as **subject contrast.**

Try this experiment to demonstrate the concept: suppose you were to make an exposure of two objects having the same thickness, but of dissimilar atomic numbers, for example, a 1-inch stack of bandages and a 1-inch stack of coins. What happens? Of course, there is a dramatic difference in contrast on the radiograph, with the coins appearing almost white, and the bandages very dark—a very short scale of contrast. The difference occurs because the coins have a much higher atomic number than do the bandages; or put another way, the contrast difference appears because of the difference in density *inherent in the subjects.*

Atomic number of the body part being examined and quality of radiation as determined by kilovoltage, filtration, target material, and collimation all affect subject contrast.

Last, the contrast inherent in radiographic film is referred to as **film contrast.** There are many types of film, each with design parameters intended to perform a certain type of function. For example, a film designed for short-scale, high-contrast bone work will be vastly different from that of a typically wide-exposure latitude, long-scale film used for portable radiography.

Obviously, the technologist cannot control film contrast—each film's characteristics are inherent. But awareness of a given film's contrast attributes is vital, especially because most departments use a variety of film for a variety of tasks. Remember, too, that outside influences such as processing stability, fog level, and sources of radiation also have an impact on film contrast.

Radiologic contrast is the sum of film contrast and subject contrast.

KILOVOLTAGE PEAK (KVP)

Kilovoltage is the primary controlling factor of radiographic contrast. As kVp is increased, more body tissue is penetrated, and therefore a wider variety of densities is recorded on film. When there are many shades of gray present on the image, there is less difference from one shade of gray to the next; therefore, contrast is reduced. The more shades of gray demonstrated, the longer the scale of contrast. A longer scale of contrast is sometimes referred to as an increased **gray scale.**

In the range of kilovoltage associated with diagnostic radiology, which can be approximately defined as the range from 50 to 140 kVp, the photoelectric effect (photon absorbed) and the Compton effect (scatter radiation) are the primary x-ray interactions with matter. Scatter radiation diminishes radiographic contrast, because it does not affect the entire image uniformly. Scatter radiation has a greater effect on the whiter areas of the radiograph than the darker areas, because some exposed areas have reached their blackness potential, and cannot get darker, irrespective of kilovoltage used. Above 80 kVp, the Compton effect is the primary x-ray interaction, which reduces short-scale contrast. Therefore, the higher the kilovoltage used, the longer the scale of contrast.

BEAM RESTRICTION

Beam restriction, whether with collimation or with devices such as cones or diaphragms, restricts the area of tissue interaction. Decreasing field size decreases scatter radiation production, producing a shorter scale of contrast. A skilled technologist can dramatically improve radiographic contrast with the conscientious application of collimation.

GRIDS

The purpose of a grid is to decrease the amount of scatter radiation reaching the film, thereby increasing radiographic contrast. A grid's scatter radiation reduction capability is dependent on grid ratio and number of lines per inch. Grids will be discussed in greater detail later in this chapter.

FILTRATION

Modern x-ray units are generally equipped with 2.5-mm aluminum (Al) equivalent filtration, consisting of 1.5-mm inherent filtration from the glass envelope and collimator, and an additional 1-mm added filtration. Radiographic tubes operated above 70 kVp must have at least 2.5-mm Al equivalent, according to National Council for Radiation Protection and Measurements regulations.

Standard filtration hardens the x-ray beam by eliminating low-energy photons that would otherwise reach the patient, but photons of this energy level do not have sufficient energy to reach the image receptor. Therefore, filtration has no significant effect on radiographic contrast. Compensating filters such as wedge or trough filters primarily have an impact on image density, not contrast.

ANATOMIC AND PATHOLOGIC FACTORS

The body is composed of a variety of tissue types and thicknesses. The attenuation properties of the part under examination have a dramatic effect on radiographic contrast. Structures with high atomic numbers—bone, for example—tend to produce high contrast, whereas an area like the abdomen is comprised primarily of soft-tissue organ structures, with comparatively low atomic numbers that produce low contrast. The radiographer must consider these factors when selecting technique, using a kilovoltage range that is appropriate for the part under examination.

Pathologic conditions have a similar effect on contrast. Consider, for example, two common but quite different conditions of the bone: osteoarthritis and osteoporosis. Patients who have arthritis develop dense osteophyte formations that increase contrast, whereas patients who have osteoporosis, usually women, have demineralized bone, a condition that lowers radiographic contrast.

QUESTIONS FOR CONTRAST

select the best answer

1. Using the same type film for all exposures, which of the following techniques will produce the longest scale of contrast?

   (A) 20 mAs, 80 kVp
   (B) 40 mAs, 70 kVp
   (C) 80 mAs, 60 kVp
   (D) 160 mAs, 50 kVp

2. Scatter radiation _____ radiographic contrast; and its impact may be affected by the use of _____

   (A) increases, collimator
   (B) decreases, filter
   (C) increases, cone
   (D) decreases, grid

3. What adjustment of technical factors would a patient who has ascites (an abnormal accumulation of intraperitoneal fluid containing protein and electrolytes) require?

   (A) Increase mAs
   (B) Decrease FFD
   (C) Increase kVp
   (D) Increase filtration

4. The purpose of filtration relative to contrast is:

   (A) filtration lengthens the scale of contrast.
   (B) filtration shortens the scale of contrast.
   (C) filtration reduces low-energy photons to ensure adequate contrast.
   (D) filtration is unrelated to contrast.

5. Two chest radiographs of a small patient are made. Radiograph number 1 is collimated to 14 × 17. Radiograph number 2 is collimated so that it demonstrates a 2-inch border around the edge of the film. Which of the following statements is true concerning the comparison between the two radiographs?

   (A) Radiograph number 1 demonstrates higher contrast than radiograph number 2.
   (B) Radiograph number 2 demonstrates higher contrast than radiograph number 1.
   (C) The two radiographs will produce equal scales of contrast.
   (D) Not enough information is provided to answer the question.

▶▶ ANSWERS TO CONTRAST

1. The answer is (A). Long-scale contrast is associated with low mAs, high kVp technique. Strictly speaking, all of the listed techniques would produce the same film density, but with a progressively shorter scale of contrast as mAs increases and kVp decreases.

2. The answer is (D). Scatter radiation decreases radiographic contrast, primarily affecting the whiter areas of the film, because the black portions have already reached maximum density potential. The effect of scatter radiation on film may be decreased by the use of grids, which clean up scatter radiation created by the patient before it reaches the film.

3. The answer is (C). In order to properly penetrate

the abdomen and produce a diagnostic film, a patient who has ascites would require an increase in kVp. Increasing kVp as the sole factor of technical adjustment will lengthen the scale of contrast.

4. The answer is (D). Standard filtration hardens the x-ray beam by eliminating low-energy photons that would otherwise reach the patient, but photons of this energy level do not have sufficient energy to reach the image receptor. Therefore, filtration has no significant effect on radiographic contrast.

5. The answer is (B). Decreasing field size decreases scatter radiation production, which produces a shorter scale of contrast. A skilled technologist can dramatically improve radiographic contrast with the conscientious application of collimation.

C. Recorded Detail

Recorded **detail** may be defined as the amount of visual **clarity** or **resolution** on the processed radiograph. Recall that resolution may be measured by means of a resolution test pattern, and is expressed in line pairs per millimeter (1lp/mm). There are a variety of test patterns available. The test device consists of lines or patterns of lines, which when exposed are demonstrated on the radiograph. The film is examined, and the number of discrete line pairs, that is, the number of pairs that are observed individually, and not blended into one, is recorded.

When evaluating a radiograph for recorded detail, the technologist must consider two important factors. The first factor is **image sharpness,** which refers to the visibility of structural borders of the part being examined. Lack of image sharpness is sometimes referred to as **penumbra.** Factors that control image sharpness are called **geometric factors,** and include focal spot size, object-to-image receptor distance (OID), source-to-image receptor distance (SID), patient motion, and intensifying screen speed. The second important factor is **visibility of detail,** which describes the ability to visually determine detail on the radiograph. Detail visibility is described in terms of factors that detract from it. For example, film fog resulting from light or radiation exposure as well as excess scatter radiation degrade image detail, and are therefore factors in determining visibility of detail. Devices that improve visibility of detail are those that promote scatter radiation reduction, that is, grids and beam restriction devices such as collimators and cones.

Distortion is the misrepresentation of image size by **magnification, shape, elongation,** or **foreshortening.** The primary causes of distortion are improper tube-part-image receptor alignment, or inherent object distortion.

OBJECT-TO-IMAGE RECEPTOR DISTANCE (OID)

OID, also known as **OFD** (object-film distance) is a term that describes the location of the part being examined in relation to the image receptor or film. To demonstrate this concept, consider the example of a hand placed 4 inches from the x-ray cassette. Turn on the x-ray illuminator on the tube head. What happens? The light projects a shadow on the cassette larger in size than that of the true size of the hand. In this instance, the x-ray beam has a similar effect on the developed image. Like light, as the x-ray beam travels from its source, it is divergent. The divergent beam strikes the hand and continues to diverge until depositing the image on film. The image now demonstrates magnification and unsharpness. Therefore, the rule is, as OID increases, magnification increases, and recorded detail decreases.

X-ray examinations performed using the bucky tray also demonstrate some degree of magnification, because the distance between the tabletop and bucky tray increases OID. Depending on the manufacturer, tabletop/bucky tray distance varies between 6 and 13 cm. The radiographer can minimize the magnification effect caused by fixed OID by positioning the part being examined as closely as possible to the image receptor. For example, an orbit examination performed in the supine position places the orbits approximately 20 cm from the tabletop. Taken in conjunction with the tabletop/bucky tray distance, such an examination may result in magnification of the orbits of up to 50%. Performing the same examination in the prone position reduces the magnification to only 10%, by placing the orbits closer to the image receptor. As you will see, increasing SID and using the smallest allowable focal spot as determined by heat loading capacity also decrease the effects of increased OID.

SOURCE-TO-IMAGE RECEPTOR DISTANCE (TFD AND FFD)

The effect of **SID** on detail can also be demonstrated using the previous example. For the sake of demonstration, turn on the x-ray illumination with the hand again placed 4 inches from the cassette. What happens when you move the illumination closer to the hand? The image becomes more magnified and less distinct. Conversely, if we move the light farther away, the projected shadow becomes less magnified and more distinct. The effect of SID on detail is the same. Like the previous example, x-ray behaves similarly to light. Therefore, as SID (also called focal film distance [FFD] and target film distance [TFD]) increases, recorded detail increases, and magnification decreases. Practical application of this concept is especially useful when performing examinations in the nonstandard mode, such as that encountered during portable, surgical, or trauma radiography, when the examination is tailored in order to suit the limitations of the environment.

FOCAL SPOT SIZE

Just as density is controlled *primarily* by mAs, and contrast is controlled *primarily* by kVp, focal spot size is considered the principal determinant for radiographic detail. If the x-ray beam were to originate from a point source, detail would be recorded with remarkable clarity, assuming that all other factors, such as tube part alignment and appropriate technique, were correct. In actuality, however, no source point of radiation exists. Instead, the x-ray beam is emitted from a square or rectangular area that varies

in size from approximately 0.3 to 2 mm on a side, which is called the **focal spot.** Because the ideal situation in terms of recorded detail would be a single point source, it makes sense that the smaller the focal spot, the better the recorded detail. Put another way, recall that increasing focal spot size increases geometric unsharpness and decreases detail.

Because the x-ray beam does not originate from a point source, a blurred area called **penumbra** results on the radiograph. Obviously, penumbra is undesirable, because it reduces detail. **Figure 4-2** demonstrates how focal spot size affects penumbra.

The substantive area of the anode bombarded by electrons is called the **actual focal spot,** whereas the **effective focal spot** is the size of the focused area as it would be viewed from the film's perspective, looking up toward the emerging x-ray beam.

The single greatest obstacle to use of small focal spots is heat buildup. When the small focal spot is selected at the control panel, electron bombardment is directed to a smaller area of the target than when using a large focal spot. If heat is delivered in sufficient quantity over a short enough period of time, localized melting of the target or anode pitting and cracking may occur, which will shorten tube life span. The smaller the focal spot, the greater the heat units produced, whereas the larger the focal spot, the greater

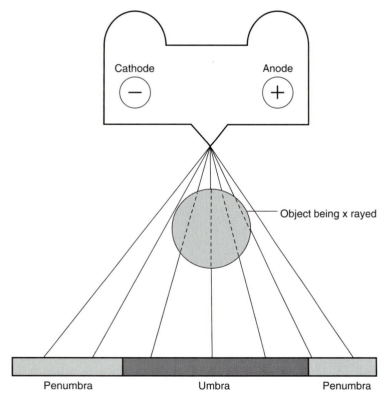

FIGURE 4-2. Penumbra is geometric unsharpness on the radiograph. In this instance, penumbra is the result of the measurable size of the focal spot. Note that penumbra is greater at the cathode end.

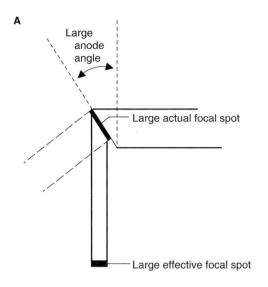

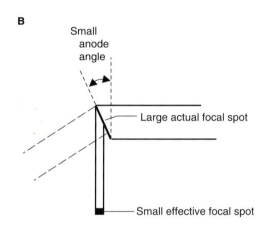

FIGURE 4-3. *View A* demonstrates large anode angle, with both large effective and actual focal spots. *View B* demonstrates how decreasing anode angle can maintain a large actual focal spot to facilitate heat dissipation while yielding a comparatively small effective focal spot to optimize detail.

the area for heat dissipation, and the less likely tube cooling overload will occur. The optimum situation is to use the smallest focal spot possible without risking tube damage from exceeding tube cooling limits.

To some degree, the dilemma posed by heat unit buildup in conjunction with small focal spots can be overcome by decreasing the angle of the anode. Decreasing the anode angle maintains a large actual focal spot while decreasing the effective focal spot **(Figure 4-3).** X-ray tubes that are designed in this way are known as **fractional x-ray tubes,** because effective focal spot is a fraction of the size of the actual focal spot. Fractional x-ray tubes have target angles that

range from 7 to 10 degrees, and demonstrate improved recorded detail over that of conventional tubes, without endangering the x-ray tube by exceeding anode heat tolerance.

Unfortunately, decreasing target angle also accentuates the anode heel effect. For example, a typical exposure made using a 40-degree FFD and a 14 × 17 image receptor will demonstrate a 2-inch border of unexposed film on the anode end of the radiograph. Compensation for the anode heel effect may be made by increasing FFD, but remember, increasing FFD also requires increasing technical factors in order to maintain adequate density and increases patient dose.

FILM-SCREEN COMBINATIONS

The characteristics of intensifying screens and film type have a profound impact on recorded detail. It would be impractical to discuss all the variants relative to intensifying screens and film by manufacturer, because there are literally hundreds of film and screen types, each with their own unique set of traits. There are, however, fundamental categories of characteristics relating to both film and screens that the radiographic technologist must understand.

A film's sensitivity to light is known as its **spectral response.** This is important to realize, because both film and screen type may be categorized according to the type of light they are sensitive to. Old-style calcium tungstate screens emit blue-violet light, and are only properly matched with standard blue-violet light–sensitive silver halide film. On the other hand, rare earth screens are generally coupled with green light–sensitive film, but can be matched with film that is sensitive to both blue-violet and green light. The correct combination of light sensitivity in a film-screen system is known as **spectral matching.**

Spectral matching is especially important in radiology departments that use more than one screen type. An improper spectral match will result in decreased image density and detail due to decreased screen speed. If the technologist is not aware of the underlying cause of decreased density, he or she may increase technique to compensate, thus needlessly exposing the patient not only to a repeat exposure, but also to one that results in a higher dose.

Precautions in the darkroom are important as well. Blue light–sensitive film is used with an amber safe light, which emits light wavelengths above its spectral response. However, amber light will fog green light–sensitive film, and so a red safe light, which emits light of an even longer wavelength than amber, is used instead. Red safe lights may also be used with blue light–sensitive film.

Screen film, that is, film that is designed for use in conjunction with intensifying screens, is by far the most commonly employed film for diagnostic radiology. A film's sensitivity, or **speed,** is a factor of its emulsion thickness. The thicker the emulsion, the faster the film; but thicker film emulsions and larger silver crystals produce images of less detail than film with thinner emulsions. When screen film combinations are considered as a whole, however, the impact of the intensifying screen has a much greater influence on recorded detail than does the film. Most screen film is coated with silver halide containing emulsion on both sides, which provides twice the speed of a single-emulsion film, even if the single-emulsion film were to be made twice as thick.

Another related problem associated with faster film speed relative to recorded detail is **quantum mottle.** As speed of the system increases, the mAs required for some exposures decreases dramatically. In some cases, the exposure is so minimal that not enough photons are produced to adequately expose the image, which results in the grainy appearance known as quantum mottle.

As previously mentioned, intensifying screens enhance the action of x-ray photons by producing light when exposed. The light produced is either blue-violet or green, depending on the type of **phosphor** used in manufacturing the screen. Approximately 98% of the image-producing energy that exposes the film emulsion comes from light, with only a small percentage of x-ray energy contributing to forming the latent (unprocessed) image.

The manufacturing process for intensifying screens involves grinding the phosphor material into fine powder that is mixed with a binding substance. This mixture is then spread onto a durable plastic layer, and the resulting product is known as the **active layer.** The thicker the active layer is made, the faster the screen speed. Hence, with a thick active layer, less intensive exposure factors are required to produce a given exposure, but less detail is recorded on film.

The ability of a given phosphor to convert x-ray energy into light is known as its **conversion factor.** The greater the conversion factor, the greater the speed of the screen. Phosphors possessing higher atomic numbers, such as rare earth elements, have higher conversion factors than do phosphors with comparatively low atomic numbers, such as calcium tungstate. Similarly, screen speed and size of the phosphor used are directly related. As phosphor size increases, so does screen speed.

The ability of the screen's reflective backing to di-

▶ **TABLE 4-3.** Factors That Affect Screen Speed and Detail

When these factors increase:	Speed is . . .	Detail is . . .
Phosphor size	Increased	Decreased
Phosphor sensitivity	Increased	Decreased
Active layer thickness	Increased	Decreased
Reflectivity of backing	Increased	Decreased
Conversion efficiency	Increased	Decreased

rect light toward the film emulsion is a function of screen speed. The more light reflected, the greater the screen speed.

Loss of recorded detail occurs as the degree of light **diffusion** (spreading over a comparatively larger area) increases. Remember, thicker emulsions are used to increase screen speed. But as emulsions grow progressively thicker, the film emulsion is exposed by light that is progressively farther from it. As distance increases, so does light diffusion. **Table 4-3** presents factors that affect screen speed and detail.

Recorded detail also decreases when improper **screen film contact** occurs. Poor screen film contact may result from warped or damaged screens or cassettes, and also from foreign bodies present inside the cassette. Poor contact permits greater light diffusion; consequently, detail decreases (blurring increases). Larger cassettes are more likely to have poor screen contact.

Screens should be periodically evaluated for proper contact by using the wire mesh. To perform the test, a cassette is placed on the x-ray tabletop and the wire mesh device rests on top of the cassette. A typical extremity type exposure is then made, and the developed film examined. Blurred areas on the film demonstrate areas of poor screen contact. These screens should either be discarded or sent for repair.

MOTION

Motion of either the patient or the x-ray equipment itself during the exposure appears as image blurring on the radiograph; therefore, motion significantly degrades recorded detail. Motion is categorized as **voluntary** or **involuntary.**

Voluntary motion is movement by the patient of the part under examination during the exposure. Generally speaking, this type of motion does not represent a deliberate effort on the patient's part to make the examination difficult; rather, it can usually be attributed to poor instructions to the patient from the technologist. In order to reduce voluntary motion, then, clear instructions must be given to the patient concerning suspended respiration and movement. If patients understand their responsibilities, they will almost always comply. After all, they are in your care in order to get well. Involuntary motion consists of actions that are beyond the control of either the technologist or the patient, and include the motion of the beating heart; peristaltic action, as with the esophagus or small bowel; or muscle spasms. The single best method to reduce the effects of involuntary motion is the use of the shortest possible exposure times. With relatively small parts such as extremities, it's easy to attain short exposure times simply by using the highest possible mA station in conjunction with a short exposure. The situation is more difficult with larger body parts, however, because heat loading concerns come into play.

A typical abdominal examination, for example, may use 300 mA, 0.5 sec, and 70 kVp. Increasing technique to 600 mA would reduce exposure time to 0.25 second; however, these factors may exceed the heat loading capacities for one-time exposure on a given machine, depending on the design of the unit. One could also raise the kVp by 15% in this example, but this technique revision would lengthen scale of contrast.

Many physicians feel that abdominal radiography technique should not exceed 70 kVp, because higher kVp technique lengthens the scale of contrast, making visualization of kidney and ureteral stones difficult. In addition, optimum opacification of iodinated contrast material, as is used with excretory urography, occurs in the range of 60 to 70 kVp, and should therefore not be exceeded, or else the effect of the contrast agent will be minimized.

Motion of the x-ray equipment, as when the tube head is accidentally bumped just before exposure, will also produce motion artifact and therefore should also be eliminated.

Occasionally, motion is used deliberately in order to blur certain incidental structures and delineate important ones. For example, the rib and lung markings often obscure clear visualization of the thoracic spine in the lateral position. In order to offset the effects of these unwanted structures, a technique is used whereby a low mA (usually 25 or 50 mA), a low kVp (usually 60 to 70 kVp), and a long exposure time, together with instructing the patient to maintain slow, even breathing during the exposure, are used. With this technique, the patient's breathing over the course of the relatively long exposure time will blur the lung parenchyma and ribs, while clearly visualizing the spine.

QUESTIONS FOR RECORDED DETAIL

select the best answer

1. If all other exposure factors are stable, then of the following factors, which is MOST important concerning recorded detail?
   (A) Grid ratio
   (B) Exposure time
   (C) Screen speed
   (D) kVp

2. The effect of TFD on recorded detail can be best described by which of the following statements?
   (A) TFD has no effect on detail.
   (B) Increased TFD increases detail.
   (C) Decreased TFD increases detail.
   (D) A 40-inch TFD is the optimum TFD for diagnostic radiography.

3. In order to produce a radiograph of greatest detail, the kidneys should be examined in which of the following positions?
   (A) Anteroposterior (AP)
   (B) Posteroanterior (PA)
   (C) Lateral
   (D) Left posterior oblique

4. A fractional x-ray tube achieves an improvement in recorded detail by:
   (A) increasing anode angle.
   (B) decreasing anode angle.
   (C) increasing heel effect.
   (D) using fractional exposure times.

5. The single best method the technologist can use to decrease voluntary motion is:
   (A) short exposure times.
   (B) long exposure times.
   (C) good communication.
   (D) fast screens.

▶▶ ANSWERS TO RECORDED DETAIL

1. The answer is (C). All of the factors listed have the potential to have an impact on detail; improper grid ratio, exposure time, and kVp would primarily affect density and scale of contrast. However, screen speed is directly related to

recorded detail: as screen speed increases, detail decreases.

2. The answer is (C). As TFD increases, the body part under examination is exposed to less divergent, more perpendicular rays, which results in decreased penumbral blurring and magnification. Using TFD as a controlling factor in detail is impractical, however, for two primary reasons: first, increasing TFD also requires an increase in exposure factors, resulting in increased patient dose; second, many grids have an optimal focusing distance, and exceeding this distance results in unwanted grid cutoff.

3. The answer is (A). Recorded detail is greatest using the least object-film distance. In this example, you were asked to produce a hypothetical kidney radiograph; therefore, you must determine which of the listed positions places the kidneys closest to the film (has the least OFD). Because the kidneys are located posteriorly, the AP projection places them closest to the film and is therefore best in terms of detail.

4. The answer is (A). A fractional x-ray tube is one that uses a comparatively steep target angle of 7 to 10 degrees, which increases detail by reduction of effective focal spot, while maintaining a fairly large actual focal spot. The small effective focal spot reduces penumbra, whereas the large focal spot permits greater heat loading. A negative factor associated with such tubes is an increase in the anode heel effect, and associated decrease in film coverage ability.

5. The answer is (C). Although using short exposure times and fast screens will reduce the likelihood of involuntary motion producing motion artifact, clear, concise patient instruction is the most important factor in the technologist's ability to reduce voluntary motion.

D. Distortion

Distortion is defined as a misrepresentation of the actual appearance of the object being radiographed. The object may have a disproportionate appearance in either **size** or **shape.**

An object whose size is distorted is said to be **magnified.** Magnification occurs as a result of increased object-to-image-receptor distance (OID, OFD) and source-to-image-receptor distance (SID, TFD). The relationship between object distance and magnification is direct; that is, as OID increases, magnification increases. However, the relationship between SID and magnification is inverse: as distance from the source to the image receptor increases, magnification decreases. In general, thick objects are magnified, and thin objects are not, because with a thick object the OID changes considerably across the object.

Distortion of shape may be further classified as image **elongation** or **foreshortening.** The effects of tube-part-film alignment on distortion are complex, and must be discussed individually. Elongation and foreshortening occur when the plane of the object and the plane of the image are not parallel. Inclining a tubular, flattened, or wedge-shaped object at a steeper angle in relation to the film while maintaining beam and film alignment will result in a foreshortened image, whereas inclining the same type of object and angling the tube so as to place the beam perpendicular to the long axis of the object will produce an elongated image **(Figure 4-4).** The same sort of distortion will occur if the x-ray tube is angled improperly relative to the object plane. Spherical and cubical objects have no identifiable long axis; therefore, their orientation in relation to the film is unimportant.

One method of minimizing the effects of foreshortening and elongation is utilization of **Ceiszynski's law of isometry,** which states that if a specialized angle equal to one half of the angle formed by the part and the film is used for tube angulation, then distortion will be eliminated or greatly minimized. This type of angle is known as an **isometric angle.** Ceiszynski's law can be demonstrated clearly using the AP projection of the sacrum as an example. In the standard AP position, the patient lies supine on the table, with the sacrum forming an angle of 30 to 35 degrees to the film. If a 15-degree cephalic tube angulation is used, however, geometric distortion of the sacrum will be nearly eliminated.

Shape distortion is unavoidable to some degree, because the position and shape of various body parts are the direct cause of some object unsharpness. This **inherent geometric unsharpness** occurs when the corporate body part under examination contains components that lie in different planes.

For example, an intravenous urogram (IVU, IVP) examines three key components: kidneys, ureters, and bladder. These components are contained within the framework of a standard abdominal film, and enhanced with iodinated contrast. However, these three parts lie in slightly different planes: the ureters are anterior to the kidneys, and the upper poles of the kidneys are more posterior than the lower. The position and shape of the urinary bladder are influenced by age, sex, and degree of distention. Generally speaking, in male patients the urinary bladder is anterior to the rectum, whereas in female patients the cervix

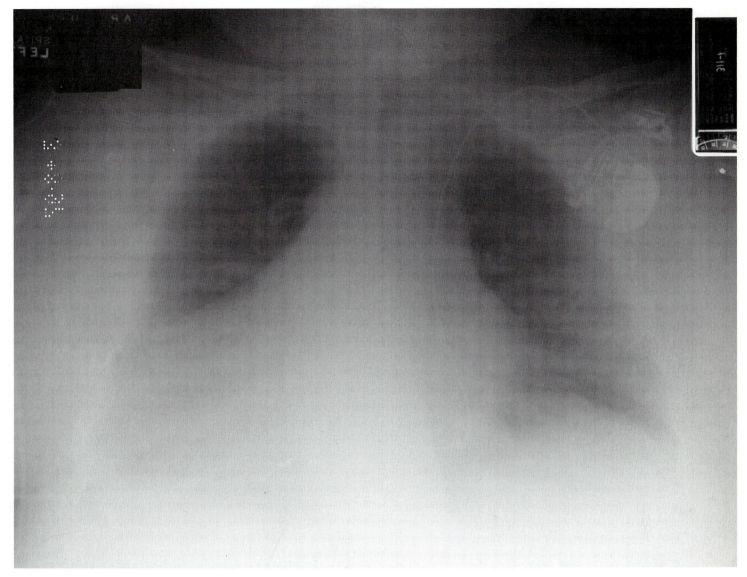

FIGURE 4-4. Upright portable AP chest examination demonstrates elongation, particularly noticeable in ribs. Note upward projection of clavicles due to improper cephalic angulation of tube.

and vagina intervene between the urinary bladder and the intestine. Because these structures must all be parallel to the x-ray tube and the image receptor in order to be accurately recorded, some distortion of the recorded image will occur. The shape of any structure placed at an angle in the body relative to the central ray (CR) will also be distorted on the film. In addition, when the edges of the object lie outside the axis of the divergent beam, blurring will occur, along with changes in optical density that relate to thickness of the part.

Alignment of the object to the CR and image receptor is critical. If any of three components are im-properly aligned, then shape distortion (foreshorten-ing, elongation) will occur. Distortion associated with tube, receptor, and object alignment is of particular concern during trauma and portable radiography ex-aminations, when nonstandard use of distance, tube placement, and film placement is required in order to obtain an image. It is relatively common for shape distortion to play an important role in radiography of fractures, where two views at right angles must be obtained in order to determine fracture alignment. The technologist must pay particular attention to tube-part-film alignment in order to produce a radio-graph as free of distortion as possible; otherwise, the degree of malalignment of the fracture could be misrepresented.

Distortion may also be used to clinical advantage, as when demonstrating the relationship of the sacroiliac (SI) joints to the pelvis. Where standard AP positioning fails to reveal this relationship, a 35-degree cephalic tube angulation elongates the pelvis and demonstrates the SI joints clearly. Similarly, standard AP and PA views of the rectosigmoid colon produce a foreshortened image of the area. Angling the tube 35-degree cephalic in this case elongates the rectosigmoid colon in a manner that increases visualization, thereby facilitating more accurate diagnosis.

QUESTIONS FOR DISTORTION

select the best answer

1. What type of image misrepresentation, if any, occurs if a wedge-shaped object is tilted relative to the film and the central ray is angled so it is perpendicular to the long axis of the object?

   (A) Blurring
   (B) Elongation
   (C) Foreshortening
   (D) No geometric unsharpness occurs

2. The most likely cause of radiographic elongation is:

   (A) FFD.
   (B) OFD.
   (C) grid cutoff.
   (D) tube angulation.

3. You are sent to the intensive care unit to obtain portable radiographs of a patient's femur. The patient is in traction. Because of the cast and the limitations of the environment (traction, location of the bed), you are unable to minimize OFD. The best method of reducing magnification in this instance would be:

   (A) increase FFD.
   (B) decrease FFD.
   (C) cephalic tube angulation.
   (D) caudal tube angulation.

▶▶ ANSWERS TO DISTORTION

1. The answer is (B). Elongation and foreshortening occur when the plane of the object and the plane of the image are not parallel. Inclining a tubular, flattened, or wedge-shaped object at a steeper angle in relation to the film while maintaining beam and film alignment will result in a foreshortened image, whereas inclining the same types of objects and angling the tube so as to place the beam perpendicular to the long axis of the object will produce an elongated image.

2. The answer is (D). Although there are instances where the three-dimensional shape of the part being examined relative to the tube and film alignment will contribute to elongation of the part, the most likely cause of any appreciable radiographic elongation is tube angulation. Improper OID and FFD are factors that relate to magnification (size) distortion. Grid cutoff is manifested as unilateral loss of density.

3. The answer is (A). FFD and image magnification are inversely proportional; therefore, in this clinical situation, it would be wise to use a longer FFD in an effort to decrease magnification. Remember, however, that as distance increases, technique must also increase in order to maintain adequate density.

E. Film, Screen, and Grid Selection

FILM CHARACTERISTICS

Modern medical x-ray film consists of four primary parts: a flexible film base, an adhesive layer, the film emulsion, and a protective coating. The **film base** must provide a rigid support for the emulsion coating. It consists of durable **polyester plastic** of a consistency that facilitates smooth transport through the automatic processing system. The base material contains blue dye whose primary purpose is to alleviate the radiologist's eyestrain. The dye, along with environmental light exposure received during production, produces a measurable density called **base fog.**

Processing the film produces an additional amount of fog, which is roughly equivalent to the base fog. Measured together by densitometer, this density is referred to as **base plus fog.** Base plus fog should not exceed a 0.2 densitometer reading.

The thin **adhesive layer,** sometimes called the **subcoating,** is applied to both sides of the base to ensure consistent adhesion of the film emulsion to the base.

The **film emulsion,** consisting of a homogeneous mixture of **silver halide crystals and gelatin,** is the portion of the film that actually interacts with x-ray and light photons. The clear gelatin serves primarily as a mechanical support for the silver halide, holding the crystals uniformly in place. It is clear and porous, in order to transmit light and allow processing chemicals to interact with the silver halide during processing. Gelatin also swells during developing, becoming porous and soft, and rehardens during the fixing process.

The silver halide crystal is the crucial ingredient of the emulsion, and is sensitive to both light and x-ray photons. A typical silver halide crystal consists of approximately **95% silver bromide** and **5% silver iodide.**

Upon exposure to light and x-ray photons, which in a clinical situation will be **remnant radiation** exiting the patient and light emission from intensifying screens, the silver bromide ions emit electrons. The electrons then move to a center of sensitivity on the crystal called the **sensitivity speck.** The negatively charged electrons attract the positively charged silver ions, and their interaction causes a conversion of the silver halide crystal to black metallic silver.

The energy deposited on the emulsion is laid down in a pattern resembling the part of anatomy being radiographed. This pattern is referred to as the **latent image.** It is known as a latent because the image is undetectable until the emulsion is exposed to processing chemistry. The conversion of the latent image to a **visible** or **manifest image** is seen as black metallic silver on x-ray film.

In order to protect the thin (approximately 1/100 of an inch) emulsion layer from the hazards of handling and processing, a durable **protective coating** consisting of clear, hard gelatin is coated on top of the emulsion in a process that involves passing the film through a trough containing the gelatin, chilling the mixture to a gel, drying it, and adding an additional nonabrasive coating.

FILM CONTRAST, FILM LATITUDE, AND EXPOSURE LATITUDE

Although each manufacturer closely guards the particular components of its film emulsion, thus preventing specific discussion of their film's makeup relative to the type of image produced, the technologist must understand that the manner in which a given film responds to a given set of exposure and processing factors is directly dependent on the film's manufacturing process. Differing **film contrast, film latitude, and exposure latitude** will be demonstrated on film, depending on the type of process and composition of emulsion used.

Film contrast is a given film's ability to record a range of densities. Film contrast may be either short scale, or high contrast, with relatively abrupt changes from black (as for gas or air) to white (as for bone, or

contrast-enhanced organs), or long scale, low contrast, which demonstrates a wide range of densities from black to white, with numerous shades of gray in between.

Film latitude describes the film's capacity to record a range of densities, whereas **exposure latitude** refers to the film's potential to allow for exposure technique error, while still producing an acceptable radiograph. For a given film, high kVp, low mAs technique will produce a greater exposure latitude than will high mAs, low kVp technique.

Remember, film contrast is directly related to film and exposure latitude. A film that has a long scale of contrast will have a correspondingly wide latitude, whereas short scale, or high-contrast film, possesses a narrow latitude.

The quantitative study of a film's characteristic response to exposure and processing is known as **sensitometry.** Two precise instruments are required for sensitometric study. A **sensitometer** uses a high-quality light source to expose a stepwedge or stepwedge-like representation on an unexposed film, while a **densitometer** is used to measure degrees of density change demonstrated by the stepwedge on the processed radiograph. Proper calibration of the densitometer is crucial; a reading taken when there is no film under the sensor should yield a measurement of 0.00.

Densitometer readings are plotted on a graph in order to generate a graphic representation of the range of densities produced relative to a given exposure, which is known as a **characteristic curve.** The measurement is also known as an **H&D curve,** named after Hurter and Driffield, two British photography students who were the first to describe the curve in 1890.

Characteristic curves consist of three main portions: the **toe, straight line portion,** and **shoulder (Figure 4-5).** The vertical axis of the curve describes exposure, whereas the horizontal axis measures exposure time. In order to limit the graph to an easily readable size, exposure is expressed logarithmically. **Film speed** is determined by the right-to-left positioning of the curve on the graph. Because the horizontal axis describes exposure time, the farther left the curve is positioned, the faster the film speed.

The **toe** measures the minimal density recorded on film following exposure, and takes into account the film's base plus fog. A reading of the toe portion will generally be only slightly higher than that of the base plus fog. The toe is referred to by some manufacturers as D_{min}.

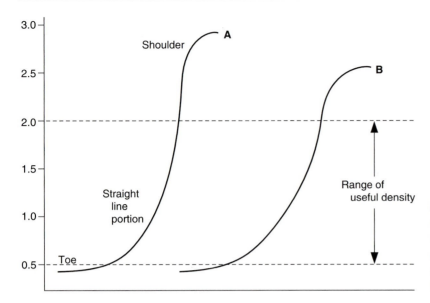

FIGURE 4-5. Characteristic curves consist of three main portions: toe, straight line portion, and shoulder. The straight line portion, or average gradient (slope) of the curve, describes the range of useful density for a given film.

The **straight line portion,** or **average gradient** (slope) of the curve describes the range of useful density for a given film. The generally accepted range of diagnostic densities occur between 0.25 and 2.5. The steeper the average gradient, the faster the film, and the higher the contrast. Fast, high-contrast film possesses less exposure latitude, or room for error, than that of slower, low-contrast film, but requires lower exposure factors, and hence, lower patient dose to produce a given density.

The **shoulder,** or highest portion of the characteristic curve, demonstrates the point at which maximum density, or D_{max}, occurs. Exposures made beyond this point do not produce diagnostically useful information. In fact, just beyond the maximum point, the curve begins to descend. This point on the curve describes the **solarization point,** where additional exposure produces reversal of the image.

The solarization point is used to advantage in the manufacture of duplication film. A film designed for duplication is exposed to the solarization point, so that when the emulsion is exposed by ultraviolet light, an x-ray image is placed on it, and image reversal occurs, producing a copy of the original image.

QUESTIONS FOR FILM CHARACTERISTICS

select the best answer

1. A logarithmic density of 1.5 would be found on which portion of an H&D curve?

   (A) Average gradient
   (B) D_{max}

   (C) D_{min}
   (D) Shoulder

   Using the characteristic curve shown in Figure 4-5, answer the following questions:

2. Film A demonstrates which of the following characteristics compared with film B?

   (A) Slower with less exposure latitude
   (B) Faster with less exposure latitude
   (C) Faster with more exposure latitude
   (D) Slower with more exposure latitude

3. Which of the following qualities describe film B compared with film A?

   (A) Requires more exposure and has lower contrast
   (B) Requires more exposure and has higher contrast
   (C) Requires less exposure and has higher contrast
   (D) Requires less exposure and has lower contrast

4. The term base plus fog describes:

   (A) unwanted exposure of film to light.
   (B) unwanted exposure of film from scatter radiation.
   (C) inherent manufacturing and processing density.
   (D) contributing environmental exposure factors, such as radon.

5. Which portions of the H&D curve represent densities that are outside the useful density range?

(A) Straight line and toe
(B) Toe and shoulder
(C) Straight line and shoulder
(D) There are no densities on the curve that are outside the range.

▶▶ ANSWERS TO FILM CHARACTERISTICS

1. The answer is (A). The straight line portion, or average gradient of a characteristic curve, describes a given film's range of useful density. The generally accepted range expressed as a logarithm is between 0.25 and 2.5.
2. The answer is (B). When an H&D curve is used to represent more than one film, the film farthest to the left is fastest. Film B, however, demonstrates a more gentle slope, which is characteristic of a film with greater exposure latitude, or one that allows for greater error in technique. Contrast and latitude are inversely proportional.
3. The answer is (A). Film B is slower than film A, and therefore would require more exposure to produce a given density. Film B also has a more shallow gradient, which is representative of a film with lower, or longer scale contrast.
4. The answer is (C). A blue tint is added to the film base by the manufacturer to alleviate eyestrain. This tint has a small density. Along with environmental exposure during manufacturing, film is shipped with an inherent density called base fog. An additional density, approximately equal to that of base fog, is added during processing. The sum of the factors equals base plus fog. Base plus fog should not exceed 0.2 by sensitometric measurement.
5. The answer is (B). The straight line portion of the H&D curve represents the useful density range. The toe represents base plus fog, or D_{min}, whereas the shoulder describes maximum density, or D_{max}. The area past the shoulder describes the solarization point, at which further exposure causes image reversal.

FILM-SCREEN COMBINATION

Recall that intensifying screens capture remnant radiation exiting the patient and convert the x-ray energy into light, which exposes the medical x-ray film. The efficiency of a screen-film combination is based on several factors.

The interaction of x-ray with intensifying screen phosphors produces a phenomenon known as **luminescence.** If the intensifying screen continues to emit light after excitation by x-radiation ceases, this phenomenon is called **phosphorescence,** or **screen lag.** Screen lag is an undesirable property, because it produces unwanted density on the film. If, however, light emission ceases in conjunction with termination of the x-ray exposure, the process is called **fluorescence.**

PHOSPHOR TYPE

From previous discussion you know that intensifying screens may be categorized into two primary categories according to the type of phosphor used. Traditional calcium tungstate screens emit light primarily in the blue-light spectrum, and are much less efficient than green light–emitting rare earth screens. The comparative increase in efficiency (speed) of rare earth screens over calcium tungstate screens is based on two factors: the **absorption** and **conversion to light** properties of each type of screen. These factors are expressed as a ratio and are called the **absorption/conversion ratio** for the purpose of determining **screen speed.**

For example, calcium tungstate screens absorb approximately 20% to 40% of the remnant radiation, of which roughly 5% is converted into light. On the other hand, rare earth screens absorb approximately 60% of the remnant radiation, converting 15% to 18% of it into light energy.

Remember that film type must be matched with screen type (blue light–emitting with blue light–sensitive, and so on), or a 50% loss of screen speed occurs.

RELATIVE SPEED

Manufacturers have adopted an arbitrary means for defining screen speed, which is a screen's capacity to produce density at a given exposure. The faster the screen, the more density produced. A calcium tungstate screen matched with a blue light–sensitive conventional x-ray film is labeled as a **100-speed system.** This type of combination, sometimes referred to as a **par speed system,** is used as a baseline from which other combinations are measured. For example, a 200-speed system is roughly twice as fast as a 100-speed system; a 300-speed system is three times as fast; and so on. **Table 4-4** demonstrates useful conversion factors for various speed systems.

It is important to note that the **thickness of the phosphor layer** also plays an important role in determining screen speed. The thicker the phosphor layer, the faster the screen speed.

Before the advent of rare earth screens, screen

▶ **TABLE 4-4.** Conversion Factors for Various Speed Systems

Screen Speed	Screen Type	mAs Conversion Factor	Density Produced Relative to 100 Speed
3.3	Direct exposure / no screen	30X	$\frac{1}{30}$
25	Ultraslow detail	4X	$\frac{1}{4}$
50	Fast detail/extremity cassette	2X	$\frac{1}{2}$
100	Par/medium speed	1	1
200	High speed	$\frac{1}{2}$	2
300	High-plus (blue light–emitting rare earth type)	$\frac{1}{3}$	3
400	Rare earth (green light–emitting)	$\frac{1}{4}$	4
800	High-speed rare earth	$\frac{1}{8}$	8
1200	Ultra–high-speed rare earth	$\frac{1}{12}$	12

thickness was equal on both sides of the x-ray cassette. However, because rare earth screens absorb light much more efficiently, using screens of equal thickness became problematic, because the front screen would absorb a disproportionate amount of light, leaving little for use by the rear screen. Hence, rare earth intensifying screens are asymmetric; they are constructed thinner in front than in the rear, in order to blacken both sides of the film emulsion equally.

Phosphor crystal size is also a factor in screen speed; the larger the crystal, the more light is transmitted, and hence the faster the screen speed; but as crystal size increases, so does image blurring. A combination of crystal sizes is used in most phosphor layers.

A phenomenon known as **light crossover** occurs when light passing through one side of the film emulsion to the other side results in a decrease of image sharpness (detail). Some film screen combinations permit as much as 30% of transmitted light to cross over. Light crossover is increased by thicker phosphor layers. Because some crystals are situated more posteriorly, or deeper in the layer, light has farther to travel to reach the film emulsion. As light travels, it widens, forming a "halolike" effect that further increases image blurring.

Manufacturers are working to decrease the amount of crossover that occurs. Some companies add dye to the film base to minimize crossover, whereas others have used **tabular** or **T grain** technology, a method that decreases crossover while enhancing image clarity by adding a specialized dye to the film emulsion itself.

The cutting edge of intensifying screen development is known as **zero crossover technology.** Currently, it is used primarily in conjunction with chest radiography. With the zero crossover process, an orange-colored dye is added to the film that completely prevents crossover from one film emulsion to the other. The dye washes off in the developer rack of the processor. The film-screen combination actually produces two images that are seen as one on the finished radiograph. The anterior side of the receptor records the vascular markings of the chest, and consists of a high-contrast film emulsion exposed by a thin, high-detail screen. The posterior aspect of the receptor is roughly six times faster than the anterior side, and it records the mediastinal structures on film. It is composed of an ultrawide latitude film emulsion exposed by the thicker posterior intensifying screen.

An **undercoat layer** is added to modern screens, which can be either light reflecting or light absorbing, depending on the desired effect. If the undercoat reflects light back toward the film, the result is increased density on the radiograph, because the reflected light increases system speed. Remember, though, an increase in speed produces a decrease in detail.

An **overcoat layer** is added to protect the screen from handling damage. **Figure 4-6** shows the typical intensifying screen construction.

SINGLE- AND DOUBLE-EMULSION FILM

Most modern x-ray film is of **dual-emulsion** construction; that is, it has an emulsion coating on both sides of the film base. A relatively thin film base is used with dual-emulsion film to increase the clarity of the superimposed images. Dual-emulsion film produces twice the density of that of a single-emulsion film, even if the single-emulsion film were to be made twice as thick. This characteristic reduces both patient dose and deterioration of the x-ray tube from excessive heat loading. There are, however, several draw-

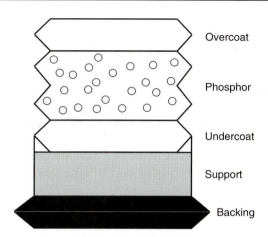

FIGURE 4-6. Typical intensifying screen construction. The support is the base of the intensifying screen. The added backing prevents curling. The undercoat fixes the phosphor layer to the support, while the overcoat acts as a protective layer.

backs to dual-emulsion film (discussed next); these should be considered when making film selection.

When the need for detail outweighs the advantages of dual-emulsion film, a single-emulsion film is often substituted. For example, the quality of such examinations as mammography and extremity imaging is directly dependent on extremely high resolution. So important is the detail element of these films that many departments use only single-emulsion film in conjunction with a solitary detail speed-intensifying screen as their standard protocol for this class of examinations.

Another disadvantage of dual-emulsion film is loss of clarity due to crossover. A **single-emulsion system,** which uses a fine grain single-emulsion film exposed by a single intensifying screen, eliminates the difficulty of crossover altogether. Single-emulsion films use a special backing called **antihalation**

backing that minimizes light scatter radiation in the cassette.

Another consideration relative to choice between single- and double-emulsion systems is known as the **parallax effect.** The parallax effect occurs when a tube angulation of greater than 10 degrees is used in conjunction with a dual-emulsion film. The angulation of the tube causes a separation of images from the front to the back emulsion, as shown in **Figure 4-7.**

SPECIAL APPLICATIONS

There are other, nonstandard types of film that the technologist should be aware of. Single-emulsion film's role is used when detail is the prime consideration for choice of film, but the exact opposite situation also exists. There are clinical situations that demand that the film used allows as much room for error as possible. Such is the case with portable radiography. There are so many variables involved with this clinical setting that it becomes imperative that the film-screen combination used for this task possesses an extremely wide exposure latitude. Obviously, ultrawide latitude film-screen combinations must sacrifice some contrast and detail in order to realize sufficient gains in allowance for exposure error.

Copying original films onto **duplicating film** for physician or legal referral is a common practice in most radiology departments. Duplicating film is of single-emulsion design, and is exposed by a duplicating machine. The machine produces ultraviolet light that travels through the existing film to produce a copy. Once the duplicating film is exposed, it is processed as a normal radiograph. Duplicating film is **solarized;** that is, it is already exposed to its maximum potential. Thus, the longer the film is exposed to ultraviolet light, the lighter the film becomes.

Certain examinations, such as full-length vascular

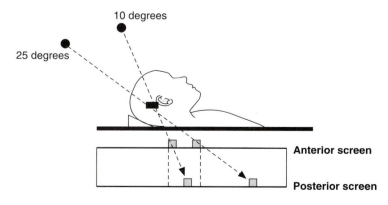

FIGURE 4-7. The parallax effect. Note the separation of objects increases as tube angulation increases.

studies, and radiography of the entire spine (scoliosis), employ **gradient screens** to overcome the difficulty of differing tissue thicknesses that occur naturally when multiple body parts are examined. The screens are arranged inside the cassette in a series of ascending speeds, with the high-speed end used for the thickest body part, such as the lumbosacral portion of the spine, or the femur portion of the leg, and the low-speed end positioned nearest the thinnest body part. Optimally, these cassettes should be wall-mounted and labeled as to which screen is where, so that no confusion arises about screen placement during the examination. Obviously, placing the cassette upside down will result in a film too dark at one end and too light at the other.

CONVERSION FACTORS FOR GRIDS

A **grid** is a scatter radiation absorbing device used with radiography of body parts that are approximately 10 cm or greater. Grids are constructed of alternating lead strips and radiolucent interspace material of either plastic or aluminum, and are placed between the patient and film cassette. The design of the grid allows the useful portion of the beam to pass unobstructed between the lead strips, while the scatter radiation (the radiation that has changed direction as a result of interaction with the patient) is absorbed by the lead strips. The term **cleanup** is often used as a synonym for the scatter radiation–absorbing power of a given grid. *The primary purpose of a grid is to improve contrast by reducing scatter radiation.*

There are a number of ways by which grids are classified. One way is according to their function; they may be either **stationary** or **moving. Stationary grids** are the simplest type. They are composed of vertical lead strips and radiolucent filler material. Examples of stationary grids include grid cassettes, slip-on grids, wafer grids, and crosshatch grids. The primary disadvantage associated with stationary grids is visible **grid lines** on the radiograph. Grid lines are produced when the primary beam is absorbed by the lead strips, leaving white lines of no density on the radiograph.

The difficulty of the presence of grid lines was solved by the development of the **moving grid,** sometimes called **the bucky grid,** or the **Potter-Bucky diaphragm.** The names for these devices are derived from the physicians who developed them. Dr. Gustave Bucky developed the first grid in 1913, which was a **crosshatch** type grid, composed of two sets of lead strips that intersected and aligned on the long and short axes of the grid. The first crosshatch grid was crude by today's standard; it produced a fairly coarse-appearing image. But Dr. Bucky discovered an important radiographic principle still in use today: that tube angulation is not possible with crosshatch grids because even the slightest angle produces **grid cutoff,** an image-degrading phenomenon that will be discussed more completely later.

In 1920, Dr. Hollis Potter developed the concept of moving the grid during the exposure, and making the grid strips thinner in order to eliminate grid lines on the radiograph. Dr. Potter's Potter-Bucky diaphragm was heralded as one of the most significant advances in the then fledgling field of radiology. His work still stands as important today.

There are three basic types of moving grids. The first two, the **single stroke grid,** and the **reciprocating grid,** have been largely replaced by the third and most modern type, the **oscillating grid.**

The single stroke grid is powered by a spring-loaded, manually cocked mechanism, which moves laterally in both directions while exposure is made. Exposure times are limited, because the mechanism cannot accommodate shorter times than approximately 0.2 second. In addition, on some models, the technologist must set the grid movement time as well as the exposure time.

The reciprocating grid also moves laterally in both directions, but is motor driven. There is no need to reset the reciprocating bucky after each use, as is the case with the single stroke grid.

The oscillating grid is positioned within a metallic frame, and is held in place on each of the four corners by spring devices. When an exposure is about to be made, the grid is pulled to one side by a strong electromagnet, which releases the grid when the exposure begins. The grid oscillates in a circular fashion, which is the most effective motion for elimination of grid lines.

Another method of grid classification is by **grid ratio.** Grid ratio is a numeric statement of grid efficiency expressed as the height of the lead strips over the width of the interspace. As grid ratio increases, the lead strips increase in height; however, the interspace width remains the same. Grid ratio provides an effective means of determining that grid's contrast improvement capability. Generally, the higher the grid ratio, the more contrast improvement.

However, this statement must be considered along with other important information about the grid. For example, each grid is manufactured with a certain number of **lines per inch.** Most modern grids are usually 100 to 200 lines per inch, but some still in use will be in the range of 60 to 80 lines per inch. Grids with more than 100 lines per inch are sometimes called **fine line grids.** In order to manufacture fine line grids and maintain the grid ratio, the lead strips are made thinner and shorter. Although fine line grids provide the advantage of virtually invisible grid lines, they are not as effective at cleanup as a comparable standard grid. For example, a 12:1 200-lpi fine line grid is only approximately as effective as an 8:1 or 10:1 100-lpi grid. A grid may also be classified according to the orientation of its lead strips. Grids that have lead lines aligned in the same direction are called **linear grids.** Linear grids may be either **parallel** or **focused.**

Parallel grids are the simpler type of linear grid; they are usually low-ratio devices with lead strips assembled vertically across their width. The use of parallel grids is somewhat limited according to field size and FFD, because of the divergent nature of the x-ray beam. As the beam diverges, some of the image-contributing radiation is intercepted by the parallel grid lines, which causes a loss of density on both sides of the cassette. This bilateral loss of density is an important phenomenon known as **grid cutoff.** Because of grid cutoff, positioning with a linear parallel grid is critical. The center axis of the primary beam must correspond precisely to the center of the grid, or grid cutoff will occur.

The lead lines in a **focused grid (Figure 4-8)** are angled uniformly in both directions so they correspond with a predetermined point in space known as the **grid focus** or **grid radius.** When the angled

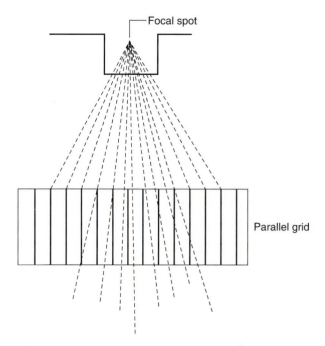

FIGURE 4-9. Grid cutoff using linear parallel grid. The divergent beam is intercepted by the lateral lead strips, causing grid cutoff.

strips are aligned so that their planes converge toward the tube focal spot, the grid then has a grid radius or grid focus equal to the distance from the focal spot to the surface of the grid. Grids will be marked as to their intended grid radius, along with information concerning the grid ratio and lines per inch. If an exposure is made at other than the correct SID, grid cutoff will occur.

As previously mentioned, grid cutoff occurs when the grid is improperly positioned relative to the central axis of the x-ray beam **(Figure 4-9).** There are five clinical situations that the technologist should be familiar with in order to prevent grid cutoff.

An **off level grid** occurs when the grid does not lie in a lane perpendicular with the central axis of the x-ray beam. The cause may either be that the grid itself is angled relative to the beam, or, as is the case more frequently, that the tube head is angled improperly relative to the center of the grid.

Grid cutoff also occurs if the beam is perpendicular to the grid, but laterally decentered. As with off level grids, an **off-center grid** generally occurs because of an improperly placed tube head, rather than grid mis-positioning. An off-center grid causes a lack of density on one side of the film.

An **off-focus grid** occurs when an improper FFD is used in conjunction with a focused grid. An off-

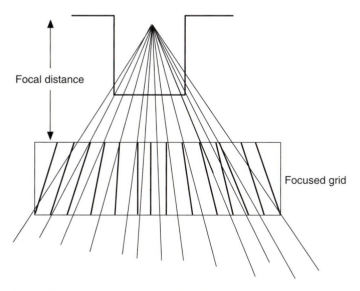

FIGURE 4-8. A focused grid. Note that the lead strips are coincident with the divergent beam across the entire width of the grid.

focus grid causes loss of density at the periphery of the film. It should be noted that more positioning latitude is possible with low-ratio grids than with high-ratio grids.

The causative factor involving the **upside down grid** artifact is obvious. Grids are always marked as to which side is the tube side of the device. When the grid is used in reverse position, only the central portion of the beam reaches the detector, leaving the lateral portion of the film unexposed. As with off-focus grids, the higher the grid ratio, the more pronounced the effect.

The fifth grid type, a crosshatch grid, is sometimes constructed by using two grids of the same ratio placed one on top of the other, with their grid lines at right angles. If the grid lines are improperly placed, that is, so that they overlap each other instead of being perpendicular, a **"moiré"** artifact, which is a wavelike or rippled appearance on the film, occurs.

It is significant to note that grid artifacts primarily occur with stationary, rather than moving grids. Most modern x-ray rooms are equipped with both table and upright bucky grids, which will not operate when off-center or off-distance errors occur. The operator will receive an "exposure hold message" when attempting to make the exposure, which will require a correction of the error before proceeding.

Although size and shape of the body part under examination obviously influence the choice of grid, the relationship between kVp range and grid ratio selection is also important. The higher the ratio of the grid, the higher the kVp range the grid will effectively clean up. The availability of a given size and ratio grid will depend on the size and budget of your radiology department. In general, at kVp ranges below 90 kVp, grid ratios of up to 8:1 are used, and above 90 kVp, grid ratios exceeding 8:1 are used.

Patient dose is also of course a factor in deciding what size and ratio grid to use. For example, it can be argued that the difference in cleanup ability between a 12:1 and a 16:1 grid ratio is rather small, but the increase in patient dose needed to produce a radiograph of adequate density is significant. Some radiology departments have standard grid protocols in place, indicating which grid to use for a given examination, whereas other departments leave the choice to the technologist.

A few other terms relating to the application of grids should be noted. **Contrast improvement factor (k)** is a numeric expression of radiographic contrast between a grid and a nongrid study. Analysis of both films is based on **average gradient,** a measurement obtained using a sensitometer and densi-

tometer. As a baseline, note that a contrast improvement factor of 1 is indicative of no improvement. In general, grids have contrast improvement factors ranging between 1.5 to 2.5, with higher grid ratios having higher contrast improvement. The formula for obtaining contrast improvement factor is as follows:

$$k = \frac{radiographic\ contrast\ with\ grid}{radiographic\ contrast\ without\ grid} \quad (8)$$

In an ideal world, all primary radiation would be transmitted, and all scatter radiation would be absorbed by the grid. However, some of the primary beam is absorbed as well. The ratio of the transmitted primary beam to that of the transmitted scatter radiation is known as **grid selectivity.** Selectivity is expressed mathematically as the Greek letter sigma (Σ) and is influenced by grid ratio and lead content of the grid. The formula for grid selectivity is:

$$\Sigma = \frac{primary\ radiation\ transmitted}{scatter\ radiation\ transmitted} \quad (9)$$

When a grid is employed, exposure factors need to be adjusted upward so that adequate radiographic density is maintained, because the grid absorbs both primary and scatter radiation. Unfortunately, there is not a hard-and-fast rule that can be employed to make the conversion, because the subject of grid conversion factors is the cause of some debate in the radiologic community. One author, the esteemed Quinn B. Carroll, who wrote *Fuchs's Principles of Radiographic Exposure, Processing and Quality Control,* states: "This can be a controversial subject, and there seem to be as many formulae for grid conversion techniques as there are authors."

Bearing this in mind, the following conversions can be useful. The most common grid ratios for the table or upright bucky are 8:1, 10:1, and 12:1. These ratios can be compensated for by adjusting mAs three to four times higher than for a nongrid technique. When using nongrid instead of grid technique, the conversion is inverse; instead of three to four times higher, the mAs is adjusted to one third or one fourth of the original technique. Of course, these are simply rules of thumb; you should obtain the specific information that applies to your workplace.

When changing from one grid ratio to another using the mAs adjustment method, the technologist can construct the following ratio based on the suggested mAs conversion factors presented in **Table 4-5:**

$$\frac{grid\ ratio\ changing\ to:\ (conversion\ factor)}{grid\ ratio\ changing\ from\ (conversion\ factor)} \quad (10)$$

▶ **TABLE 4-5.** mAs Conversion Factors

Grid Ratio	mAs Conversion Factor
4:1, 5:1, 6:1	2
8:1	3
10:1	3.5
12:1	4
15:1, 16:1	5

For example, to change techniques from a 4:1 grid to an 8:1 grid, you would:

$$\frac{TO}{FROM} = \frac{8:1\ grid\ (increase\ technique\ 3\times)}{4:1\ grid\ (conversion\ factor)} = \frac{3}{2} \quad (11)$$

Using this method, you would increase mAs 3/2, or 1.5 times the original technique. To reduce grid ratio, the same method is used.

$$\frac{TO}{FROM} = \frac{8:1\ grid}{12:1\ grid} = \frac{3}{5} \quad (12)$$

In this instance, the mAs would be reduced by 3/5.

Another method that is used to make technical adjustments concerning grids is called the bucky factor. As you will see, the bucky factor is similar in nature to the mAs conversion factor in that it is a numeric expression of mAs adjustment. As with previously described methods, it is used when substituting a new grid ratio for an old one, or when changing technique from nongrid to grid technique, or vice versa.

The bucky factor is derived from the ratio of the remnant radiation incident to the grid over the remnant radiation transmitted through it **(Table 4-6)**. In other words:

$$B = \frac{incident\ remnant\ radiation}{transmitted\ remnant\ radiation} \quad (13)$$

▶ **TABLE 4-6.** Bucky Factor

Grid Ratio	Bucky Factor
No Grid	1
5:1	2
6:1	3
8:1	4
10, 12:1	5
16:1	6

Try this sample problem to practice using the bucky factor. An AP tabletop knee examination is performed using 5 mAs, 70 kVp, and 40 inches SID. The patient is large, and a significant amount of image degrading scatter is produced by this technique. In order to clean up scatter, a 10:1 bucky examination is performed instead. If all other factors remain consistent, what new technique should be used in order to reduce scatter and maintain density?

You can use this derivation of the formula based on Table 4-6:

$$\frac{mAs_1}{mAs_2} = \frac{bucky\ factor_1}{bucky\ factor_2} \quad (14)$$

Substituting,

$$\frac{5}{x} = \frac{1}{5} \quad (15)$$

QUESTIONS FOR CONVERSION FACTORS FOR GRIDS

select the best answer

1. Of the following, which are characteristics unique to a focused grid?
   1. Canting
   2. Radius of infinity
   3. Grid radius
   4. Grid ratio
   (A) Choices 2 and 3
   (B) All of the aforementioned
   (C) Choices 1 and 3
   (D) Choices 1 and 4

2. Compared with an 8:1 grid, a 16:1 grid exhibits which of the following characteristics?
   (A) Greater cleanup, less positioning latitude
   (B) Less cleanup, greater positioning latitude
   (C) Greater patient dose, greater positioning latitude
   (D) Greater selectivity, less patient dose

3. An examination of the abdomen is performed using a 12:1 oscillating bucky with the tube placed 2 inches off center toward the right side of the patient. The resulting radiograph will demonstrate:
   (A) overall loss of density.
   (B) unilateral right-sided loss of density.
   (C) unilateral left-sided loss of density.

(D) loss of density on the anode side of the tube.

4. If a stationary focused 12:1 grid with a focal range of 36 to 42 inches is used to make an exposure at 72 inches FFD, the resulting radiograph will demonstrate:

(A) unilateral right-sided cutoff.
(B) unilateral left-sided cutoff.
(C) loss of density bilaterally.
(D) that only a narrow center portion of the film is exposed.

5. Using the bucky factor, adjust the technique of an exposure of 50 mAs, 75 kVp, and a 10:1 grid to nongrid tabletop technique. The new correct factors will be:

(A) 10 mAs, 85 kVp.
(B) 10 mAs, 75 kVp.
(C) 25 mAs, 75 kVp.
(D) 75 mAs, 75 kVp.

▶▶▶ ANSWERS TO CONVERSION FACTORS FOR GRIDS

1. The answer is (C). In a focused grid, the process of tilting the lead strips so that they are aligned toward the focal spot of the x-ray tube is known as canting. Grid radius is the distance from the grid at which lines drawn from the lead strips converge toward the focal spot. Most grid radii occur in a range that allows some room for error. Because the majority of examinations are performed at either 40 inches or 72 inches, grid radius ranges are found from approximately 36 inches to 42 inches and 66 inches to 74 inches. The lines in a parallel grid are not canted; therefore, parallel grids have a radius of infinity—as distance from the grid is increased, the beam remains parallel.

2. The answer is (A). The greater the grid ratio, the more accurate must be the positioning in order to avoid grid cutoff. A 16:1 grid would require greater patient dose than an 8:1 grid, but would be superior in cleanup ability. Selectivity is the ratio of transmitted primary radiation to transmitted scatter radiation and is related to the lead content of the grid. Two grids can be of the same ratio but have differing lead content. In general, heavier grids have high selectivity and high-contrast improvement factors.

3. The answer is (C). If the x-ray tube is positioned off center in relation to the bucky, the result will

be a loss of density on the side of the radiograph away from the tube. In the previously mentioned example, the tube is positioned toward the right side of the patient, so grid cutoff occurs on the left.

4. The answer is (C). If a radiograph is made with an improper focal film range, for example, using a 72-inch FFD with a 40-inch focal range, the result is a bilateral loss of density. Generally, 1- to 2-inch segments on either side appear underexposed. If a grid is used upside down, only x-rays parallel to the center of the grid reach the detector, therefore exposing only a narrow center portion of the grid.

5. The answer is (B). The bucky factor grid conversion method uses a table of conversion factors. The bucky factor for a 10:1 grid is 5; therefore, when converting from grid to nongrid, the correct technical adjustment is to divide the mAs by 5. Kilovoltage is not adjusted.

F. Technique Charts

A technique chart is a simple reference tool that technologists can use to correctly select technical factors for commonly performed examinations in a given exposure room. There are various methods of constructing the charts, but regardless of the method used, several constants must be maintained in order to assure their efficacy.

First of all, it is important to stress that the exposure factors listed on the chart will produce a diagnostic radiograph only if all the conditions for that particular exposure are met. If the chart lists an AP hand radiograph at 1 mAs and 50 kVp at 40 inches, for example, and the exposure is made at 52 inches, the radiograph will suffer the consequences for not fulfilling the conditions—it will be underexposed.

This may seem to be an obvious point to some students, but how often I have heard the lament from students: "But I used what was on the chart!" The radiologic clinical situation is a dynamic one. You will constantly be faced with adapting technique for anatomic considerations, range-of-motion limitations of the patient, available film, processing conditions, and so on. It is crucial that you train yourself now to think of the technique chart for the purpose it was intended—that of a helpful guide.

A quality control program involving calibration of the x-ray units and processing machines must be in place. If either of these two elements is functioning out of their known control values, then the technique chart will not be valid.

CALIPER MEASUREMENT AND VARIABLE KVP CHARTS

As the name implies, the variable kVp technique chart uses a fixed mAs and a baseline kVp and average thickness for a given body part. The technologist increases or decreases kVp level according to part thickness. Using this method, the technologist employs metallic calipers to measure the part being examined, selects the fixed mAs, and then adjusts the kVp 2 ± kVp for every 1 cm difference in part thickness. The thicker the part, the more kVp will be required, as beam attenuation increases proportionally with part thickness. The variable kVp technique chart is not widely employed today; simply changing the kVp in order to increase density both lengthens the scale of contrast and increases the level of scatter radiation.

FIXED KVP

With fixed kVp charts, an optimum kVp level is assigned to each body part, and mAs is used to compensate for variance in size of the part. Generally, each part is further classified as small, medium, or large, with a specific kVp corresponding to each size. Some charts define part size as a range, for example, small might equal a size from 13 to 15 cm; medium, 16 to 18 cm; and so on. Using this method would, if strictly interpreted, require caliper measurement; however, in actual practice the technologist simply decides what size the patient is based on experience.

The fixed kVp chart is most often associated with the use of automatic exposure controls (AED). Whether with an ion chamber or phototimer device, an optimum kVp is selected at the control panel, and the exposure is terminated by the AED.

ANATOMIC AND SPECIAL CONSIDERATIONS

Used properly, a well-constructed technique chart will produce the correct optical density and appropriate scale of contrast on the radiograph. But the technologist must not become overly dependent on the chart. He must learn to manipulate exposure factors in accordance with the clinical situation, because various anatomic and clinical variables will change the baseline exposure settings.

For example, part thickness may change according to positioning; when thickness changes, so must exposure factors. One very common example of variance in part thickness is the supine and erect abdominal examination, also known as the flat and upright abdomen or, when accompanied by a PA chest radiograph, as an acute abdominal examination. In this case, the upright radiograph requires an increase in technical factors compared with that of the supine examination because the abdominal contents shift position caudally and attenuate more of the primary beam when the patient is moved from supine to erect position. Note also that this increase could not have been determined by simple caliper measurement, because the abdomen measures approximately the same whether flat or upright.

Contrast media also plays an important role in technical factor selection. Consider again a plain AP abdominal radiograph. Suppose the technique chart listed 30 mAs and 80 kVp as the correct technique for an average-sized patient. Now think about adding contrast media to this situation. If one were to examine the same abdomen with a barium-filled stomach, a very different technique must be used. Barium requires a minimum of 100 to 110 kVp in order to be adequately penetrated. Obviously, one must reduce mAs significantly when increasing kVp from 80 to 110, if density is to be maintained. Similarly, if iodinated contrast were to be introduced into the same abdomen, the kVp must be lowered to 70 or lower in order to avoid overpenetration of the iodine contrast, which would require an increase in mAs.

Another common clinical variable that necessitates manipulation of exposure factors from the baseline is associated with emergency room and orthopedic patients—the cast. Casts are external medical devices constructed of either plaster of Paris or fiberglass layers wrapped in a circular pattern around an injury site, most commonly a fracture.

Because casts increase thickness of the part under examination, technique must be increased also. Although cast construction varies widely, a rule of thumb for technique adjustment is increase mAs two times for fiberglass and dry plaster, and increase mAs three to four times for wet plaster.

One interesting variant of a standard short arm cast that has bearing on a discussion of technique differentials is known as the "sugar tong" splint, so called because its shape resembles the dining implement. The sugar tong consists of a U-shaped length of plaster that extends the length of the forearm from wrist to elbow, covering the dorsal and volar aspects of the forearm, and held in place by wrapping an ace bandage around its length. Depending on the severity of the injury, some physicians may prescribe an additional length of splint to extend to approximately the midhumerus, thus effectively constructing a long-arm sugar tong.

Because a significant amount of swelling accompanies a new fracture injury, it is impractical to apply a standard cast, because as the swelling recedes, the cast will no longer fit, and the effectiveness of immobilization is reduced. Therefore, the sugar tong is used in place of a standard cast when the injury is new. The splint provides sufficient fixation of the injury to allow early healing to take place, and is replaced with a standard cast after 7 to 10 days.

Radiography of the wrist and forearm through the sugar tong is somewhat of an anomaly, because the PA projection must penetrate through two layers of plaster, one on each aspect of the forearm, but the lateral projection is not through plaster. Normal wrist radiography requires a doubling of mAs from PA to lateral projections, but not so in the case of the sugar tong. The PA radiograph must be exposed at increased technique; usually two to four times as much mAs is used, depending on the thickness of the plaster and the relative wetness or dryness of the material, but the lateral film can be exposed at the same technique as the PA—in some cases, even slightly less than the PA projection.

A complete discussion of pediatric radiography is outside the scope of this text; however it should be mentioned that as a general rule, the radiographer should always select the shortest exposure time and, except in rare cases, use the fastest intensifying screen possible when performing examinations of children, in order to decrease the likelihood of motion artifact and possible re-exposure of the patient.

AUTOMATIC EXPOSURE CONTROL

Exposure rooms that are equipped with automatic exposure devices are generally associated with Fixed kVp technique charts. In this case, an ideal kVp or kVp range is selected for each body part, and the exposure is terminated once correct exposure has occurred. With some AEDs , the operator selects a body part and body size at the control panel, and the kVp and mAs are automatically read out on the liquid crystal display (LCD) of the panel. It is worth mentioning that what is really selected in this case is kVp, mA, and a maximum time (S), after which the exposure will terminate. In most cases, the preset maximum time is sufficient, and the exposure is stopped before the max time is reached; however, in cases of large patients, a more lengthy exposure may be required to adequately penetrate the part being examined. If this "backup" time is not increased before making the exposure, then the AED will shut down prematurely, resulting in an underexposed radiograph.

QUESTIONS FOR TECHNIQUE CHARTS

select the best answer

1. The use of calipers is required for which type of chart?

   (A) Fixed kVp
   (B) Variable kVp
   (C) AED controlled chart
   (D) Fixed distance chart

2. The AED accounts for all of the following exposure factor variables EXCEPT:

   (A) distance.
   (B) part thickness.
   (C) pathology.
   (D) positioning.

3. Which of the following sets of exposure factors would be most appropriate to use for a right anterior oblique (RAO) projection of the esophagus?

   (A) 10 mAs, 110 kVp
   (B) 50 mAs, 70 kVp
   (C) 25 mAs, 80 kVp
   (D) 100 mAs, 65 kVp

4. Which of the following is a special consideration that requires a decrease in exposure factors?

   (A) Congestive heart failure
   (B) Osteoporosis
   (C) Pleural effusion
   (D) Osteoarthritis

5. Evaluation of the patient chart before performing an acute abdominal series for a 50-year-old male diabetic patient reveals the presence of abdominal ascites. In order to account for the presence of this condition, the most appropriate technical adjustment from the listed exposure factors of 50 mAs, 70 kVp, 40 inches FFD would be:

   (A) no technical adjustment.
   (B) increase FFD to 72 inches.
   (C) increase exposure factors.
   (D) decrease exposure factors.

▶▶ ANSWERS TO TECHNIQUE CHARTS

1. The answer is (B). As the name implies, the variable kVp technique chart uses a fixed mAs, a baseline kVp, and average thickness for a given body part. The technologist increases or decreases kVp

level according to part thickness. Using this method, the technologist employs metallic calipers to measure the part being examined, selects the fixed mAs, and then adjusts the kVp ± 2 kVp for every 1 cm difference in part thickness.

2. The answer is (D). AEDs work on the principle of preset values equaling exposure values. Whenever the predetermined charge (in the case of a phototimer) has been reached, or the level of ionization has been reached (as with an ionization chamber), the exposure terminates. The AED will account for part thickness, distance, and density increasing or decreasing patient pathology; however, improper positioning over the AED sensor will result in an under- or overexposed radiograph.

3. The answer is (A). The RAO projection is most commonly associated with a barium-filled esophagus. The patient is positioned in the right prone oblique position, with the left hand holding a cup of barium and the drinking straw placed in the patient's mouth. The patient is instructed to drink continuously, and a high kVp, low mAs exposure is made as the patient swallows the barium.

4. The answer is (B). Osteoporosis is a condition characterized by demineralization of bony structures, and is especially common among women over age 60. The loss of bone density requires a reduction in normal exposure factors in order to prevent overexposure of the radiograph. Congestive heart failure and pleural effusion are consistent with the presence of abnormal amounts of fluid in the chest, which require an increase in normal exposure factors, and osteoarthritis is characterized by dense osteophyte formation, which also may require an increase in technique in order to produce an adequately exposed radiograph.

5. The answer is (C). Ascites is an abnormal accumulation of intraperitoneal fluid containing large amounts of fluid and electrolytes. It generally becomes clinically detectable by auscultation, percussion, or palpation when more than 500 cc of fluid has accumulated. The presence of ascitic fluid requires an increase in technical factors (mAs or kVp, depending on the situation) in order to penetrate the increased attenuation of the abdominal cavity.

G. Manual Versus Automatic Exposure Control

The goal of any methodical approach to exposure factors is the same: to produce consistently high-quality

radiographs that are reproducible at the same settings. But because you will encounter both automatic and manual exposure control in the workplace, it is necessary to compare them with respect to the means by which each attains the common goal.

For any given radiology department, both manual and automatic exposure settings are formulated according to known film and screen speeds, FFD, grid ratio and radius, type of generator (single- or three-phase), and processing conditions used with a particular examination. Any change in these factors will obviously affect the efficacy of either method.

To briefly summarize, AEDs have sensors that stop the exposure after a predetermined, known correct exposure has been achieved, and are used almost exclusively in conjunction with tabletop and wall bucky setups. Tabletop exposure techniques, as are used for example with extremity radiography, must be manually set, because no AED can be placed in such a way as to terminate the exposure after the desired density is reached on a tabletop cassette.

There are two primary types of AED. The ionization chamber is located beneath the x-ray tabletop but above the x-ray cassette. The device shuts down the exposure when the correct amount of ionization has been reached. The phototimer, on the other hand, consists of a small fluorescent screen located beneath the cassette. Remnant radiation exposes the film and exits the rear of the cassette, causing the screen to fluoresce, and in turn charging a photomultiplier tube. The photomultiplier tube has preset values that terminate the exposure once the preestablished charge level has been attained.

Manual exposure techniques use varying levels of mA, time, and kVp as the primary variables that are manipulated in order to achieve the desired density and scale of contrast on the radiograph. Specific information regarding the effects of these variables is discussed in greater detail earlier in this chapter.

An AED is equipped with a master density control. The means of representing various changes in density on the control panel varies according to manufacturer, but in general each incremental change represents a 25% change, plus or minus. For example, some machines may give the choice of desired density as −1/2, −1/4, N(normal), +1/4, +1/2, and so on, whereas others may read −3, 2, −1, N, +1, +2, and +3.

There may be occasions when the available master density on the AED will not provide an appropriate setting for the desired radiographic effect; the radiologists may ask for an extremely overpenetrated chest radiograph, for example, as in the case of a metastatic survey, or may ask for a soft-tissue lateral cervical spine study, in order to evaluate the trachea of a pediatric patient. In these and like instances, manual technique is required.

Each AED has a limit as to its shortest possible exposure time, sometimes referred to as minimum reaction time. If the technologist attempts an examination of a fairly low-density object that will reach the desired exposure before the minimum reaction time, the radiograph will be overexposed, because it is not possible to terminate the exposure quickly enough. This situation is another instance in which manual exposure technique is the preferred method.

With AEDs, positioning of the patient is much more critical relative to radiographic quality than with manual technique. The AED is equipped with sensors, the number and location of which again vary according to manufacturer. One popular configuration involves three sensors, one centrally located and two laterally located.

Chest radiography is one example of a type of examination that almost always is performed using an AED. With this scenario, the lateral two sensors are selected for the PA view, one corresponding to each lung field. The left lateral chest view is then obtained using the lateral sensor only, which corresponds to the appearance of the chest in this position. One might encounter a three-sensor AED selector on the x-ray control panel that looks like this:

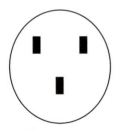

Common methods of selecting this type of AED include a knob that can be turned in order to select one, two, or all three sensors, or a pushbutton system by which one pushes the desired sensors on the control panel itself.

The technologist must correctly select the sensor or sensors that correspond to the part being examined, and the part under examination should be placed directly over the ionization chamber or photocell in order for the density and scale of contrast to be correct. For example, if a PA chest study is being performed, and only the center cell is selected, then the radiograph will be overexposed. In this case more radiation than is necessary to penetrate the chest in the PA position will reach the sensor in the lateral

position, because the chest is thicker laterally than front to back. Similarly, if an AP knee study is performed using one or both outside sensors, the AED will terminate the exposure too quickly, resulting in an underexposed film. In this example, the knee is placed centrally in relation to the film, and there is nothing laterally to attenuate the primary beam, so the preset amount of ionization or charge is achieved prematurely.

Moreover, if the part under examination is incorrectly positioned in relation to the sensor, that is, placed too far mediolaterally, or too superio-inferiorally, the exposure on film will be incorrect, either too dark or too light, depending on the clinical situation.

Therefore, remember that even though the exposure is considered automatic, structural knowledge of the anatomy and adequate positioning skills must be applied in order to produce quality radiographs.

QUESTIONS FOR MANUAL VERSUS AUTOMATIC EXPOSURE CONTROL

select the best answer

1. Which of the listed devices incorporates a fluorescent screen and is located behind the x-ray cassette?

   (A) Phototimer
   (B) Photomultiplier
   (C) Ion chamber
   (D) Cutie pie

2. Increasing kVp from 70 kVp to 110 kVp for a phototimed PA chest examination will result in which of the following effects?

   1. Longer scale of contrast
   2. Increased exposure latitude
   3. More scatter production

   (A) Choice 1 only
   (B) Choices 1 and 2 only
   (C) Choice 3 only
   (D) All of the aforementioned

3. What will happen to radiographic quality if the TFD is increased from 40 inches to 72 inches using an ion chamber type AED?

   (A) Density will decrease
   (B) Contrast will shorten
   (C) Magnification will decrease
   (D) Density will increase

1. The answer is (A). A phototimer is a type of AED that consists of a fluorescent screen located behind the x-ray cassette, which in turn charges a photomultiplier tube that terminates the exposure once a predetermined level of charge has been reached. An ion chamber is another AED device, and a cutie pie is a portable ion chamber used as a radiation survey instrument when exposure levels are in excess of 1 mR/hr.

2. The answer is (D). Increasing kVp on any exposure, whether manually or automatically exposed, will have the effect of producing more scatter radiation and lengthening the scale of contrast present on the radiograph.

3. The answer is (C). By definition, an AED compensates for an increase in TFD by lengthening exposure time. Contrast is primarily governed by kVp selection, which may be changed by the radiographer according to the desired scale of contrast. The higher the kVp, the longer the scale of contrast. Increasing TFD will decrease magnification, although this is not a function of an AED.

II. FILM PROCESSING AND QUALITY ASSURANCE
A. Film Storage

As the field of diagnostic imaging moves toward digital filmless systems, the topic of film processing and quality assurance as we know it will decrease in importance. However, the transition to digital film systems is one requiring a significant monetary commitment, and most radiology departments are shifting incrementally toward the change rather than adopting a wholesale approach. For the moment, therefore, student technologists must acquaint themselves with technology that is now important but that will be considered only from a historical perspective in 10 or 15 years.

Radiographic film must be properly stored and handled in order to maintain optimum quality. An unprocessed film should be clear, except for a slight blue tint manufacturers add to the film base in order to alleviate eyestrain; the film should be free of artifacts of any type. Remember, artifacts are unwanted faults or blemishes on the processed radiograph. Their appearance may stem from a number of causes, some which will be discussed in this section, and the rest later in this chapter.

Film boxes must be stored in an upright position, because stacking the boxes one on top of the other will result in pressure artifacts. These aberrations on the x-ray images have the appearance of fog, and are the result of the sensitive central portion of the film emulsion being exposed to the cumulative weighted pressure of stacked boxes.

Caution must be used in handling of the film. Clean hands are a must in the darkroom; lotions and creams are to be avoided. Gentle fingertip lifting technique is applied when removing the film from the cassette and placing it on the feed tray of the automatic processor. Even slight bending or creasing of the emulsion will result in an artifact, with the appearance of a fingernail or line. This particular type of artifact is often incorrectly attributed to damage inflicted by a fingernail, but it is actually a manifestation of the film's inherent sensitivity to pressure. (See Figure 4-15 [C]).

Temperature of the film storage area must be maintained at no more than 68°F (20°C), because storage temperatures in excess of this temperature will result in increased film fog. Humidity of the storage area is crucial as well, because humidity below 40% will increase the percentage of static artifact, and humidity greater than 60% will likely cause reduced contrast and increased fog.

Static artifact may also occur when technologists slide the film in and out of the cassette, so this practice should be avoided. The precipitating factors for static artifact are fairly simple. Whenever two dissimilar surfaces such as film and intensifying screens are pressed together and separated, a static charge develops. The static charge becomes significant when, as with film and screens, the surfaces are nonconductive, and the humidity is low. A static charge emits light that exposes the film, usually with a tree or branchlike appearance. In order to minimize these artifacts, screens may be treated with an antistatic solution, and low humidity may be offset with the use of a commercial humidifier although, as previously mentioned, relative humidity in the darkroom should not exceed 60%.

Radiographic films are stored and handled in a white light–free environment. If films are exposed to low level, diffuse white light, as might be associated with a minor light leak in the darkroom, then increased levels of film fog will be the result. If bright white light exposes the film, then gross blackening of the film will occur. Some darkrooms incorporate an electronic interlocking device that prevents opening of the film storage bin when the darkroom door is opened, or if the white room light switch is turned on. Light leaks may be observed by completely darkening the darkroom and visually inspecting it after dark adapting one's eyes. If the radiology department includes a nuclear medicine department, care must be taken to avoid bringing radioactive materials into proximity with unprotected boxes of film. Even though these materials are wrapped to prevent occupational exposure, long-term storage of radioactive nuclides near film is sufficient to cause significant levels of fog.

The film bin itself is sufficiently lead-lined so as to prevent radiation from adjacent exposure rooms exposing the film unintentionally. The fog level of unprocessed diagnostic x-ray film is approximately 0.2 mR, so lead thickness in storage bins and shelves where film is stored must be sufficient to protect film from exposure levels above this level.

Safelights are specialized light fixtures that provide a relatively safe means of darkroom illumination while the technician is handling and developing the unprocessed radiograph. The light radiated from a safelight is of a spectral quality and intensity that does not expose medical x-ray film if the film is handled in its presence for less than approximately 1 minute. The word "safe" is used cautiously here, because no darkroom illumination is safe if not used properly. This is particularly true of clinically exposed x-ray film, which is eight times as sensitive to light than is unexposed film. No safelight will provide protection from exposure if the film is left in its presence too long. The type of safelight used must be correctly matched with the type of film being used. Traditional film exposed by calcium tungstate screens is sensitive to the blue-violet end of the light spectrum; therefore, a safelight that only permits light in the yellow-red portion of the spectrum, such as the Wratten 6B safelight filter, a filter used in conjunction with a 7.5- or 15-watt frosted light bulb, or the Kodak GBX all purpose filter, can be used with this type of film. On the other hand, film used in conjunction with rare earth intensifying screens, such as Kodak ortho-green (OG) film, is sensitive primarily to green light, which is closer to the red end of the spectrum than is blue-violet. Therefore, OG film is more sensitive to the yellow-red of the light emitted by the Wratten 6B. The GBX safelight is designed to emit only the lowest portion of the red spectrum, and indirectly illuminates the film, because its light is directed toward the ceiling and directed downward; so this safelight can be used with OG film.

The walls and ceiling of the darkroom should be painted with a light-colored gloss finish paint so as to provide maximum reflection of available light, be-

cause increased reflectivity of the darkroom wall and ceiling surfaces increases the effectiveness of the safelight.

QUESTIONS FOR FILM STORAGE

select the best answer

1. The practice of stacking multiple boxes of film on top of each other instead of in an upright position is not recommended because it is likely to result in:
   (A) pressure artifact.
   (B) static artifact.
   (C) tree artifact.
   (D) pi lines.

2. All of the following are possible darkroom-related causes of film fog EXCEPT:
   (A) white light leak.
   (B) film illumination by safelight over 1 minute.
   (C) humidity under 40%.
   (D) Wratten 6B filter used with rare earth screen film system.

3. Of the following colors emitted by radiologic accessories, the color LEAST likely to fog orthochromatic film would be:
   (A) amber.
   (B) green.
   (C) blue-violet.
   (D) red.

▶▶ ANSWERS TO FILM STORAGE

1. The answer is (A). Film boxes must be stored in an upright position, because stacking the boxes one on top of the other will result in pressure artifacts. These aberrations on the x-ray images have the appearance of fog, and are the result of the sensitive central portion of the film emulsion being exposed to the cumulative weighted pressure of stacked boxes. Static artifact usually has a treelike appearance and is the result of too low humidity and improper film handling. Pi lines are related to the automatic processor and appear as minus density areas on film.

2. The answer is (C). Humidity must be maintained between 40% and 60% in order to maintain film supplies free of image degrading artifact. If humidity falls below 40%, the likelihood of static

artifact increases, whereas humidity greater than 60% is likely to lead to increased fog levels. The Wratten 6B safelight filter is used with film exposed by calcium tungstate screens, but film illumination even by proper safelighting will lead to film fog if the film is held under the safelight too long. White light leaks lead to gross blackening wherever the light falls on the film.

3. The answer is (D). Orthochromatic film is spectrally matched with green light–emitting rare earth intensifying screens and should only be used with a safelight that emits the darkest red portion of the light spectrum. Blue-violet light is emitted by calcium tungstate screens, and amber light is fine for use with this type of film.

B. Cassette Loading

Proper care and storage of cassettes is an integral part of the radiology quality assurance program. As with all components in a quality assurance program, care of cassettes should be documented in order to assure ongoing quality is maintained. Cassettes should be stacked vertically according to size and speed, with a clearly understood labeling system either on the cassette itself or the storage area referring to screen speed. In this way, correct spectral matching of film and screen speed can be achieved with ease. Recall that incorrectly matched film and screen speed results in a loss of density on film and increases repeat radiograph rates. Repeat radiographs are undesirable because of increased patient dose, increased cost, and decreased efficiency.

As with film, stacking cassettes on top of one another, handling the cassettes in a rough manner, or slapping them haphazardly in the passbox are poor practices that increase the likelihood of both internal and external damage. Rough handling may lead to poor film/screen contact. The wire mesh test should be performed on a regular basis in order to evaluate screen film contact. To perform the test, obtain a small piece of wire mesh, such as is commercially available, place the mesh on top of the cassette and make a low, extremity-like exposure of approximately 5 mAs and 40 kVp at 40 inches. Any blurred areas on the resulting radiograph are areas of poor contact that require repair.

Cassettes should be visually inspected both inside and out on a regular basis. Regular cleaning should be done with a commercially prepared solution, and followed with regular application of antistatic solution. The antistatic solution is of particular importance both in low humidity areas and winter months.

Aside from the previously mentioned screen artifacts, dust and lint on the screen itself will produce pinhole artifacts, which are minute specklike areas of minus density on the radiograph.

Additionally, cassettes should be numbered or labeled so that they produce a small label on the radiograph. In this way, artifacts may be eliminated by maintenance, or sent for repair when necessary.

QUESTIONS FOR CASSETTE LOADING

select the best answer

1. Pinhole artifacts are the result of:
   (A) dropping the cassette.
   (B) dust and lint on the intensifying screen.
   (C) defective manufacturing of film.
   (D) humidity over 80%.

2. Spectral mismatch with cassette, film, and intensifying screen can result in:
   (A) loss of density on the radiograph.
   (B) increased patient dose.
   (C) increased cost of care.
   (D) all of the aforementioned.

ANSWERS TO CASSETTE LOADING

1. The answer is (B). Dust and lint on the screen itself will produce pinhole artifacts, which are minute specklike areas of minus density on the radiograph. Pinhole artifacts are easily eliminated by regular cleaning of intensifying screens with a commercially prepared solution.

2. The answer is (D). If the type of film being used in a cassette is not matched correctly with correct screen speed, that is, OG film with rare earth screens, loss of density occurs on the film, resulting in a necessary repeat exposure, increased patient dose, and increased cost to the radiology department for the examination.

C. Radiographic Film Identification

Legally, medical x-ray film must have the following information clearly identified:

- Patient name /ID number
- Name of facility
- Right or left marker
- Date of examination

Optional information that may be included on the radiograph includes:

- Time of examination
- Ordering or admitting physician
- Date of birth or patient age

Portable radiographic examinations are generally identified with additional information, including patient position, that is, supine, upright, or decubitus; technical factors; technologist's initials; and time of day. As with any patient who undergoes multiple examinations on the same day, portable examinations should prominently display time of day on the radiograph so that ready comparisons may be made with previous films. Multiple examinations, particularly of the chest and abdomen, are commonplace among the intensive care population, who often have central lines, feeding or nasogastric tubes, endotracheal tubes, or other supportive devices placed at the bedside, and proper placement of these medical devices may need to be confirmed by portable radiograph.

There are two primary types of film identification systems. The most commonplace involves a moving lead blocker on a cassette that is inserted into a daylight film ID camera that places patient information on the film. Another, older type of system is used in the darkroom. A 3 × 5 card with patient information is placed in the device, commonly called a flasher; the film is removed from the cassette and inserted in the device, and the flasher is depressed, placing the information on the film.

QUESTIONS FOR RADIOGRAPHIC FILM IDENTIFICATION

select the best answer

1. All of the following are legal requisites for film identification EXCEPT:
   (A) date of birth.
   (B) name.
   (C) right or left marker.
   (D) name of institution.

2. Which of the following criteria are considered to be vital information to be included in a portable radiographic examination?
   (A) Patient position
   (B) Time of day
   (C) Technical factors
   (D) All of the aforementioned

▶▶ ANSWERS TO RADIOGRAPHIC FILM IDENTIFICATION

1. The answer is (A). Although the patient's date of birth or age is commonly included on the radio-graph, it is not legally required. It is interesting that patient date of birth is also one of the most common means of positively identifying a specific patient, especially when the patient has a common name. Most hospital computer data bases can search according to various data fields, with date of birth being one of the most important identifiers. Other important search fields include mother's maiden name, date of service, and social security number.

2. The answer is (D). Time of day must be listed on portable examinations so that appropriate comparisons can be made with previous examinations. The radiologist must know the patient position in order to accurately interpret the radiograph, particularly with respect to air and fluid levels. Technical factors are crucial, because another technologist can note the technique used for a certain radiograph and use the same factors on the following examinations, thus ensuring technical cohesion of the examinations. Important technical factors include mAs, kVp, distance, and type of screen/film combination.

D. Automatic Film Processor

The process of film development is the transformation of the latent or unseen image to a manifest or visible one. The automatic processor is a device that mechanically transports the exposed film through a series of chemical baths while providing agitation (moving the film in the chemical), regulation of chemical temperatures, and automatic chemical replenishment. The three primary phases of automatic processing are develop, fix, and wash.

The developer is the chemical agent that converts the latent image into a manifest one. Before the action of chemicals can take place on the exposed film, a wetting agent must be applied to the film in order to swell and expand the emulsion. In automatic processing, the wetting agent is the developer solution. Water is the solvent for all automatic processing solutions.

The developer consists of five primary ingredients: developing agent, activator, restrainer, preservative, and hardener.

The action of the developing agent upon exposed silver bromide crystals that changes the crystals into black metallic silver is called reduction. In reduction, the positive ionic silver is neutralized when the developing agent surrenders an electron and reduces the silver ion. The reduction process is described chemically as:

$$Ag^+ + e^- \rightarrow Ag \qquad (16)$$

The principal reducing agents for rapid automatic

processing are hydroquinone, a slow-acting chemical that is responsible for the blackest tones on the radiograph, and the faster-acting phenidone, which works to produce the gray tones on film. On an H&D curve, hydroquinone influences the shoulder of the curve, and phenidone influences the toe.

In order for the reducing agents to penetrate the gelatin emulsion, the processing chemistry is made alkaline by sodium or potassium carbonate. These chemicals are referred to as the developer solution activator or accelerator.

The developer solution is subject to oxidation over time, a process that reduces its effectiveness. Therefore, a preservative known as sodium sulfite, or cycon, is added to the developer to slow oxidation. Additionally, the hood on the processing unit itself helps to prevent aerial oxidation, which is oxidation that occurs as a result of exposure to room air.

Without the action of potassium iodide or potassium bromide acting as a restrainer, agents that restrict the action of hydroquinone and phenidone, the developing agents would also affect the unexposed silver crystals, producing film fog.

The high temperatures of rapid processing result in excessive swelling of the film emulsion unless the chemical glutaraldehyde is added to the solution as a hardener. Insufficient or depleted hardener often results in processor transport downtime, because a film with too swollen an emulsion will get caught in the rollers and jam the machine. Films that emerge from the machine still damp may also be a sign of improper levels of hardener.

The purpose of the fixer solution is to clear the film of unexposed silver bromide crystals. The chemical fixing agent is ammonium thiosulfate. Fixer is sometimes referred to as the clearing agent. Fixer solution is acidic; it functions to neutralize residual action by the developer. Acetic acid provides the needed acidic medium for the solution and is referred to as the fixer activator. The fixer solution also contains a hardening agent that serves to reharden the emulsion and protect the finished radiograph from abrasions. The fixer hardening agents are potassium alum and aluminum chloride. As is the case with developer, the fixer also contains the preservative sodium sulfite to prevent oxidation.

The wash solution is plain water. It functions to rid the radiograph of residual chemicals that could discolor the radiograph over time. Agitation of the radiograph in the wash aids in this process.

COMPONENTS AND SYSTEMS

The transport system of the automatic processor conveys the film through the various solutions by a system of rollers that are in turn propelled by a series of chains, sprockets, and gears. The transport system assures that the film remains in solution for the proper length of time and provides constant agitation of the film over its surface. The primary components of the transport system are feed tray, deep racks, crossover racks, turnaround assemblies, and receiving bin.

Film enters the processor at the feed tray. The dimensions of the feed tray permit a standard 14 × 17 film to be introduced into the processor crosswise. As the film enters the system, a sensor, or microswitch, initiates replenishment of film chemistry, which continues until the film is entirely past the sensor. It is important that the film be sent through in this manner, because sending the film in lengthwise will result in overreplenishment and increased density on the radiograph.

The crossover racks are located between each of the three solution tanks (developer, fixer, and wash) and the dryer section. They are situated outside the solution and serve as a link between the sections. Crossover racks should be cleaned daily because they rapidly accumulate crystalline solution that can mar film quality. The terminal set of rollers on each processor section applies squeegee action to the film in order to eliminate excess solution.

The turnaround section consists of guide shoes or deflector plates that serve to change the direction of the film from downward to upward motion. Improperly seated guide shoes leave characteristic guide shoe marks, a repetitive linear artifact that indicates the need for guide shoe adjustment (**Figure 4-10**).

When performing routine processor cleaning, it

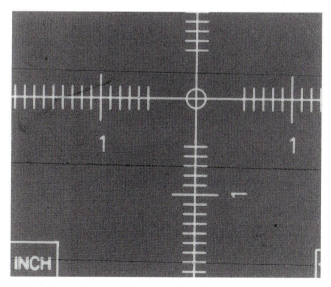

FIGURE 4-10. Guide shoe marks on a test radiograph.

is vital that both crossover and deep racks are properly reseated or film will almost certainly jam in the machine the next time it is run. Although exact temperatures vary according to the manufacturer, solution temperature is quite warm, usually approximately 92° F. Once the machine is shut down, solutions cool, and condensation forms on the inside lid of the processor, which can dilute or contaminate solutions if it is permitted to drip down into the main tanks. Therefore, it is advisable to leave the lid open approximately 1 inch during downtime so that moisture can escape.

As the film travels through each tank, chemistry is carried away with it, diminishing the level of the solution tank. The processor replenishment system infuses the correct amount of replacement chemistry, thereby maintaining a constant level and concentration of solution. Incorrect or insufficient replenishment may be the source for several processor problems. Inadequate replenishment results in decreased immersion time and inadequate density on the finished film, and incorrect developer replenishment may also lead to inadequate hardener reaching the film. A film with too soft and swollen an emulsion may jam inside the racks.

Automatic processors are equipped with a thermostat-controlled temperature regulation system that maintains solution temperature at approximately 92° to 95°F. Of the three solutions, developer temperature is most crucial, because even minor fluctuations can produce visible density changes on the radiograph.

The replenishment system works in conjunction with the recirculation system. The recirculation system functions primarily to provide agitation that maintains solution contact against the film emulsion, filters debris, and maintains solution concentration and temperature.

The wash and dryer systems of the automatic processor function together to ensure that the radiograph maintains sufficient archival quality. The wash removes residual chemistry, primarily residual fixer, which, if allowed to remain on the film surface, will yellow the film and degrade the image over time. The wash process is enhanced by agitation provided by the recirculation system. The processor dryer operates at approximately 120° to 130° F, blowing warm, dry air over the film surface to dry and shrink the emulsion to its finished state. Maintenance of proper temperature is essential, because excessive temperatures will result in brittle film, and inadequate temperature will result in film that is too damp.

MAINTENANCE

The two primary advantages of automatic film processing over that of manual processing are decreased total time to produce a finished radiograph and improved consistency of results. In order to maintain consistency, however, preventive maintenance must be performed on a regular basis.

At start up time, crossover racks should be cleaned with a gentle cloth and warm water to remove residual chemistry. Manual inspection of deep solution racks and replenisher tanks should also occur at this time. Frequently, low tanks are indicative of a systemic problem with the equipment, and responsible parties should be notified if the problem persists. The feed tray and receiving bin should be wiped clean with a gentle cloth and commercially prepared antistatic solution, and four unexposed 14 × 17 films should be run through the machine to pick up any debris left on rollers. Unexposed films are used because exposed film may contain residual fixer. Sensitometric testing, which is discussed fully earlier in this chapter, should be performed, and the results should be recorded at this time. When the machine is shut down, crossover racks should be recleaned, and the lid should be left open approximately 1 inch to permit moisture to escape.

Even with a conscientious preventative maintenance program, malfunction of the automatic processor can lead to noncontributory observable effects on the radiograph, and the technologist should be acquainted with their various causes. As previously mentioned, improperly positioned or sprung guide shoe marks leave a characteristic mark on the film, usually on the leading or trailing edge of the radiograph. Pi lines, so called because they occur at 3.14-inch intervals, are the result of a dirty or stained roller. Most rollers are 1 inch in diameter; therefore, 3.14 inches represent one revolution. Improperly mixed or contaminated processor chemistry results in chemical fog, which is similar in appearance to radiation-induced film fog—a uniform, image-degrading gray over the entire radiograph. Irregular or dirty developer tank rollers can cause pressure during development, which results in wet pressure sensitization, an artifact that appears as small circular areas of increased density on the image. Chemical stains may appear in varying colors on the radiograph, including blue, purple, yellow, and green. The general name given all chemical type stains is dichroic, which is a term that means in two colors. The curtain effect occurs when chemicals are not properly squeezed off rollers, and chemistry runs up or down the radiograph, producing a characteristic curtainlike appearance **(Figure 4-11)**.

The key measurement of a processor maintenance program is sensitometry. Recall that sensitometry is accomplished with the sensitometer, a precise instrument that exposes a stepwedge image on the quality

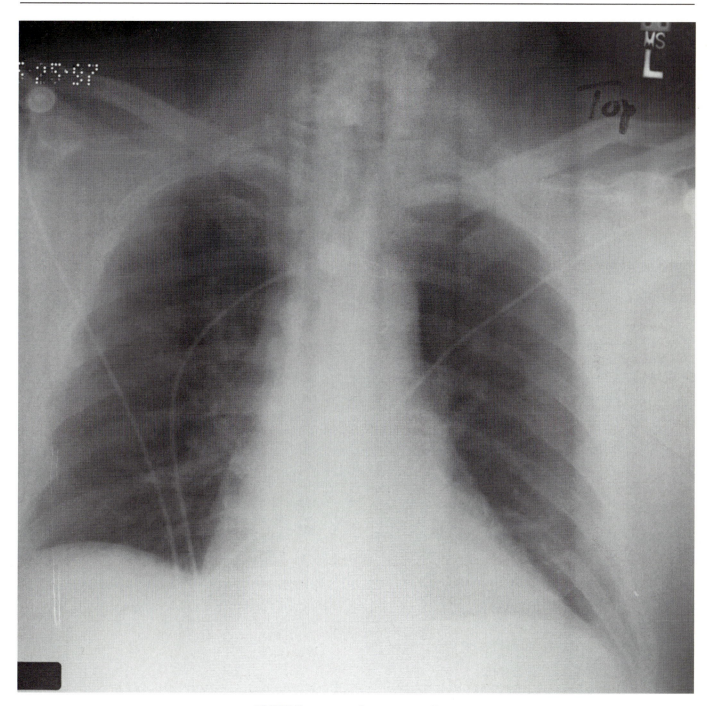

FIGURE 4-11.   The curtain effect.

control film, and a densitometer, an instrument that reads the various steps and gives numeric density data concerning each. These data are then compared to baseline data, logged, and then changes in temperature or chemistry are made, if necessary. A specific box of film is designated for quality control purposes only in order to maintain as pristine a film condition as possible.

SYSTEM MALFUNCTION

The causes of automatic processor system malfunction can be categorized into simple groups. Transport malfunctions occur when the film hangs at some point in the system and fails to drop into the receiving bin. The technologist may be alerted to this problem by an audible clicking as the film passes repeatedly over a crossover rack, or the film may become lodged in a deep rack or the dryer assembly, which will not produce a sound. In either case, it will soon become apparent that a film is missing.

Inadequate replenishment leads to insufficient hardener concentration in the developer solution. Without adequate chemical hardening, the film emulsion remains swollen and will stick to rollers. If the problem remains undetected while numerous films are being run, entire examinations can be ruined, and repeat examinations are necessary.

The cycle of film through the processor is precisely timed. When multiple films are being run, the leading film must reach a given point in the system before another may be fed in; that point is signaled either audibly or visibly, which indicates the go-ahead for the next film. Films introduced into the system too rapidly will overlap and jam. Overlapped films can adhere to each other and will not be properly processed, which prevents their use for diagnosis even if they are "rescued" by manually pulling them from the jammed area. Misaligned crossover or deep racks will also cause transport system jams.

Damp films can be attributed to the dryer assembly; the temperature may be set too low, or the dryer motor may be faulty. Inadequate hardener in developer or fixer concentration may also lead to damp films.

Inadequate or excessive density can also be processor-related. Elevated developer temperature or solution concentration increases the action of the reducing agents phenidone and hydroquinone, causing dark films. Too low developer temperature or concentration causes light films.

Darkroom-related fog may result from improper safelight conditions, light leak, or improper storage conditions. Outdated film may also be fogged. Last, processor solutions that are mixed with other solutions, as when fixer is splashed in developer, are said to be contaminated. Contaminated developer results in overall film fog.

QUESTIONS FOR AUTOMATIC FILM PROCESSOR

select the best answer

1. Of the following, which could be described as ideal storage conditions for medical x-ray film?
   (A) Greater than 70°F, less than 70% humidity
   (B) Between 70°F and 80°F, and less than 70% humidity

   (C) Less than 70°F, between 40% and 60% humidity
   (D) Between 40°F and 60°F and greater than 70% humidity

2. All of the following information must be included on every radiograph EXCEPT:
   (A) age or birth date.
   (B) right or left marker.
   (C) patient name or ID number.
   (D) name of institution.

3. The chemical responsible for clearing the film of unexposed, undeveloped silver bromide crystals is:
   (A) potassium bromide.
   (B) ammonium thiosulfate.
   (C) hydroquinone.
   (D) sodium sulfite.

4. Which of the following functions performed by an automatic processor is carried out by the recirculation system?
   (A) Removing residual chemicals from emulsion
   (B) Keeping fresh solution in contact with emulsion
   (C) Recirculating air
   (D) Contributing to archival quality

5. The chemical _____ is known as a restrainer; its function is to _____
   (A) glutaraldehyde, control emulsion swelling
   (B) phenidone, produce gray tones
   (C) potassium bromide, act as an antifog agent
   (D) sodium carbonate, provide alkaline medium

6. The process of reduction can be described chemically as:
   (A) $Ag^= + Ag^+ = Ag$
   (B) $Ag + e^- = Ag^-$
   (C) $Ag^+ + e^- = Ag$
   (D) $Ag^+ + Ag^+ = 2Ag$

7. The correct range of developer temperature for a 90-second automatic film processor is:
   (A) 60°F to 75°F.
   (B) 70°F to 90°F.
   (C) 80°F to 90°F.
   (D) 90°F to 95°F.

▶▶ ANSWERS FOR AUTOMATIC FILM PROCESSOR

1. The answer is (C). Medical x-ray film must be stored at temperatures no greater than 70°F. Hu-

midity should be between 40% and 60%. Excessively low humidity increases the chance of static artifact production, whereas excessive humidity may cause overall film fog.

2. The answer is (A). Although date of birth or age is very commonly included on the radiograph, it is not required. Legally, name or ID number, name of institution, examination date, and right or left marker must be included.

3. The answer is (B). Ammonium thiosulfate is the fixing, or clearing, agent. Its function is to clear the film of unexposed, undeveloped silver bromide crystals. Sodium sulfite is a preservative used in both developer and fixer. Hydroquinone is the slow-acting reducing agent in the developer solution that builds black tones in areas of greater exposure on film.

4. The answer is (B). The recirculation system performs four primary functions. By solution agitation, it maintains solution contact with the film emulsion, and provides uniform solution concentration and temperature throughout the tanks. The system also removes debris, such as gelatin particles, from the solution.

5. The answer is (C). Potassium bromide is added to the developer in order to limit the activity of the activator to that of the exposed crystals. Without the action of the restrainer, the developing agents would interact with the unexposed crystals, producing film fog. Therefore, the restrainer is regarded as an antifog agent.

6. The answer is (C). The action of the developing agent upon exposed silver bromide crystals that changes the crystals into black metallic silver is called reduction. In reduction, the positive ionic silver is neutralized when the developing agent surrenders an electron and reduces the silver ion. The reduction process is described chemically as:

$$Ag^+ + e^- \rightarrow Ag \qquad (17)$$

7. The answer is (D). Although exact temperatures vary by manufacturer, the range for developer temperature is approximately 90° F to 95°F. Of all the solutions contained in the processor, developer temperature is most critical, because even slight variations may cause image-degrading density changes on the radiograph.

III. EVALUATION OF RADIOGRAPHS
A. Criteria for Diagnostic-Quality Radiographs

The factors that affect radiographic quality are numerous and interrelated. For any one radiographic result,

there may be multiple contributing components relative to an image-degrading deficiency, or one. Accurate critical assessment must be based not only on the empiric information, but also on a detailed understanding of the clinical situation that produced it. Therefore, learning to critically evaluate radiographs is a skill that can only be thoroughly acquired through a combination of practical experience and persistent scholarship.

DENSITY

As a starting point in the learning process, the technologist must understand the baseline criteria necessary for a diagnostic-quality radiograph. First and foremost, the radiograph must demonstrate appropriate radiographic density. Density may be defined as the degree of blackening present on the finished radiograph. Overexposure of the radiograph obliterates needed anatomic information by producing too much overall blackening, and is primarily caused by excessive radiation reaching the image receptor. Similarly, an underexposed film lacks sufficient density to display important details, and is caused by insufficient radiation exposure. For example, **Figure 4-12** (A) is an underexposed, or too-light lateral chest radiograph. The ill-defined cardiac silhouette makes diagnosis difficult. The patient was unable to completely raise his arms, which worsened the underexposed effect on the superior portion of the chest. Figure 4-12 (B) is a correctly exposed portable AP chest examination. The lung fields, cardiac silhouette, and mediastinum are well defined, with a central line in place in the region of the superior vena cava. Figure 4-12 (C) demonstrates a grossly overexposed AP foot examination. The exposure was made using a phantom, hence the visualized metallic objects. Visualization of the thinner metatarsal region of the foot is completely obscured, whereas the thicker tarsal region attenuated more of the primary beam and is partially appreciated.

CONTRAST

Radiographic contrast is defined as the difference in densities of adjacent structures on the radiograph. Contrast may be either short-scale, high-contrast, with the radiograph demonstrating sudden changes from black to white and few intermittent levels of gray; or long-scale, low-contrast, with the radiograph exhibiting a wide range of slightly differing shades of gray. **Figure 4-13** (A) demonstrates a short-scale chest radiograph produced using a 12:1 grid and an

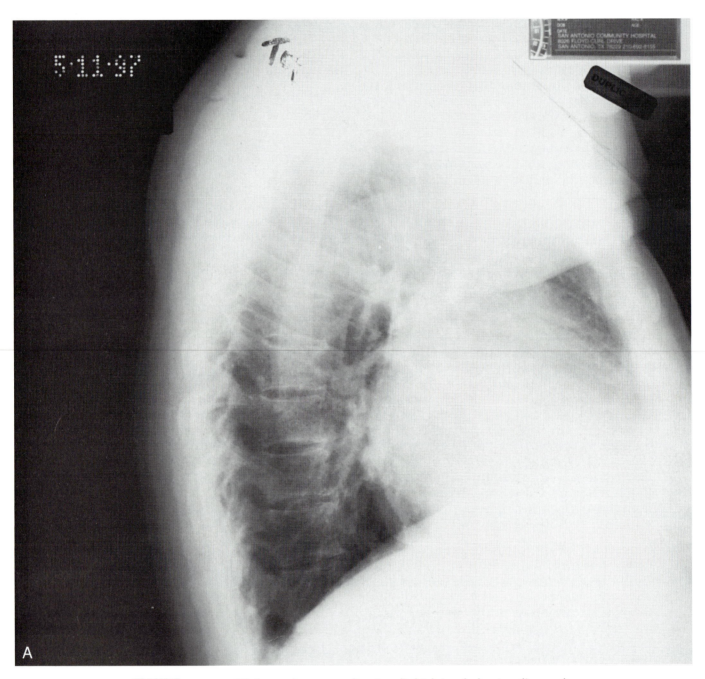

FIGURE 4-12. *(A)* An underexposed or too-light lateral chest radiograph.

AED. Although the grid provided admirable scatter cleanup, the selected kVp was inadequate; therefore, the AED compensated with a longer exposure time, yielding the inappropriately short-scale film. Most radiologists prefer a long scale of contrast for chest radiography, using 100 to 140 kVp in conjunction with a grid, or with a wide latitude film and fast screen system, as is demonstrated in Figure 4-13 (B). This portable AP chest examination is typical of the desired long scale of contrast associated with portable radiography.

RECORDED DETAIL

Recorded detail is another important image quality factor. There are two important considerations for detail: image sharpness and image visibility. Image sharpness refers to the clarity of structural lines and borders and lack of penumbra. The controlling factors for recorded detail are also referred to as geometric factors, and include FFD, focal spot size, and OFD. Secondary controlling factors include intensifying screen speed and the presence or lack of motion. A radiograph that demonstrates optimum detail uses the longest appropriate FFD, the least amount of OFD, and the smallest feasible focal spot, with tube heating overload taken into account. **Figure 4-14** demonstrates how varying screen speeds and technique can be used to demonstrate optimum detail. The patient came to the emergency room to be evaluated for trauma and was sent to the radiology department in order to rule out fracture of the nasal bones. Figure 4-14 (A) is a Waters' view of the maxillary sinus. The exposure was made in the bucky using a 40-inch FFD,

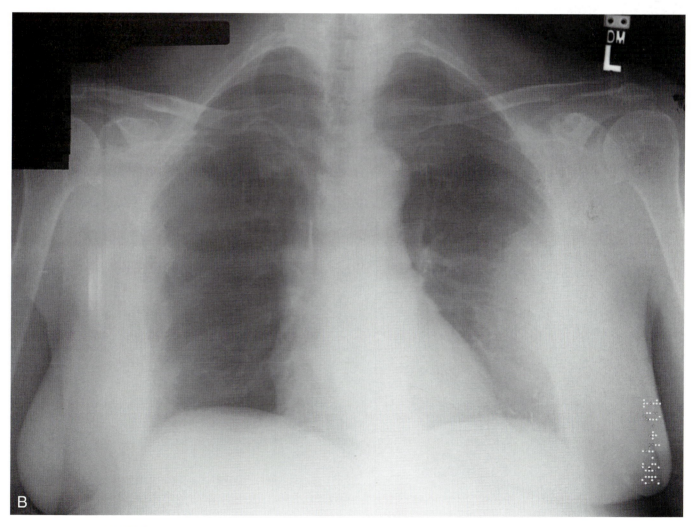

FIGURE 4-12. *(continued) (B)* A correctly exposed portable AP chest examination.

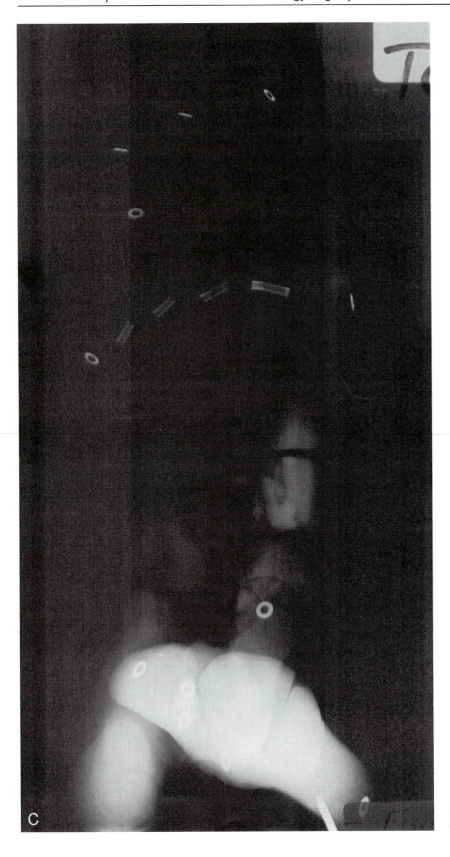

FIGURE 4-12. *(continued) (C)* A grossly overexposed AP foot examination.

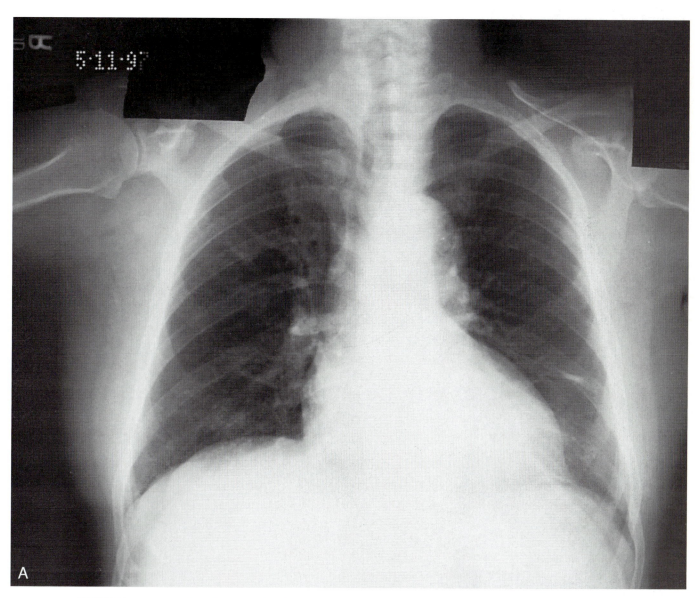

FIGURE 4-13.   *(A)* A short-scale chest radiograph produced using a 12:1 grid and an AED.

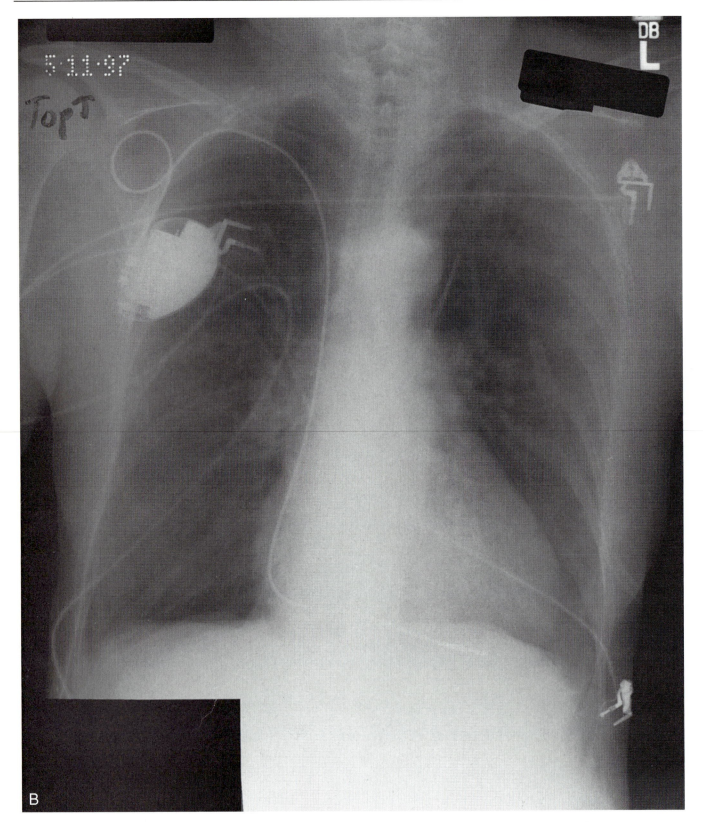

FIGURE 4-13. *(continued) (B)* This portable AP chest examination is typical of the desired long scale of contrast associated with portable radiography.

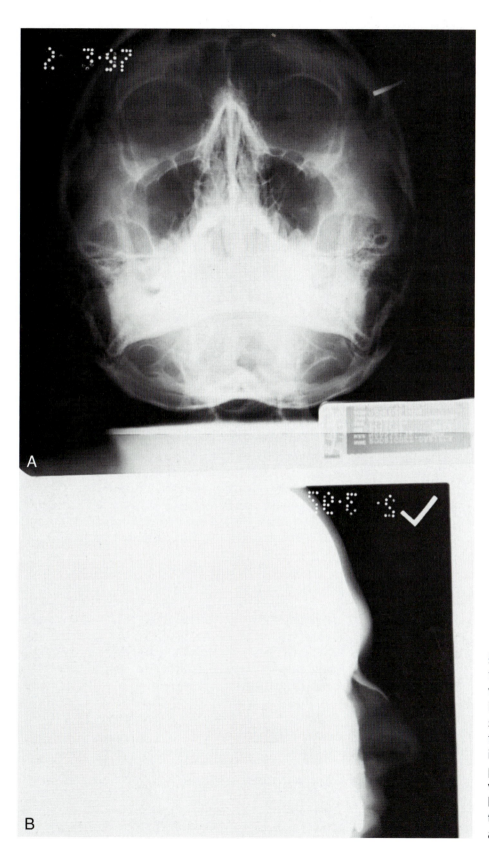

FIGURE 4-14. *(A)* Waters' view of the maxillary sinus. The exposure was made in the bucky using a 40-inch FFD, 400-speed rare earth screens, 32 mAs, and 76 kVp. This technique provides excellent visualization of the nasal bones in the PA plane. *(B)* Closely collimated lateral view of the nasal bones performed by tabletop, using a 100-speed detail cassette, 40-inch FFD, 5 mAs, and 60 kVp.

400-speed rare earth screens, 32 mAs, and 76 kVp. This technique provides excellent visualization of the nasal bones in the PA plane. Figure 4-14 (B) is a closely collimated lateral view of the nasal bones performed by tabletop, using a 100-speed detail cassette, 40-inch FFD, 5 mAs, and 60 kVp.

DISTORTION

Distortion is misrepresentation of the size or shape of the anatomic area of interest. Tube-part-film alignment and patient positioning are the primary controlling factors relative to image distortion. The primary radiographic manifestations of distortion are elongation and foreshortening. **Figure 4-15** (A) and (B) were obtained using the foot phantom. Radiograph A used a 45-degree cephalic tube angulation versus the normal 15-degree angulation, and demonstrates elongation. Radiograph B used a 25-degree caudal angulation and demonstrates foreshortening.

ARTIFACTS

Artifacts are faults or densities present on the radiograph for reasons unrelated to the normal course of the examination. They may result from poor patient instructions, improper handling of film, automatic processing, defective film or intensifying screens, or other radiographic accessories. **Figure 4-16** (A) is an upright AP chest examination. The patient was disoriented and unable to stand, so the procedure was carried out with the patient sitting upright on a stretcher. Can you see the artifact? It may not appear to you right away. Look at the cardiac silhouette. The patient's hand overlies the area of interest. In this instance, the technologist was not observing the patient carefully, and a repeat exposure had to be obtained. In addition, debris was left on the feed tray of the processor that adhered to the film and is visible over the cardiac silhouette. Figure 4-16 (B) is another example of an artifact that could have easily been prevented. In this case, the patient was permitted to leave his shirt on for the PA chest examination. Unfortunately, he had a pen in his pocket! Figure 4-16 (C) is an example of the so-called "fingernail" artifact, a spurious mark caused by rough film handling, not by a fingernail. In this case, the artifact was present in the heart; however, it was of no consequence, because the poorly positioned film required a repeat exposure anyway. Figure 4-16 (D) is a scout film for an IVP examination. The film was run too closely together with other films, which caused a processor jam. When the films were retrieved, they were stuck together, and the emulsion was scratched by pulling them apart.

GRID ALIGNMENT

The primary result of improper tube-part-grid-film alignment is grid cutoff. **Figure 4-17** demonstrates the consequences of lateral decentering on an AP hip examination. The examination was performed in the bucky at 40 inches SID, and a 14 × 17 film was used instead of the more standard 10 × 12 film in order to visualize the longer-than-normal postoperative area of interest. There is drastic loss of density on one lateral aspect of the radiograph, caused by improper lateral centering. Additionally, the superior-inferior plane of the radiograph was improperly centered relative to the area of interest, and the hip itself is not seen.

PROPER DEMONSTRATION OF ANATOMIC STRUCTURES

In order to be of diagnostic quality, the radiograph must depict the area of interest in the desired position and projection. Film size and collimation must be appropriate relative to the desired examination. For example, a PA chest examination incidentally includes the humeral heads and clavicles; however, you certainly would not want to use a 14 × 17 cassette to radiograph an injured clavicle or shoulder, nor should you needlessly expose the patient to radiation that lies outside the area of interest.

Technical factors are also a consideration. Consider the example of the chest and ribs. Although geographically these parts lie in the same region, a rib series generally uses low kVp, short-scale radiographic technique in order to best demonstrate the ribs, whereas a chest examination uses relatively high kVp, long-scale technique in order to best represent the lungs, heart, and mediastinum.

Close attention must be given tube-part-grid-film alignment in order for the desired structure to be appreciated on film.

IDENTIFICATION MARKERS

For medicolegal reasons, patient name, date, right or left side marker, and facility name must be clearly visible on each radiograph. A number of methods for pro-

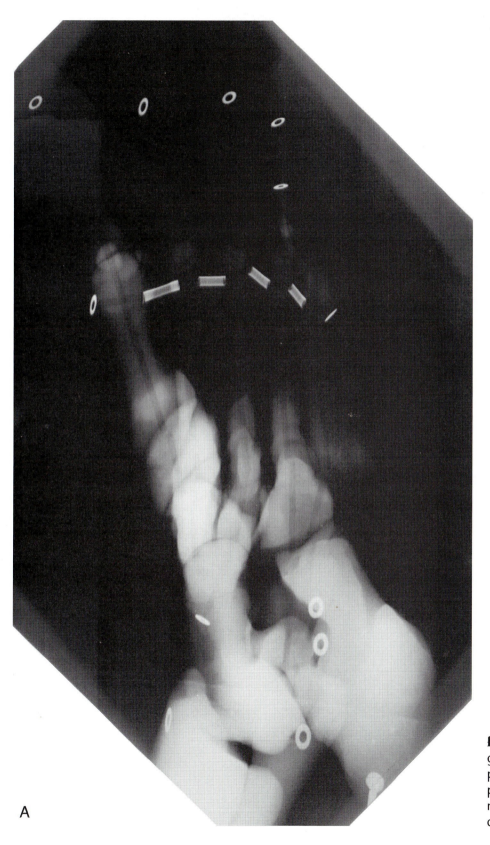

A

FIGURE 4-15. These radiographs were obtained using a foot phantom. *(A)* used a 45-degree cephalic tube angulation versus the normal 15-degree angulation, and demonstrates elongation.

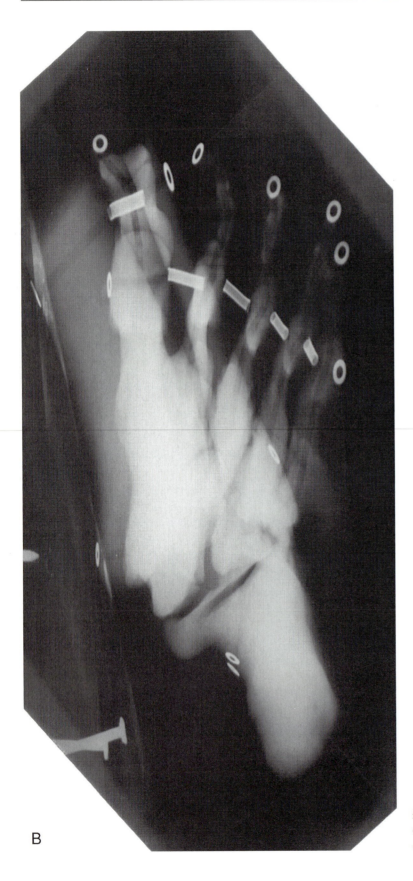

B

FIGURE 4-15. *(continued) (B)* used a 25-degree caudal angulation and demonstrates foreshortening.

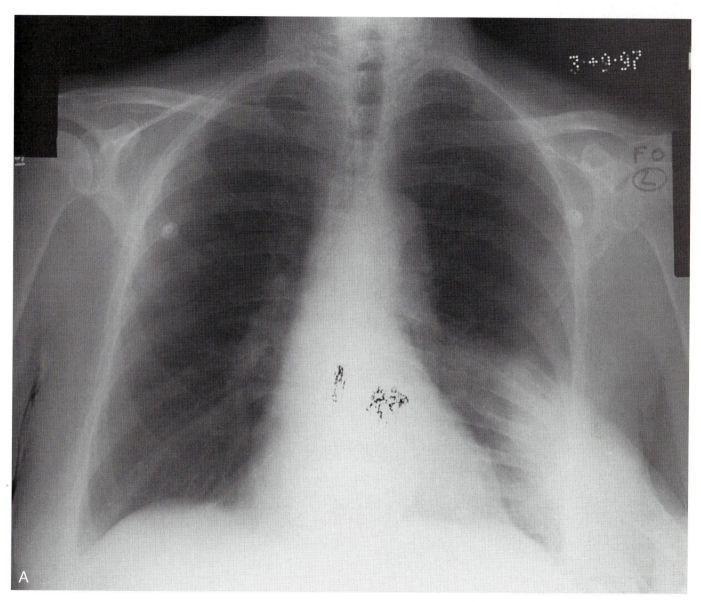

FIGURE 4-16. Artifacts. *(A)* An upright AP chest examination in which the patient's hand overlies the area of interest. In addition, debris left on the feed tray of the processor adhered to the film and is visible over the cardiac silhouette.

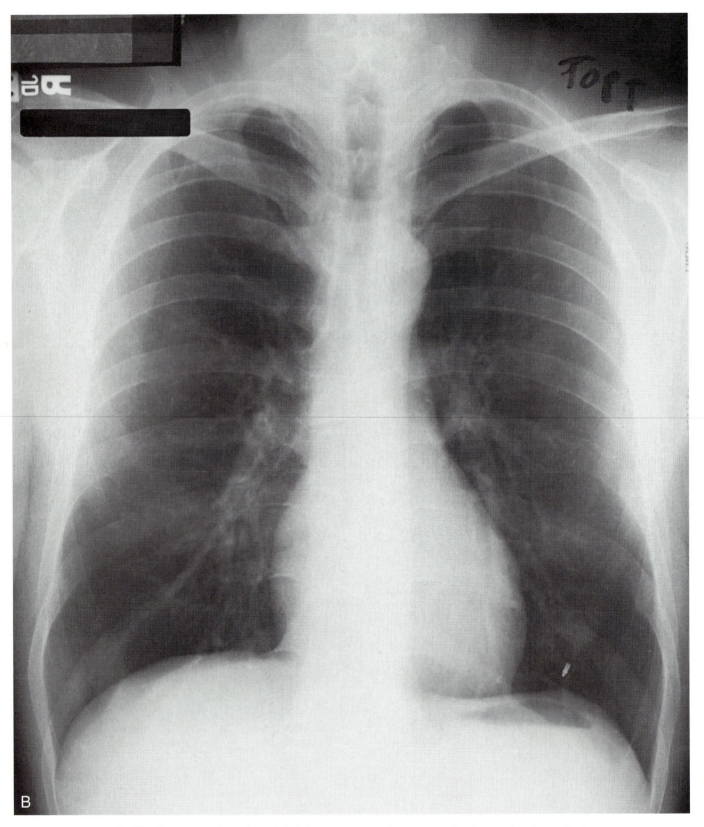

FIGURE 4-16. *(continued) (B)* Artifact created by a pen in the patient's pocket.

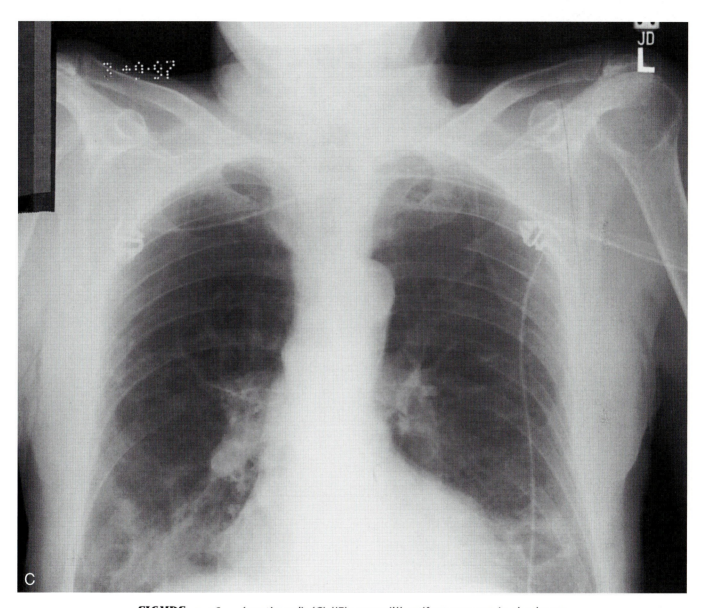

FIGURE 4-16.   *(continued) (C)* ''Fingernail'' artifact present in the heart.

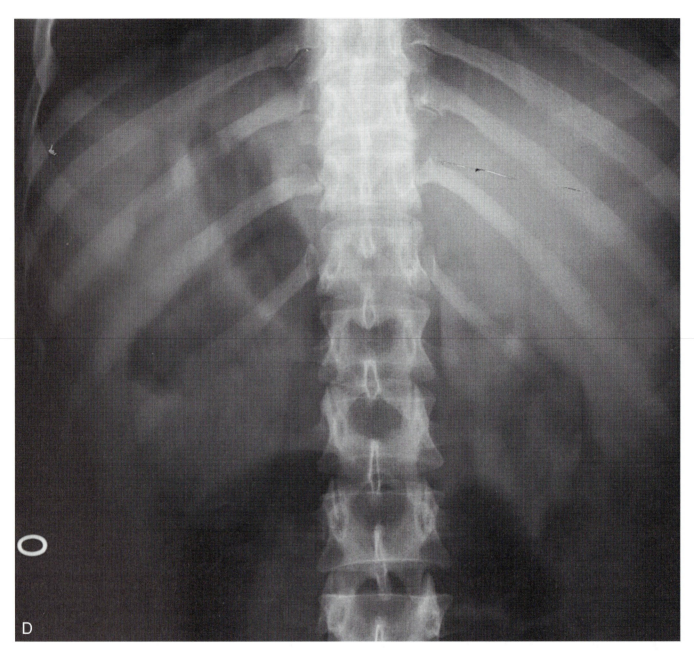

FIGURE 4-16. *(continued) (D)* Cracked emulsion on a scout film for an IVP examination; a processor jam caused some films to stick together, and the emulsion was scratched by pulling them apart.

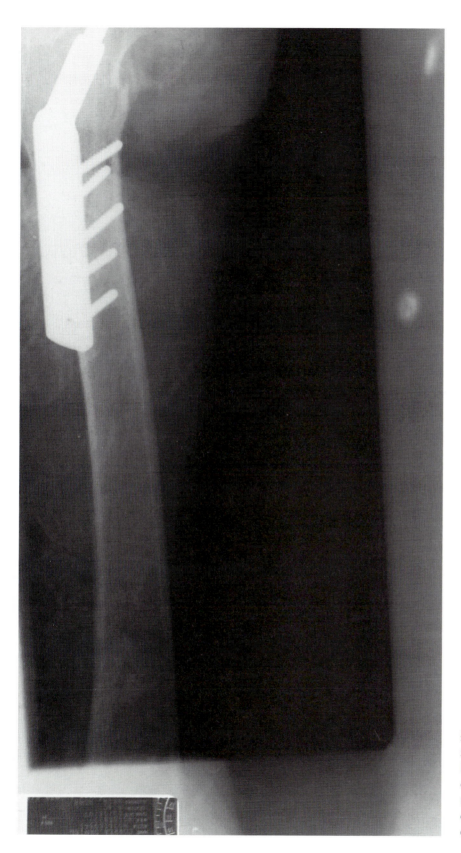

FIGURE 4-17. AP hip examination showing drastic loss of density on one lateral aspect, caused by improper lateral centering. In addition, the superior–inferior plane of the radiograph was improperly centered relative to the area of interest, and the femoral head is not seen.

viding film identification, along with a variety of commercially made products such as date stickers, are available for this purpose. Films should not pass the quality control area for reading until all legally required information is determined to be present on the radiograph.

QUESTIONS FOR CRITERIA FOR DIAGNOSTIC-QUALITY RADIOGRAPHS

select the best answer

1. **Figure 4-18 (A)** was exposed using a 100-speed screen/film system, and **Figure 4-18 (B)** was made using a 400-speed screen/film system. Which of the following statements are true concerning these foot films?
   - (A) Film (A) demonstrates better detail and required less technique than did film (B).
   - (B) Film (A) demonstrates better detail and required more technique than did film (B).
   - (C) Film (B) demonstrates better detail and required less technique than did film (A).
   - (D) None of the aforementioned are true statements.

2. All of the following statements are true concerning **Figure 4-19,** which is a portable AP chest examination taken in the ICU, EXCEPT:
   - (A) the film demonstrates a long scale of contrast.
   - (B) the film has a wide exposure latitude.
   - (C) the film exhibits proper demonstration of anatomic structures.
   - (D) the film demonstrates foreshortening.

3. The most appropriate technical correction regarding the lateral thoracic spine radiograph in **Figure 4-20** would be:
   - (A) increase mAs.
   - (B) increase kVp.
   - (C) decrease exposure time.
   - (D) increase distance.

4. The artifact that appears on the inferior aspect of the cardiac silhouette in **Figure 4-21** is most likely related to:
   - (A) poor screen film contact.
   - (B) low humidity.
   - (C) incorrect stacking of film boxes.
   - (D) rough handling.

5. The terms that best describe the scale of contrast in the portable AP chest radiograph in **Figure 4-22** is:
   - (A) short-scale, low kVp.
   - (B) short-scale, high kVp.
   - (C) long-scale, low kVp.
   - (D) long-scale, high kVp.

6. The AP chest radiograph in **Figure 4-23** required a repeat exposure because of:
   - (A) motion.
   - (B) technique.
   - (C) artifact.
   - (D) distortion.

▶▶ ANSWERS TO CRITERIA FOR DIAGNOSTIC-QUALITY RADIOGRAPHS

1. The answer is (B). A 100-speed system is slower than a 400-speed system and requires more technique to produce the same approximate density on film. The slower the film and intensifying screen speed, the greater the detail recorded on the image receptor.

2. The answer is (D). Virtually all film used in conjunction with portable radiography, and in particular with portable chest radiography, has wide exposure latitude. As is the case with this radiograph, in general this type of screen/film combination exhibits a long scale of contrast. This examination is properly positioned relative to the area of interest, and in particular does not demonstrate evidence of poor tube-part-film alignment, as would be the case with a film that demonstrated foreshortening or elongation.

3. The answer is (A). The radiograph is underexposed. The primary controlling technical factor for density is mAs. Increasing kVp would increase density; however, it will also lengthen the scale of contrast, which is an undesirable effect relative to this examination. Decreasing exposure time might be desirable in conjunction with an increase in mA, because it would decrease the likelihood of patient motion; however, as a solitary technical change, it would decrease density. Increasing distance would decrease magnification but also decrease density.

4. The answer is (B). Figure 4-21 demonstrates an example of a static artifact, commonly attributed to low-humidity conditions.

5. The answer is (D). Portable chest radiography is typically performed with a low mAs–high kVp technique—using film that has wide exposure latitude—and produces a long scale of contrast.

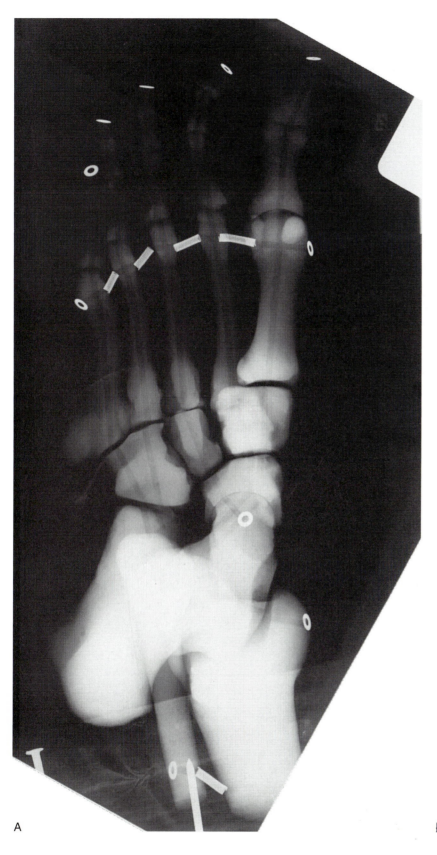

A

FIGURE 4-18.   *(A)* See Question 1.

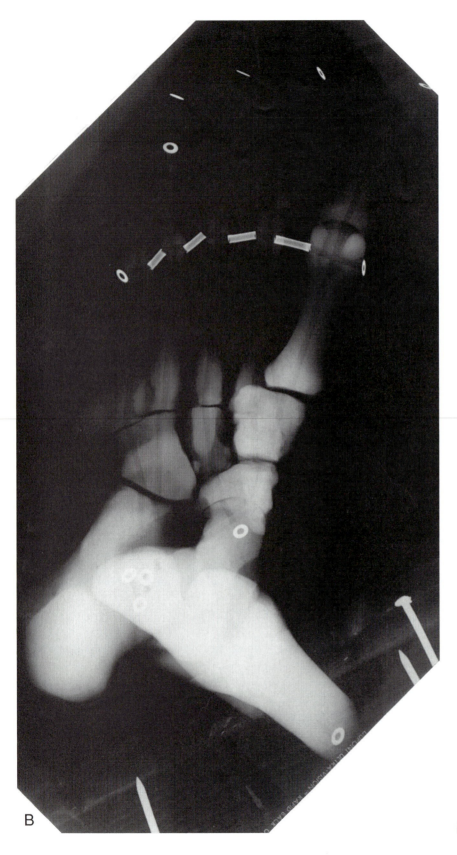

B

FIGURE 4-18. *(continued) (B)*

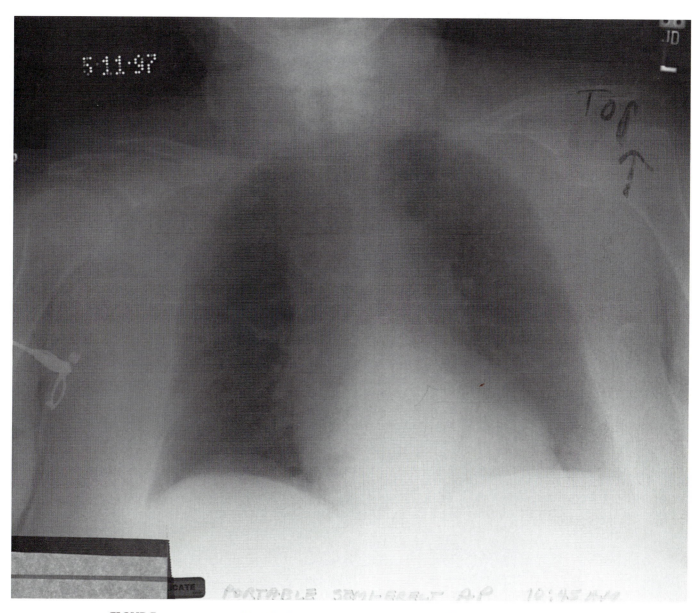

FIGURE 4-19. Portable AP chest examination taken in the ICU. See Question 2.

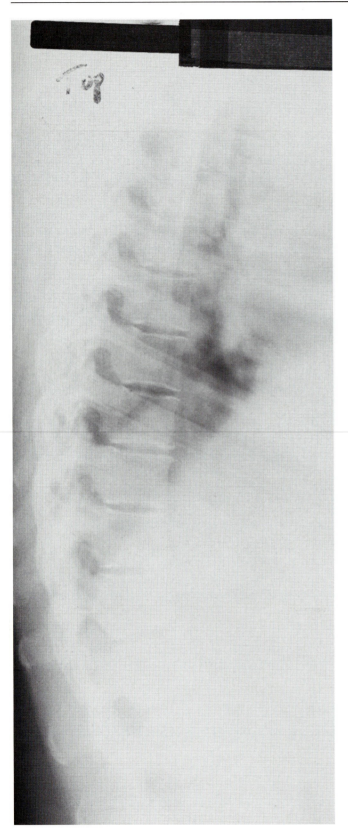

FIGURE 4-20. Lateral thoracic spine radiograph. See Question 3.

6. The answer is (C). The intensifying screen used in making this exposure was dirty, causing multiple specklike areas of opacity. Additionally, the radiograph demonstrates the "curtain effect," a processor-related artifact described earlier in this chapter.

B. Causes of Poor Radiographic Quality: Improving the Suboptimal Image

Given the factors or combinations of factors that can conceivably contribute to imaging errors, it would be impractical to illustrate them all here. Suffice it to say that the technologist must learn to recognize the nature of imaging errors and their corresponding causes, and then demonstrate an ability to correct them. It is helpful, however, to understand that the causes and corrective actions relative to the suboptimal image may be categorized into groups. Technical factors represent the first and perhaps most comprehensive group of imaging components. Primary considerations in this group include the mAs–density relationship; the inverse square law; the 50-15 rule; the effect of distance variance on grids; grid ratio, radius, and type; film and intensifying screen speed and its relationship to density and detail; and filtration.

Patient positioning represents another important group, and will be discussed completely in the next chapter. Important positioning information contained in this chapter, however, includes the effects of OID, SID, and tube-part-grid-film alignment on varying image receptors. Various patient considerations, such as the presence or absence of pathology and the patient's ability to cooperate with the requirements of the requested examination, as with suspension of respiration or cessation of movement, must also be taken into account. Processing conditions account for another significant portion of suboptimal images, and variables such as developer, fixer, and dryer temperature; cleanliness of processor rollers and tanks; correct safelighting; and proper storage of film and accessories must be considered. Last, the technologist must be able to identify and correct an extensive group of image-degrading artifacts.

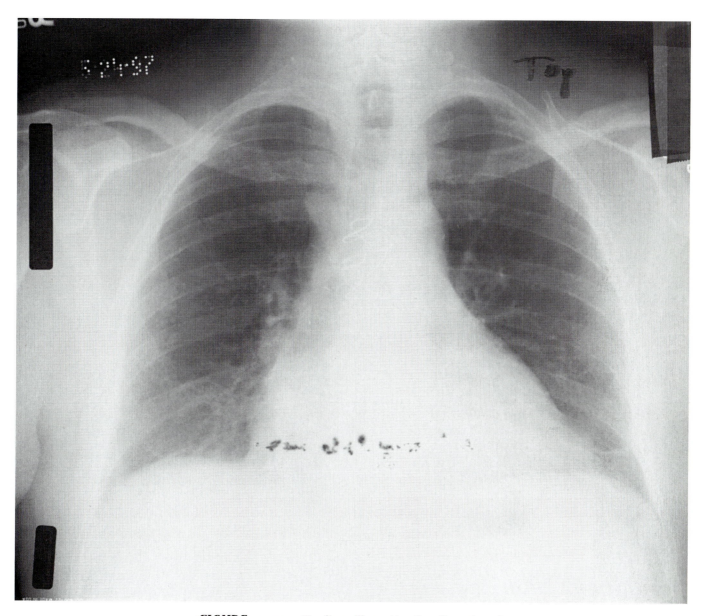

FIGURE 4-21.   Cardiac silhouette. See Question 4.

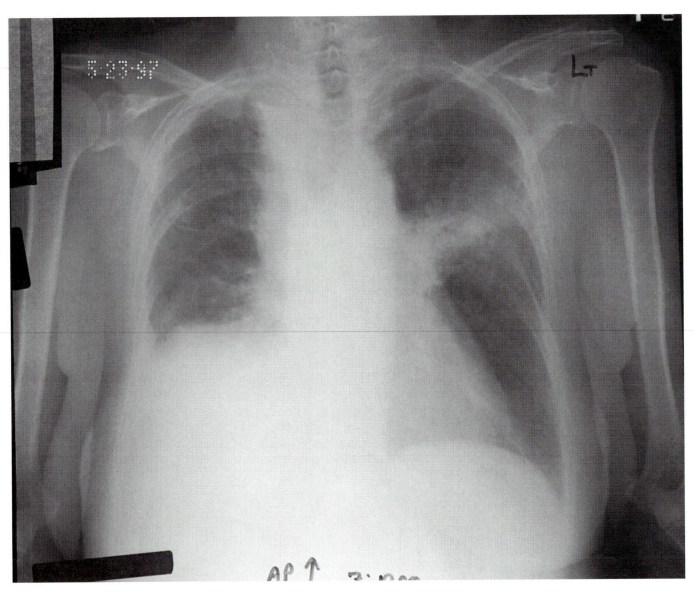

FIGURE 4-22. Portable AP chest radiograph. See Question 5.

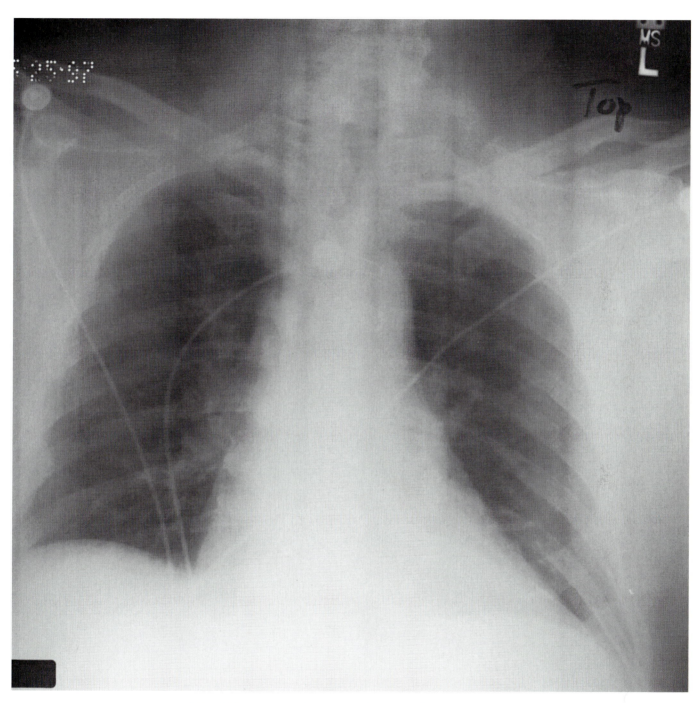

FIGURE 4-23.   AP chest radiograph. See Question 6.

END-OF-CHAPTER EXAMINATION

►► QUESTIONS

Select the best answer

1. Which of the following primary exposure factors describes the amount of current flowing through the x-ray tube?

   (A) kVp
   (B) mA
   (C) S
   (D) OID

2. Refer to **Figure 4-24,** which depicts the effects of beam divergence on an AP abdominal radiograph. The circles in the abdomen represent hypothetical lesions. Which of the following statements are true concerning lesion C?

   (A) Lesion C is foreshortened and magnified compared to A and B.
   (B) Lesion C is elongated and magnified compared to A and B.
   (C) Lesion C is elongated but less magnified than lesion B.
   (D) Lesion C is foreshortened and is the least magnified of the three lesions.

3. Which of the following systems are responsible for chemical agitation in a 90-second automatic film processor?

   (A) Dryer and transport
   (B) Transport and replenishment
   (C) Recirculation and replenishment
   (D) Transport and circulation

4. All of the following situations may cause AED backup time selection malfunction EXCEPT:

   (A) an extremely thin patient.
   (B) kVp selection too low.
   (C) mAs selection too low.
   (D) additional 1-mm Al filtration.

5. If an upright bucky cervical spine examination were to be carried out using 25 mAs at 40 inches, how much mAs would be required using 72 inches?

   (A) 81 mAs
   (B) 50 mAs
   (C) 100 mAs
   (D) 12.5 mAs

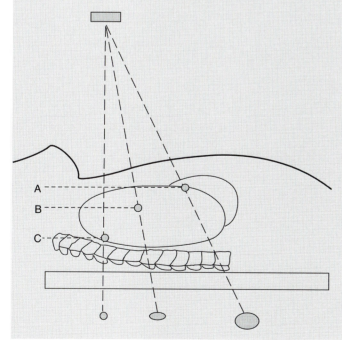

FIGURE 4-24. Effects of beam divergence and OFD on a lateral chest radiograph. See Question 2.

(Continued)

6. Sodium carbonate is a commonly used chemical in automatic processing; it may be found in the _____ tank, where it performs its function of _____
   - (A) fixer, reducing agent
   - (B) developer, activator
   - (C) fixer, restrainer
   - (D) developer, preservative

7. **Figure 4-25** is an upright AP radiograph of the ribs below the diaphragm, exposed at 30 mAs, 64 kVp, and 40 inches SID. The film is underexposed. Which of the following sets of exposure factors would best improve the diagnostic quality of the film?
   - (A) 60 mAs, 64 kVp, 40 inches SID
   - (B) 60 mAs, 64 kVp, 72 inches SID
   - (C) 30 mAs, 70 kVp, 40 inches SID
   - (D) 45 mAs, 64 kVp, 40 inches SID

8. Improper stacking of film boxes in the film storage area is likely to cause:
   - (A) static artifact.
   - (B) tree artifact.
   - (C) pressure artifact.
   - (D) fingernail artifact.

9. The term grid radius is used in conjunction with which of the following accessory devices?
   - (A) Focused grid
   - (B) Unfocused grid
   - (C) Parallel grid
   - (D) Crosshatch grid

10. In order to maintain the same density, changing from a 100-speed film/screen system to a 400-speed film system requires which adjustment in exposure factors?
    - (A) Increase mAs X2
    - (B) Decrease mAs 50%
    - (C) 15% increase in mAs
    - (D) 75% decrease in mAs

11. Which of the following examinations would be likely to employ single-emulsion radiographic film?
    - (A) Chamberlain-Townes view of skull
    - (B) Surgical lateral hip
    - (C) Mammography
    - (D) PA chest

12. All of the following are undesirable characteristics pertaining to intensifying screens EXCEPT:
    - (A) luminescence.
    - (B) phosphorescence.
    - (C) screen lag.
    - (D) crossover.

13. The relationship between recorded detail and OFD can be best described by which of the following?
    - (A) OFD and detail are directly proportional.
    - (B) As OFD decreases, detail decreases.
    - (C) OFD and detail are inversely proportional.
    - (D) OFD and detail are unrelated image factors.

14. Which of the following combination of factors would produce the greatest detail?
    - (A) 100-speed system, 2.5-mm focal spot
    - (B) 100-speed system, 1.0-mm focal spot
    - (C) 200-speed system, 2.5-mm focal spot
    - (D) 300-speed system, 2.5-mm focal spot

15. **Figure 4-26** is an overexposed PA chest examination. Using a fixed kVp, variable mAs technique chart, the technical correction for this examination would be:
    - (A) decrease mAs 15%.
    - (B) decrease kVp 15%.
    - (C) decrease mAs 50%.
    - (D) increase FFD 50%.

16. Compared with high kVp, low mAs technique, high mAs, low kVp technique produces:
    1. greater patient dose.
    2. shorter scale of contrast.
    3. less exposure latitude.
    - (A) Choice 2 only
    - (B) Choices 2 and 3 only
    - (C) Choice 3 only
    - (D) all of the aforementioned

17. A densitometer reading on the unexposed portion of a collimated, processed radiograph of the knee should produce a reading of no more than:
    - (A) 0.2.
    - (B) 2.0.
    - (C) 20.0.
    - (D) 0.002.

(Continued)

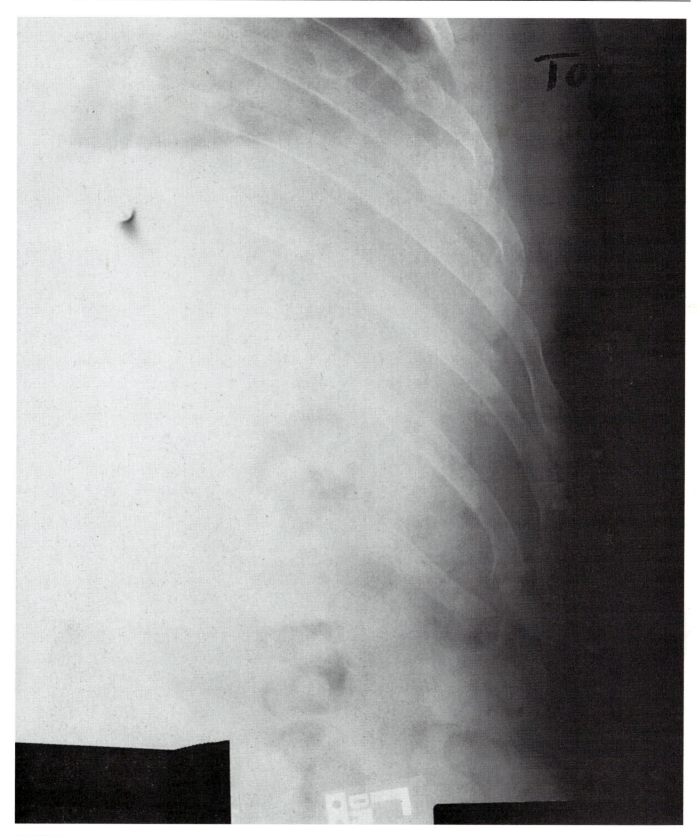

FIGURE 4-25. Upright AP radiograph of the ribs below the diaphragm. See Question 7.

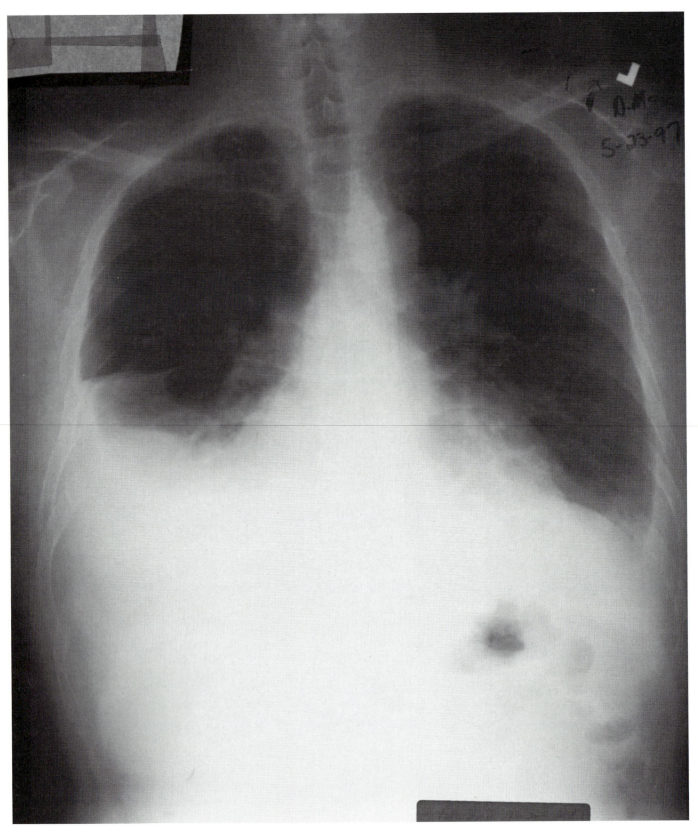

FIGURE 4-26. PA chest examination. See Question 15.

18. The D_{max} portion of a characteristic H&D curve can be found on which of the following?

    (A) Straight line portion
    (B) Toe
    (C) Head
    (D) Shoulder

19. Use the following grid conversion factors **(Table 4-7)** to compute technique. A Chamberlain-Townes view of the skull is taken using a 6:1 focused grid, 20 mAs, 70 kVp, and 40 inches FFD. What technique would be used with a 16:1 focused grid?

    (A) 40 mAs
    (B) 30 mAs
    (C) 60 mAs
    (D) 80 mAs

20. Which of the following examinations commonly employs the use of a compensating filter?

    (A) Barium enema
    (B) IVP
    (C) Wrist
    (D) Foot

21. The radiograph in **Figure 4-27** was exposed using the center cell of an AED device, and it is overexposed. Which of the following components of the examination is the most likely cause of excessive radiographic density?

    (A) Incorrect cell selection
    (B) Patient positioning
    (C) Incorrect FFD
    (D) Patient motion

▶ **TABLE 4-7.** Grid Conversion Factors

Grid Ratio	mAs Conversion Factor
No Grid	1
5:1	2
6:1	3
8:1	4
10/ 12:1	5
16:1	6

22. **Figure 4-28** is a left lateral view of the chest, exposed using 6 mAs, 90 kVp, 40 inches FFD, and a 400-speed screen/film system. This is considered to be a reliable technique for a chest examination on a patient with this body size. Which of the following variables is the most likely cause of the slightly underexposed radiograph?

    (A) Poor inspiratory effort
    (B) Inappropriate screen/film selection
    (C) Patient pathology
    (D) Inadequate FFD

23. Of the following factors, which have significant impact in determining radiographic contrast?

    1. FFD
    2. Processing chemistry
    3. OID
    4. Film latitude

    (A) Choice 2 only
    (B) Choices 1 and 3
    (C) Choices 2 and 4
    (D) All of the aforementioned

24. Which of the following examinations should always use the shortest exposure time possible?

    (A) Barium enema
    (B) Elbow
    (C) Tibia
    (D) Chest

25. Which of the following sets of exposure factors will produce the greatest density?

    (A) 100 mA, 0.10 sec, 70 kVp
    (B) 200 mA, 0.01 sec, 70 kVp
    (C) 300 mA, 0.01 sec, 72 kVp
    (D) 600 mA, 0.005 sec, 72 kVp

26. The ratio of the height of the lead strips to the width of the interspace material in a grid is known as:

    (A) grid radius.
    (B) grid ratio.
    (C) grid cutoff.
    (D) lines per inch.

(Continued)

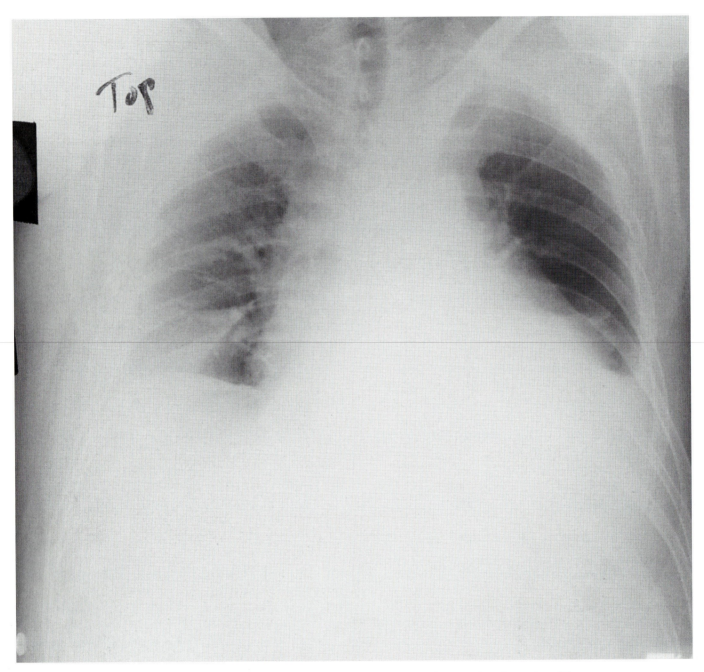

FIGURE 4-27. Radiograph exposed using the center cell of an AED device. See Question 21.

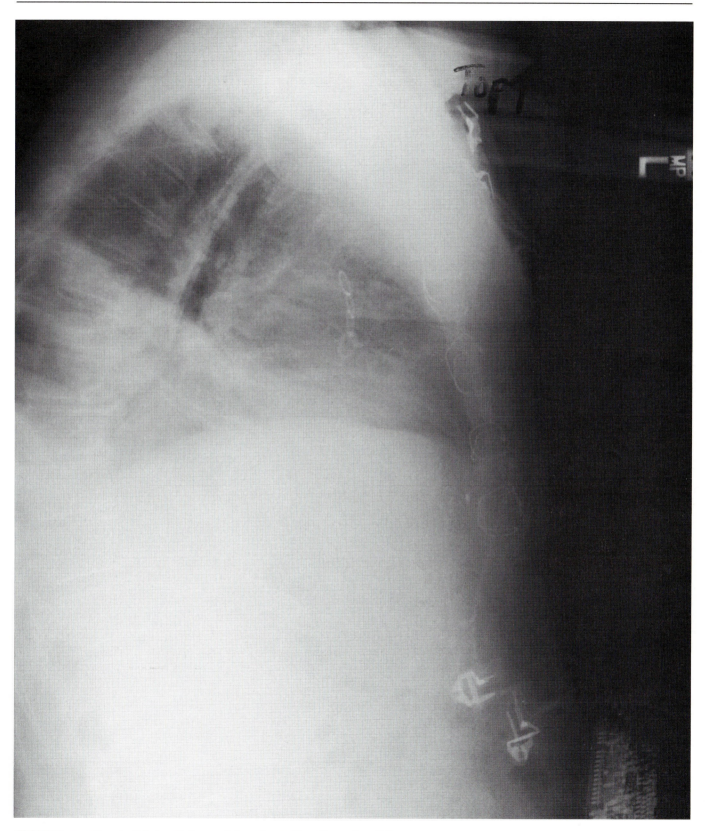

FIGURE 4-28. Left lateral view of the chest. See Question 22.

27. Which of the following chemicals found in the developer solution acts to control swelling and softening of the film emulsion?

    (A) Potassium bromide
    (B) Glutaraldehyde
    (C) Hydroquinone
    (D) Phenidone

28. Which of the following is the correct sequence of film transport through a typical 90-second automatic processor?

    (A) Fix, wash, rinse, develop
    (B) Fix, develop, wash, dry
    (C) Develop, fix, wash, dry
    (D) Develop, wash, fix, dry

29. Proper pairing of film type and intensifying screen type is known as:

    (A) spectral matching.
    (B) panchromatic matching.
    (C) spectral responsivity.
    (D) sensitometry.

30. The chief disadvantage of rare earth intensifying screens compared with traditional calcium tungstate intensifying screens is:

    (A) increased distortion.
    (B) increased quantum mottle.
    (C) increased patient dose.
    (D) increased cost.

31. A wire mesh test is used to evaluate which of the following?

    (A) Spectral matching
    (B) Screen-film contact
    (C) Afterglow
    (D) Rectification

32. Which of the following is a true statement concerning image receptors?

    (A) Fast image receptors have high levels of noise and low image resolution.
    (B) Fast image receptors have low levels of noise and low image resolution.
    (C) Slow image receptors have low quantum mottle and low patient dose compared with fast image receptors.
    (D) Slow image receptors have high image resolution and low levels of noise compared with fast image receptors.

33. All of the following are attributes of short-scale contrast EXCEPT:

    (A) high contrast.
    (B) wide film latitude.
    (C) produced by high mAs, low kVp.
    (D) few number of density differences.

34. Which of the following mobile radiographic examinations requires the use of a stationary grid?

    (A) AP chest
    (B) Sunrise view of knee
    (C) AP abdomen
    (D) Crosstable lateral ankle

35. Which of the following factors has the greatest impact on density?

    (A) FFD
    (B) Scatter
    (C) Inherent filtration
    (D) Anode cooling

36. Which of the following does NOT influence the amount of light emitted by an intensifying screen?

    (A) FFD
    (B) kVp
    (C) Thickness of the phosphor
    (D) Film speed

37. What is the grid ratio of a focused grid with 120 lines per inch and lead strips that are 2.5 mm in height, 0.25 mm thick, and are spaced 0.25 mm apart?

    (A) 8:1
    (B) 10:1
    (C) 12:1
    (D) 16:1

38. All other variables remaining constant, which of the following sets of exposure factors will produce the greatest radiographic density?

    (A) 20 mAs, 81 kVp, 36 inches FFD
    (B) 10 mAs, 93 kVp, 38 inches FFD
    (C) 40 mAs, 70 kVp, 40 inches FFD
    (D) 40 mAs, 70 kVp, 72 inches FFD

(Continued)

39. At what point is x-ray film emulsion most sensitive?

    (A) Following exposure
    (B) Before exposure
    (C) In humidity greater than 60%
    (D) At temperatures below 50°F

40. The phenomenon of variance in photon distribution between the cathode and anode end of the x-ray tube is referred to as:

    (A) inverse square law.
    (B) 50 /15 rule.
    (C) anode blooming.
    (D) anode heel effect.

41. Which of the following are important considerations concerning recorded detail?

    (A) Anode heel effect and focal spot
    (B) Filament heating and line focus principle
    (C) Heat unit production and line focus principle
    (D) Rectification and average beam intensity

42. What is the most likely result if insufficient washing occurs during processing?

    (A) Overexposed film
    (B) Underexposed film
    (C) Increased areas of fog
    (D) Decreased archival attributes

43. Look at **Figure 4-29.** Imagine that the rectangular object is a part under examination. The central ray is represented by the dotted lines, perpendicular to the solid line image receptor. Of the factors listed, which best describes the radiographic result?

    (A) Foreshortening
    (B) Elongation
    (C) 2X magnification
    (D) Blurring

44. Which of the following is NOT increased by increasing kVp?

    (A) Exposure rate
    (B) Heat units
    (C) Photon wavelength
    (D) Exposure latitude

45. Use the principle of reciprocity to substitute a new mA for the following technique: 200 mA, 0.20 seconds, and 65 kVp. Select the answer that will produce the greatest detail.

    (A) 100 mA, 0.40 sec, 65 kVp, small focal spot
    (B) 200 mA, 0.40 sec, 75 kVp, small focal spot
    (C) 400 mA, 0.10 sec, 65 kVp, large focal spot
    (D) 500 mA, 0.08 sec, 65 kVp, large focal spot

46. Of the following pathologic conditions, which one requires an increase in technique to compensate for increase in beam attenuation?

    (A) Ileus
    (B) Renal calculus
    (C) Ascites
    (D) Pneumoperitoneum

47. **Figure 4-30** is an AP portable chest examination that required a repeat examination. The most likely reason for the suboptimal film was:

    (A) chemical fog.
    (B) incorrect FFD.
    (C) incorrect mAs.
    (D) grid lines.

48. Which of the following is the most important influencing factor relative to shape distortion?

    (A) Screen speed
    (B) Film speed
    (C) FFD
    (D) Tube-part-film alignment

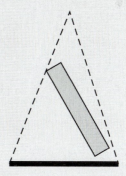

FIGURE 4-29. See Question 43.

(Continued)

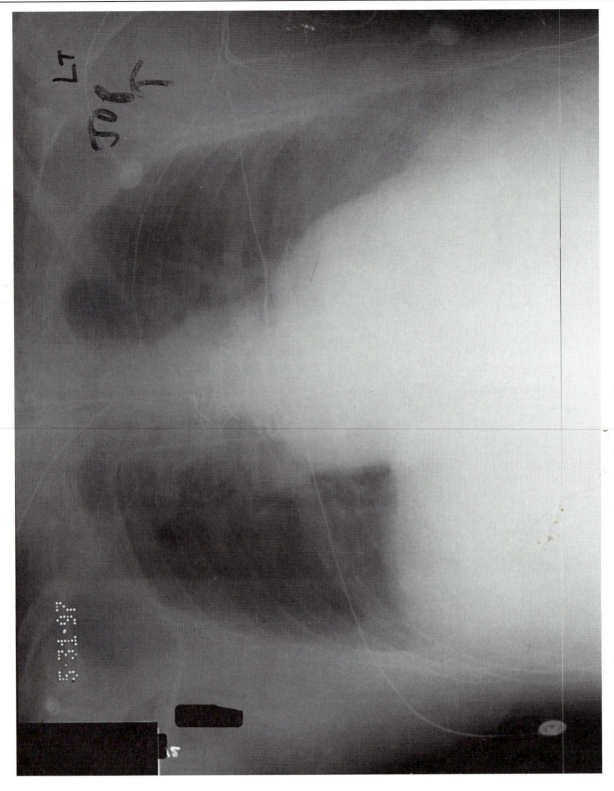

FIGURE 4–30. AP portable chest examination. See Question 47.

49. Increasing filtration from 2-mm Al to 4-mm Al has a similar effect to that of:

    (A) increasing mAs.
    (B) increasing kVp.
    (C) decreasing FFD.
    (D) using higher grid ratio.

50. All of the following should be included as part of a radiology department quality assurance program EXCEPT:

    (A) linearity.
    (B) film speed.
    (C) reproducibility.
    (D) beam alignment.

▶▶ ANSWERS TO END-OF-CHAPTER EXAMINATION

1. The answer is (B). The quantity of electrons used in making an exposure is determined by mA. The higher the selected mA, the more electrons are produced by thermionic emission at the cathode filament. Therefore, milliamperage can be described as the amount of current flowing through the x-ray tube.

2. The answer is (B). In this drawing, the central ray passes through lesion A and is more divergent through lesions B and C, with lesion C demonstrating the most elongation caused by the divergence of the beam. All of the lesions will be magnified on the radiograph because of their distance from the image receptor, with lesion C situated farthest from it and therefore demonstrating the most magnification. On the radiograph, lesion A would be the most accurate representation of the actual lesion.

3. The answer is (D). Agitation during processing ensures thorough mixing of chemistry and contact between the chemistry and film emulsion. The transport rollers are situated in such a way as to provide a wavelike motion of the film as it moves through the tank. The recirculation system keeps the wash, fixer, and developer solutions in constant motion by removing small amounts of solution from the bottom of the tank and replacing it through the top.

4. The answer is (D). Depending on the examination, an extremely thin patient may require an exposure less than the minimum achievable exposure using the AED. Selection of kVp or mAs that is too low may lengthen the required exposure time beyond the selected backup time. The use of additional 1-mm Al filtration would have little impact on automatic exposure factors.

5. The answer is (A). This problem is solved using the distance maintenance formula, which is:

$$\frac{I_1}{I_2} = \frac{D_1^2}{D_2^1} \qquad (18)$$

Substituting known values:

$$\frac{25}{x} = \frac{40^2}{72^2} \qquad (19)$$

$$1600\ X = 129,600$$
$$X = 81\ mAs$$

6. The answer is (B). Sodium carbonate is found in the developer solution; it is an activator. It is responsible for maintaining an alkaline environment (pH of 10–11.5), which enhances the action of the reducing agents, and softens and swells the film emulsion so the emulsion can work on deeper-lying silver halide crystals.

7. The answer is (A). The primary trouble with Figure 4-25 is lack of density. The best corrective measure in this instance is to double the mAs, thereby doubling the density. Increasing mAs while also increasing distance would produce an underexposed radiograph. Increasing mAs by 50% would increase density, but not enough. Increasing kVp by 10% would also produce an insufficient increase in density, and simultaneously lengthen the scale of contrast, which would be an undesirable effect for a rib examination.

8. The answer is (C). In order to avoid artifact caused by less-than-optimum storage, film boxes should always be stored vertically in a cool, dry area of between 50°F to 70°F, and 40% to 60% relative humidity, away from ionizing radiation. Pressure artifact is a direct result of stacking boxes directly on top of each other.

(Continued)

9. The answer is (A). A focused grid has lead lines that tilt more as they move away from the center of the grid so that they are in alignment with the x-ray source. The process of tilting the lead strips is known as canting. The grid radius is the focal point in space at which imaginary lines drawn from the lead strips converge. Because there is some room for error, most grid radii are listed in a range; 36 to 42 inches and 66 to 74 inches are the most common ranges.

10. The answer is (D). A 400-speed system is four times faster than a 100-speed system; therefore, only 1/4 the mAs is required to produce the same density on film. Decreasing mAs by 75% equals a mAs of 1/4 the original mAs.

11. The answer is (C). Single-emulsion radiographic film is used in conjunction with a single intensifying screen for examinations that require highly detailed images, such as extremity radiography and mammography. The film employs antihalation backing that minimizes light scattering within the cassette, thereby improving image resolution.

12. The answer is (A). Light emission by an intensifying screen excited by radiation is known as luminescence. It is the property that allows intensifying screens to play an effective role in x-ray image production. Continued emission of light after exposure to x-ray energy is terminated is known as phosphorescence, screen lag, or afterglow. Crossover is light that passes from one side of the film emulsion to the other through the film base, causing scattering of light and distortion.

13. The answer is (C). The distance between the part under examination and the film is known as object film distance (OFD), or object-to-image receptor distance (OID). As OFD increases, magnification increases, and detail decreases; therefore, these factors have an inverse relationship.

14. The answer is (A). The slowest combination of film speed, intensifying screen speed, and smallest focal spot produces the greatest detail. Care must be taken to ensure that the x-ray tube heat loading capacity is not exceeded when using a small focal spot.

15. The answer is (C). By definition, a fixed kVp chart uses an optimum kVp range for a given body part; therefore, mAs is the correct exposure factor to change when making a technical correction to this examination. This particular radiograph is grossly overexposed, and the correct adjustment would be cutting mAs in half in order to decrease density by half. Decreasing mAs by 15% would not have a significant impact on the film.

16. The answer is (D). High kVp technique is associated with a long scale of contrast. The longer the scale of contrast, the greater the exposure latitude. As kVp decreases, more mAs is required to produce comparable radiographs; as mAs increases, the quantity of radiation used increases; hence patient dose increases.

17. The answer is (A). A densitometer reading of the unexposed portion of a processed radiograph is called base plus fog. The reading should not exceed 0.2. Base plus fog is the sum of the density of the film base, environmental exposure received during the manufacturing process, and density resulting from film processing.

18. The answer is (D). A characteristic curve is a graphic representation of a film's response to exposure, and it consists of three parts. The straight line portion measures a film's useful range of densities, with densitometric readings between 0.25 and 2.5. The D_{max}, or highest point on the characteristic curve, is where maximum exposure occurs, and is referred to as the shoulder portion.

19. The answer is (A). The following formula is used to find the solution:

$$\frac{mAs_1}{mAs_2} = \frac{conversion\ factor_1}{conversion\ factor_2} \qquad (20)$$

substituting,

$$\frac{20}{x} = \frac{3}{6} \qquad (21)$$

$$3X = 120$$
$$X = 40\ mAs$$

(Continued)

20. The answer is (D). A compensating filter is an accessory device that provides uniform radiographic density on examinations that contain structures of widely divergent densities. Common examples of examinations using a compensating filter include scoliosis survey, foot, femur, and mediastinal structures of the chest. The foot filter consists of a wedge-shaped piece of aluminum or leaded plastic that attaches to the tube head in the same manner as an extension cone or cylinder. The filter is thicker at the end of the foot where the less dense toes are, and thinner where the much thicker tarsals are. A technique appropriate for tarsals is used, and the filter absorbs radiation in a manner that achieves uniform density on the radiograph.

21. The answer is (B). Note that the patient is positioned posteriorly relative to the center of the radiograph, and hence posteriorly to the correctly selected center photo cell. Over- or underexposure is a common result of improper positioning when using an AED.

22. The answer is (C). Decubitus chest radiographs are generally taken to investigate fluid accumulation in the chest; Figure 4-28 demonstrates a considerable fluid level in both lungs. Therefore, technique selection for decubitus chest examinations must compensate for the additional attenuation of the primary beam caused by the fluid.

23. The answer is (C). FFD is an image factor that primarily affects density and magnification. OID is a geometric factor that relates to magnification and distortion. Processing chemistry may adversely affect image contrast if it is improperly mixed, contaminated, or used at incorrect temperatures. Film latitude is another means of expressing scale of contrast; the longer the scale of contrast, the wider the film latitude, and hence, the greater the room for exposure error.

24. The answer is (D). The shortest possible exposure time is necessary in chest radiography in order to minimize the blurring effect of involuntary motion; in this case the beating of the heart. Other examples of involuntary motion are gastric peristalsis and muscle spasm.

25. The answer is (A). Density is primarily controlled by mAs; therefore, to solve, compute mAs. A = 10 mAs, B = 2 mAs, C = 3 mAs, D = 3 mAs. The slight difference in kVp is negligible.

26. The answer is (B). The ratio of the height of the lead strips to the width of the interspace material is known as grid ratio. As the height of the lead strips increases, grid efficiency increases. Therefore, as grid ratio increases, grid efficiency increases. The greater the number of lines per inch, the thinner and less visible they are. Grid radius refers to the correct FFD for use with a given focused grid. Grid cutoff is a phenomenon that occurs with improper centering relative to a grid.

27. The answer is (B). Glutaraldehyde is found in the developer solution and is an important hardening agent. If developer replenishment is inadequate, then insufficient hardening of the film emulsion may take place, causing damp films or film transport malfunctions. Some authors have pointed to insufficient glutaraldehyde replenishment as the single largest cause of processor breakdown.

28. The answer is (C). The path of a film through the various areas of a 90-second film processor can be summarized as: develop, fix, rinse, wash, dry.

29. The answer is (A). Each type of film and type of intensifying screen is sensitive to a given spectrum of light. Blue light–sensitive film, for example, should be used in conjunction with calcium tungstate screens, which emit light in the blue-violet spectrum. Likewise, green light–sensitive film is used in conjunction with rare earth intensifying screens. Another type of film, called orthochromatic, is sensitive to both green and blue-violet light, and is also used with rare earth screens.

30. The answer is (B). Although rare earth screens provide the major advantage of decidedly increased speed, permitting examinations at much lower patient doses, and extending x-ray tube life, there is some loss of resolution. Ultra-high film /screen combinations, in particular the 1000- to 1200-speed range, are especially likely to produce significantly higher radiographic noise (quantum mottle).

(Continued)

31. The answer is (B). Areas of blurring on a radiograph are likely related to poor screen-film contact. To perform the test, expose the cassette through the wire mesh at a low technique of 3 to 5 mAs, 50 kVp, and 40 inches SID. Any blurred areas detected on the resulting film are indicative of poor screen-film contact, and point out the need for screen replacement. Causes of poor contact include worn contact felt, broken or bent hinges and latches, warped screens or cassette, foreign objects under the screen, or sprung frame.

32. The answer is (A). As screen and film speed increases, quantum mottle or radiographic noise increases. This means that patient dose is decreased, but image resolution is also decreased. The radiographer must possess an awareness of the clinical situation and decide which of the various radiographic tools to use based on the clinical needs of the patient and the needs of the radiologist reading the film.

33. The answer is (B). High mAs, low kVp techniques generally produce short-scale, high-contrast radiographs, which are useful in some clinical situations. The shorter the scale of contrast, the less exposure latitude, or room for technique selection error, exists.

34. The answer is (C). The rule of thumb concerning grid use, whether in the radiology department or for portable examinations, is that if the part being examined is in excess of 10 cm, then the use of a grid to provide adequate cleanup of secondary and scatter radiation is required.

35. The answer is (A). Although mAs is the primary control of radiographic density, of the listed factors, FFD has the greatest effect on density because exposure rate is inversely proportional to the square of the FFD. Stated in terms of density, as FFD increases, density decreases.

36. The answer is (D). FFD and kVp directly influence the amount of energy reaching the intensifying screen and therefore affect fluorescence. The thickness of the phosphor layer is also an important factor; the thicker the layer, the more light produced. Film speed, however, does not affect screen fluorescence.

37. The answer is (B). Grid ratio is determined as the ratio of the height of the lead strips to the width of the interspace material. Lines per inch and lead strip thickness are not related to grid ratio. To solve, divide:

$$\frac{2.5 \ mm}{.25 \ mm} = 10 \qquad (22)$$

38. The answer is (A). Using the 50/15 rule, all mAs and kVp techniques in this selection are equivocal. Therefore, the exposure made using the shortest FFD will produce the greatest density: 50°F

39. The answer is (A). Once a film has been exposed to light from an intensifying screen, its sensitivity to further exposure is greatly increased. Therefore, care must be taken to ensure that film is exposed to darkroom safelighting for the absolute minimum time period.

40. The answer is (D). Variations in photon distribution and therefore beam intensity, so that beam intensity gradually increases toward the cathode end of the x-ray tube, is known as the anode heel effect. The effect is most pronounced using short FFDs, large film sizes, and steep target angles.

41. The answer is (C). Focal spot size is a crucial factor relative to recorded detail; the smaller the focal spot used, the better the recorded detail. Unfortunately, as focal spot size decreases, heat unit production increases, making it an important consideration in focal spot size selection. By angling the target, however, the line-focus principle is used, enabling the effective focal spot to remain small, while maintaining a large actual area for heating.

42. The answer is (D). The primary function of the wash tank is to remove residual chemistry from the film. If inadequate washing occurs, residual fixer on the radiograph may lead to image degradation over a period of time.

(Continued)

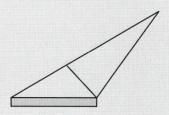

FIGURE 4-31.

43. The answer is (A). When an object is angled relative to the image receptor, but the central ray remains perpendicular in relation to it, the radiographic result is foreshortening. If the central ray were to be positioned perpendicular to the object, as in **Figure 4-31,** then the resulting radiograph would demonstrate elongation.

44. The answer is (C). Increasing kVp will have the effect of increasing exposure latitude by producing a longer scale of contrast on film. Heat units produced will increase per the formula: mAs × kVp = HU. Exposure rate will increase, because more photons will be produced at the target; however, the length of x-ray photons decreases as their energy increases.

45. The answer is (A). Choices A, C, and D all demonstrate the principle of reciprocity, which states that any combination of mA and time equaling the same mAs will produce the same radiographic density. Choice A, however, uses the 100 mA station, which is linked to the small focal spot. The smaller the focal spot, the greater the recorded detail. Choice B does not demonstrate reciprocity; rather, it illustrates the 50/15 rule.

46. The answer is (C). Ascites is an abnormal accumulation of fluid in the abdomen that increases beam attenuation; therefore, in order to maintain correct density, this condition requires an increase in exposure factors. Pneumoperitoneum is the presence of air in the peritoneum; ileus is another name for mechanical bowel obstruction; and renal calculus is another term for kidney stones. None of these conditions require a compensatory increase in technique to maintain density.

47. The answer is (A). Figure 4-30 demonstrates what can happen when film chemistry is incorrect; it is an example of a film exposed to chemical fog. Chemical fog may result from too high developer temperature, oxidized developer, or inadequate replenishment.

48. The answer is (D). Of the factors listed, the most important influence is correct alignment of the x-ray tube, the part under examination, and the image receptor. If the examination is done with a stationary grid or bucky, the alignment of the grid also becomes critical. Shape distortion may also occur naturally as a result of a given anatomic part's alignment in relation to the x-ray tube.

49. The answer is (B). Just as increasing kVp reduces the amount of low-energy photons, the primary effect of increasing added Al filtration is raising the overall energy level of the beam by filtering out low-energy photons. For both technical adjustments, the chief effect is an increase in the energy level of the x-ray beam.

50. The answer is (B). Film speed is not checked by QA; rather, the type of film/screen system used by a department is decided upon jointly by the radiologists, technologists, and management. Beam alignment must be accurate to within 2% of the FFD. Reproducibility refers to making repeat exposures at the same technique and yielding consistent beam intensity. Linearity refers to using different mA and time combinations that yield the same mAs results.

Radiographic Procedures

I. GENERAL PROCEDURAL CONSIDERATIONS
A. Patient Preparation

One of the most critical phases of any radiographic examination begins before you enter the exposure room: patient preparation. Patients inevitably base their belief in your ability as a technologist on their initial impression; it is vital that you project confident, compassionate professionalism from the start. Introducing yourself with a smile and perhaps a handshake or light touch on the arm, if appropriate, will engage the patient as a partner in the task ahead of both of you. In addition, the radiographer should assure that the room is clean; the x-ray table and accessories should be cleaned after each use with a disinfectant solution, and pillowcases should be replaced after each patient use. Assemble x-ray accessories that are needed for the examination, such as grids, cones, and lead aprons.

Following your introduction, the patient should be brought to the examining room, and a brief explanation of the procedure should be given. Eye contact with the patient is important; for the most part, the patient's facial expressions will enable you to determine if there is apprehension about some part of the examination, or questions that need to be addressed.

Generally hospital inpatients will already be attired in a hospital gown; dressing them differently for the examination is generally not an issue. Still, the technologist must be aware that certain radiopaque objects worn by the patient may need to be removed. Bras may need to be removed for chest or abdominal examinations, as well as any jewelry such as a necklace that is worn in or around the area of interest.

Partial plates or dentures should be removed for cervical spine examinations; they interfere with viewing the odontoid process of C-2. Occasionally hairpins or barrettes are worn, which will be visualized on skull and some cervical spine (C-spine) views; these objects must also be removed. Patients undergoing chest examinations who have long hair, particularly if it is styled in a manner where it is brought together in a thick band, as for "pigtails" or "dreadlocks," should have the hair removed from the area of examination by pinning it up. This type of hairstyle is infamous for appearing on radiographs as an artifact that is potentially misleading in terms of diagnosis.

Dressing of outpatients should be based on the requirements of the examination. Ideally, as little time as possible should be spent on preliminaries. If, for example, the patient who is undergoing an abdominal examination is wearing a cotton sweat suit without metallic snaps, buttons, or zippers, no changing is necessary. Similarly, if the same patient requires a knee examination, usually such attire is loose; and may be pulled high enough to permit the examination to be performed. If changing into a gown is required, the patient should be directed into the dressing room with clear, complete instructions. Nothing is more frustrating than waiting for a patient to dress on a busy day and then having them emerge dressed incorrectly. Therefore, eye contact in this situation is also important. Give instructions along these lines: "Mrs. Smith, I want to you go into this dressing room. Take off everything from the waist up, please, including your bra and your necklace, and then put on this gown, so that the opening is in the back. Tie up the openings, and then come out for your chest radiograph." The more specific the dressing instructions, the better.

B. Equipment Capabilities

The technologist must have a thorough understanding of the design capabilities and limitations of the equipment at his/her disposal relative to the task at hand. For example, if the next examination to be done is an IVU, you must then bring the patient into a room with tomographic capability, not a standard R&F room. Likewise, if there are both single-phase and three-phase rooms in your department; obese patients, who require more exposure, and pediatric patients, who generally require the shortest exposure time possible, should be examined in the three-phase rooms. Single-phase rooms should not be considered substandard, however. There are many reasons, cost being the primary one, that single-phase units are widely used. Single-phase rooms function admirably, as long as demands that are made of them are not outside the boundaries of their design.

C. Positioning Terminology

The technologist needs to thoroughly understand the terminology related to anatomy, physiology, and radiographic positioning. **Figure 5-1** is a compilation of terminology for positioning and projection, along with artistic renderings of the standard positions.

Also vital to the technologist is an understanding of terminology related to skeletal motion. These terms are discussed in pairs, because one motion is the opposite of the other. *Flexion* describes the bending motion of an articulation (joint) that decreases the angle between the related bones, whereas *extension* is bending of an articulation that increases the angle. Common examinations that relate to these terms are flexion-extension views of the lumbar and cervical spine. *Inversion* is medial, or toward the midline motion of an articulation; *eversion* is lateral, or away from the midline motion. Orthopedic surgeons often order "stress views" of a given joint, most commonly of the ankle, whereby the physician will "stress" the ankle by applying external tension to the joint, in order to radiographically document suspected torn ligaments. A positive stress view examination of the ankle shows the talus rotated away from the direction of the torn ligament.

Abduction is movement of a part away from the median sagittal plane (MSP); *adduction* is movement of a part toward the MSP. *Supination* is movement of the body so that the palm of the hand faces upward and the thumb faces away from the MSP; *pronation* is movement of the body that places the hand palm downward and the thumb toward the MSP. Standard internal and external rotation views of the upper ex-

---

STANDARD TERMINOLOGY FOR POSITIONING AND PROJECTION

Radiographic View

Describes the body part as seen by an x-ray film or other recording media, such as a fluoroscopic screen. Restricted to the discussion of a *radiograph* or *image.*

Radiographic Position

Refers to a specific body position, such as supine, prone, recumbent, erect, or Trendelenburg. Restricted to the discussion of the patient's *physical position.*

Radiographic Projection

Restricted to the discussion of the *path of the central ray.*

Positioning Terminology

  A. *Lying down*

  1. Supine   lying on the back

  2. Prone   lying face downward

  3. Recumbent   lying down in any position

  4. Decubitus   lying down with a horizontal x-ray beam

B. *Erect or Upright*

1. Anterior position   facing the film

2. Posterior position   facing the radiographic tube

3. Oblique positions

a. Anterior   facing the film

(1) *Left anterior oblique:* body rotated with left anterior portion closest to the film

(2) *Right anterior oblique:* body rotated with right anterior portion closest to the film

b. Posterior   facing the radiographic tube

(1) *Left posterior oblique:* body rotated with left posterior portion closest to the film

(2) *Right posterior oblique:* body rotated with right posterior portion closest to the film

FIGURE 5-1.   ARRT standard terminology and illustrations for positioning and projection. (© 1990 The American Registry of Radiologic Technologists. Reproduced with permission.)

Anteroposterior projection

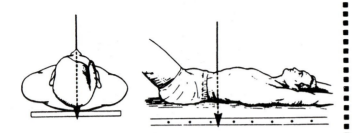

Posteroanterior projection

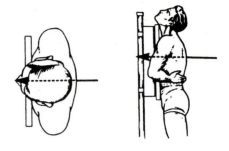

Right lateral position

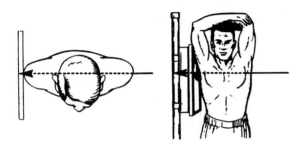

Left lateral position

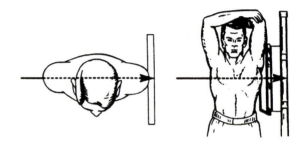

Left posterior oblique position

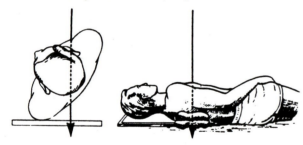

Right posterior oblique position

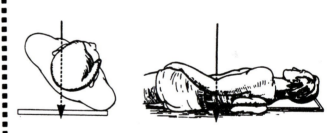

Left anterior oblique position

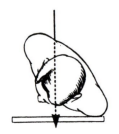
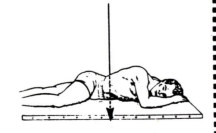

Right anterior oblique position

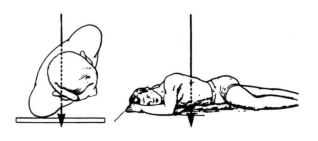

FIGURE 5-1. *(continued)*

tremity demonstrate how these terms often work together. Maximum supination of the hand rotates the humeral head in the glenohumeral articulation (shoulder) internally, which is adduction, whereas maximum pronation rotates the humeral head externally, demonstrating abduction. The final two terms are related but not opposite. *Rotation* describes movement of a body part about its long or central axis. *Circumduction* is circular motion of a limb that is small at the proximal end and wide at the distal end.

The body can be divided into an infinite number of planes. The technologist must understand these planes thoroughly in order to be effective at positioning. A plane that divides the body into right and left portions is called a sagittal plane. Although an infinite number of sagittal planes are possible, the plane most often referred to is the median sagittal plane, which divides the body equally into right and left halves. A vertical plane that separates the body into anterior and posterior parts (front and back) is called a coronal plane. Again, if the plane occurs at the midline, it is referred to as the median coronal plane. A plane that subdivides the body into superior and inferior parts, or in the case of internal organs, cuts across its long axis at right angles, is referred to as a transverse plane. **Figure 5-2** demonstrates the various planes.

Surface landmarks on the body are useful aids to positioning. These external localization points identify internal locations; for example, the iliac crest is relative to the L4 vertebra, and the manubrial or suprasternal notch is at the same level as the T2 to T3 articulation. Other external landmarks of interest and their corresponding internal locations include the mastoid process and C1, sternal angle and T4 to T5, xiphoid process and T10, anterior superior iliac spine (ASIS) and S1, and the symphysis pubis, greater trochanter, and coccyx. Some landmarks can be readily identified by visual inspection, whereas others require palpation. Palpation can be defined as a physical examination in which the technologist feels the location of surface landmarks with his/her hands. **Figures 5-3 through 5-5** demonstrate other important external landmarks.

D. Patient Respiration and Motion Control

Patient motion during the exposure results in severe degradation of the x-ray image. Involuntary motion, or movement the patient has no control over, such as muscle spasm or peristalsis, can be minimized by using the shortest possible exposure time. Remember, the reciprocity law states that if the equipment is

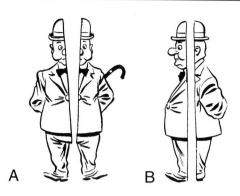

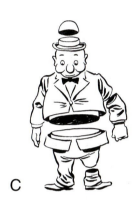

FIGURE 5-2. *(A)* Median sagittal plane. *(B)* Coronal or frontal plane. *(C)* Transverse or horizontal planes. (Reproduced with permission from John V. Basmajian, MD, McMaster University, Hamilton, Ontario.)

properly calibrated in terms of mA linearity, all combinations of mA and time produce identical radiographic density. Therefore, if 5 mAs are required for a given exposure on a patient who is having trouble cooperating for the examination, certainly do not use 100 mA and .05 sec when you can use the 500 mA station and .01 sec. Some machines even have 1000-mA stations available, in which case 1000 mA and .0005 sec could be used instead. Reassuring the patient and keeping him/her warm may also aid in controlling nervous shaking.

There are three primary tools the technologists uses regarding voluntary motion. First and foremost is good communication with the patient. The patient who understands what you are about to do and why you are about to do it will almost always be more cooperative than one who doesn't. Ill patients feel anxious and afraid; there is a sense they have lost control. By explaining the procedure and their part in it, you not only can elicit the patient's cooperation, but

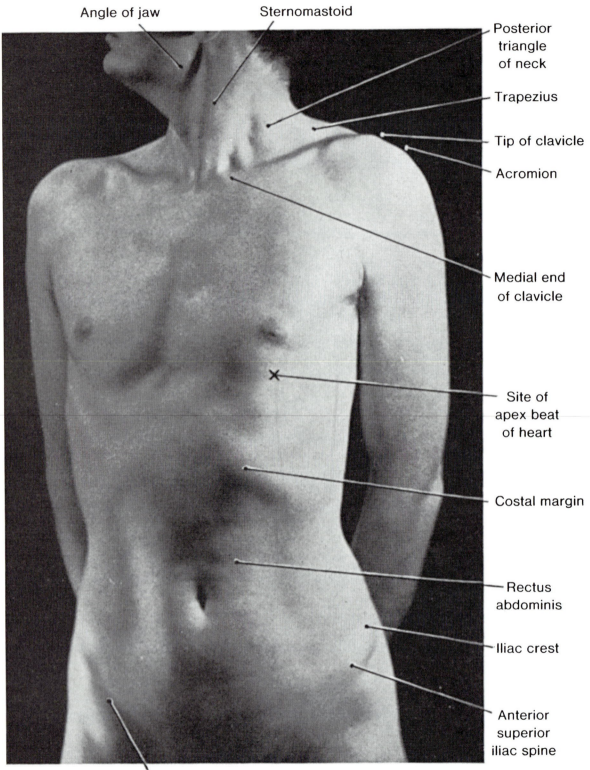

Angle of jaw

Sternomastoid

Posterior
triangle
of neck

Trapezius

Tip of clavicle

Acromion

Medial end
of clavicle

Site of
apex beat
of heart

Costal margin

Rectus
abdominis

Iliac crest

Anterior
superior
iliac spine

Groove overlying inguinal ligament

FIGURE 5-3. Surface anatomy. (Reproduced with permission from John V. Basmajian, MD, McMaster University, Hamilton, Ontario.)

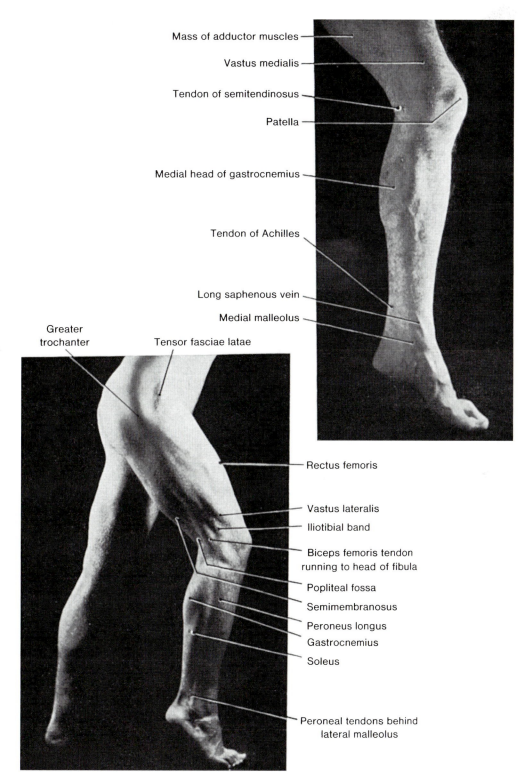

Mass of adductor muscles

Vastus medialis

Tendon of semitendinosus

Patella

Medial head of gastrocnemius

Tendon of Achilles

Long saphenous vein

Medial malleolus

Greater trochanter

Tensor fasciae latae

Rectus femoris

Vastus lateralis

Iliotibial band

Biceps femoris tendon running to head of fibula

Popliteal fossa

Semimembranosus

Peroneus longus

Gastrocnemius

Soleus

Peroneal tendons behind lateral malleolus

FIGURE 5-4. Surface anatomy. (Reproduced with permission from John V. Basmajian, MD, McMaster University, Hamilton, Ontario.)

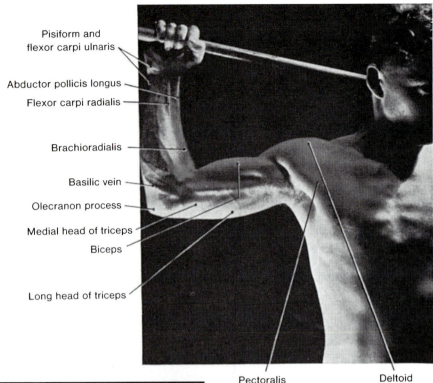

Pisiform and
flexor carpi ulnaris

Abductor pollicis longus

Flexor carpi radialis

Brachioradialis

Basilic vein

Olecranon process

Medial head of triceps

Biceps

Long head of triceps

Pectoralis
major

Deltoid

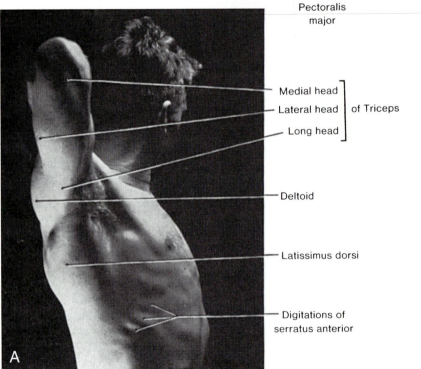

Medial head
Lateral head — of Triceps
Long head

Deltoid

Latissimus dorsi

Digitations of
serratus anterior

A

FIGURE 5-5. Surface anatomy. (Reproduced with permission from John V. Basmajian, MD, McMaster University, Hamilton, Ontario.)

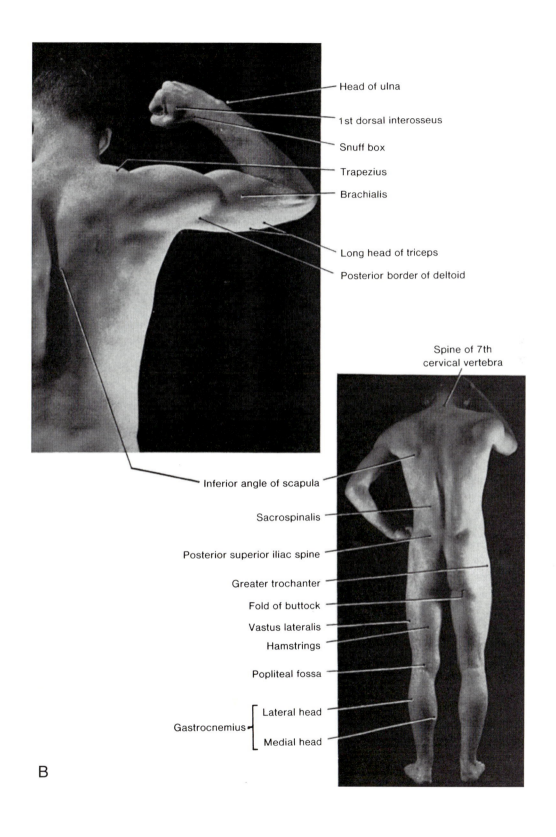

Head of ulna

1st dorsal interosseus

Snuff box

Trapezius

Brachialis

Long head of triceps

Posterior border of deltoid

Spine of 7th
cervical vertebra

Inferior angle of scapula

Sacrospinalis

Posterior superior iliac spine

Greater trochanter

Fold of buttock

Vastus lateralis

Hamstrings

Popliteal fossa

Lateral head

Gastrocnemius

Medial head

B

you can do much to restore their confidence in themselves and their surroundings.

The second technique to minimize voluntary motion is suspension of patient respiration. The key to good breathing instructions is to ensure that you are understood. Speak in a clear, well-modulated voice. It is often helpful to explain in advance to patients that you are going to instruct them to hold their breath, so they expect it. A common experience among technologists is one in which the patient is completely positioned and the technologist has returned to the control panel and says, "OK, now, Mrs. Smith. Take in a deep breath please, and hold it." Coinciding exactly with the moment the exposure is made, the patient turns from his/her position to look at the technologist and says, "Now?" The obvious result is an unusable radiograph.

Phase of respiration, whether suspension on inspiration or expiration, or variants of either, can be an important component of the examination. For example, a PA and lateral chest examination is performed on deep inspiration, so that the lung fields are well expanded. If, however, the patient has a suspected pneumothorax (air in the pleural cavity), the condition is best demonstrated with an expiration radiograph. In most cases, both radiographs are obtained. Compared with an inspiration radiograph, an expiration chest radiograph requires an increase of 6 to 8 kVp to compensate for the decreased amount of air. Inspiration and expiration examinations are also performed to rule out the presence of a foreign body (FB) and to evaluate diaphragm excursion. Diaphragm excursion is the movement of the diaphragm on inspiration and expiration, and with positional changes. The dome-shaped diaphragm contracts on inspiration, moving inferiorly and flattening out, increasing the height of the thoracic cavity as a result. During expiration, the diaphragm moves superiorly as it relaxes. Average respiratory diaphragm excursion is approximately 1.5 inches between deep inspiration and expiration. The diaphragm is at its most inferior level when a patient is upright, and most superior level when the patient is supine. Also, the presence of pulmonary markings can significantly alter density on other examinations, such as ribs, sternum, and thoracic spine, so expiration radiographs are sometimes preferable in those cases.

Last, image-degrading voluntary motion may be controlled by means of immobilization. There are numerous immobilization methods, and every seasoned technologist has his/her own personal favorites that are "tricks of the trade." Routine radiography, particularly when the patient is in pain, or has a fracture, can be greatly aided by the use of sandbags and sponges. Larger sponges can be placed behind the patient as a means of support for positions that are hard to maintain, such as RPO and LPO obliques of the lumbar spine. Various commercial devices exist that can be attached to the table and then pulled across the abdomen or chest area to hold the patient in place when the table is turned in the upright position for upright abdominal radiographs or RAO esophagus views, for example. Commercial devices are also a popular means of immobilizing pediatric patients; various types exist, ranging from ones designed for use with skull radiography to others designed for chest and abdominal examinations.

E. Technique and Positioning Variations

The clinical situation often limits a patient's ability to cooperate fully with the positioning requirements of a standard radiographic examination. A patient who has a newly fractured humerus, for example, will be unable to raise his/her arms over the head in the standard fashion for a lateral chest examination, nor will he/she likely be able to extend the arm for an axillary lateral view of the glenohumeral joint. Some patients are completely incapacitated and unable to cooperate even minimally with positioning conditions.

What is to be done with such patients? Obviously, the best radiographs possible should be obtained, but often examinations must be limited or modified, based on the patient's ability to cooperate, the radiographic information required in light of the patient's diagnosis, and the logistics of how best to obtain such information taking into account the previous factors and the limitations of available equipment.

Examinations that are ordered either to evaluate or rule out fracture are a common example of such a clinical situation. The patient's motion and ability to cooperate are hampered by pain and, in some instances, by immobilization devices such as casts, splints, or braces. In the case of removable devices, the ordering physician should be consulted before removing the device for the examination. Some orthopedic physicians use the shorthand XIP, meaning x-ray in plaster, or OOP, which means out of plaster, on the radiograph request form. The device being referred to may not necessarily be constructed of plaster; it may be fiberglass, plastic, or some other amalgam of materials, but the order refers to whether or not the physician wants the device removed for radiographic examination.

AP and cross-table lateral projections are another common method of altering the standard positioning in order to attain diagnostic radiographic results in a less than optimal clinical situation. With this method, the part under examination is placed in AP alignment, and a standard AP view is obtained. Next, the tube and film are positioned perpendicular to the long axis of the part, and the part is elevated with a pillow or sponge, so that the most inferior aspect of the part can be visualized on the film. The resulting exposure is a lateral projection of the part obtained with an absolute minimum of painful moving on the part of the patient.

In a hospital or critical care environment, many patients needing radiographic services are severely debilitated; they are unable to cooperate with even the simplest of examination requirements. In this situation, the patient will frequently be unable to stand erect. This limitation on the part of the patient is somewhat problematic in that many standard examinations—chest, abdomen, and paranasal sinus, in particular—require that the patient be in an upright erect position for the examination so that the presence or lack of air-fluid levels can be determined.

In the case of the chest and sinus, if the patient is able to sit erect in a wheelchair, the following procedure can be performed. At a 72-inch FFD, an AP radiograph of the chest is obtained by placing a screen cassette behind the patient and making an exposure at appropriate screen techniques. Of course, technique varies from facility to facility, but factors using a 400-speed system are approximately 2.5 mAs and 80 kVp, assuming that the patient is of average size. The contours of the wheelchair often make tube part film alignment somewhat askew, in which case angling the tube, usually caudally, is a helpful compensatory measure. The lateral chest radiograph can be obtained by placing the wheelchair and patient in a lateral position at the upright grid, and making a standard 72-inch FFD grid exposure. If the armpiece of the chair is removable, you should remove it, because it may interfere with visualization of the lung bases. The patient may be aided in this endeavor by placing an IV pole in front of him/her so that he/she has something to hold while raising the arms for the lateral view.

The wheelchair-bound patient may also be positioned against the upright grid or elevated x-ray table for standard views of the sinus; however, such patients are frail, and the demands of the examination, particularly the cervical flexion involved with the submento-vertex (SMV) view, may need to be modified by increasing tube angulation or accepting less-than-optimal positioning and demonstration of

structures. Portable paranasal sinus radiographs may even be ordered on a bedridden ICU patient, but such examinations are even more limited, usually being confined to a reverse (AP) Waters' view, with the head of the bed elevated, and a single cross-table lateral view. The Waters' view is generally made using a 40-inch focused grid cassette, because penetrating the dense skull in this projection requires higher kVp, which produces higher levels of scatter. The paranasal sinuses are significantly less dense in the lateral projection, however, and it is common practice to use a screen cassette for this projection because the concern of grid cutoff occurring can be eliminated without sacrifice of diagnostic information.

Lateral decubitus views, generally the left side down, or left lateral decubitus, may act as a substitute for erect abdominal films. In this case, the patient is positioned laterally on the x-ray table on top of a radiopaque pad or sponge, which, like the cross-table views, serves to elevate the part so that its most inferior aspect will be visualized on the radiograph. The tube and film, along with a 40-inch focused 14 × 17 grid, are positioned in a manner similar to that of the cross-table lateral. Because the patient is in the lateral position, the projection on film will be along the PA or AP axis, depending on which side of the patient the tube is positioned. The arms should be placed over the head or, failing that, at least above the level of the diaphragm, to avoid projecting them over the area of interest. Both sides of the abdomen should ideally be demonstrated; if free air is suspected, the side up is of most importance; if fluid collection is suspected, the side down is most important. Some authors have advocated keeping the patient in a left lateral decubitus position for 10 to 20 minutes in order to permit intraperitoneal gas to rise to the right hemidiaphragm free of superimposition of the gastric gas bubble. The side up is usually marked with a right marker to indicate which side is up to the radiologist.

QUESTIONS FOR GENERAL PROCEDURAL CONSIDERATIONS

select the best answer

1. All of the following are considered prerequisites to bringing the patient into the exposure room EXCEPT:
   (A) assuring that the room is clean.
   (B) selecting technique for the examination.
   (C) assembling needed accessories.
   (D) assuring that the patient is dressed properly and is free of radiopaque objects.

2. Which of the following are considered techniques that reduce voluntary patient motion?

    1. Explanation of the procedure
    2. Short FFD
    3. High kVp and AED

(A) All of the aforementioned
(B) Choice 3 only
(C) Choices 2 and 3
(D) Choice 1 only

3. If the standard means of obtaining a PA chest radiograph on an average-size patient is use of the two lateral cells on the unit AED, which correction is necessary for a thin patient?

(A) Select one lateral cell only
(B) Select all three photo cells
(C) Select the center cell
(D) No correction is required

4. A PA view of the hand requires which skeletal motion?

(A) Supination
(B) Pronation
(C) Inversion
(D) Eversion

5. All of the following conditions are best evaluated with both inspiration and expiration PA chest radiographs EXCEPT:

(A) foreign body.
(B) respiratory excursion.
(C) pneumocystosis.
(D) pneumothorax.

6. Which of the following techniques would be best for use with a nongrid 72-inch FFD examination of a 6-month-old infant's chest with a PA view?

(A) 400-speed system, 1000 mA, 0.001 sec, large focal spot
(B) 400-speed system, 100 mA, 0.01 sec, small focal spot
(C) 100-speed system, 500 mA, 0.01 sec, large focal spot
(D) 100-speed system, 100 mA, 0.05 sec, small focal spot

▶▶▶ ANSWERS TO GENERAL PROCEDURAL CONSIDERATIONS

1. The answer is (B). Although selecting technique before positioning the patient is considered solid clinical practice because it reduces the amount of time the patient must hold the position, it is premature to do so before entering the exposure room. The radiographer may have selected technique based on the requirements of a standard examination, only to discover after talking with the patient that the examination, and hence the technique, must be modified to suit the clinical limitations of the patient.

2. The answer is (D). Voluntary motion is motion the patient can control. The best method of reducing voluntary motion is explanation of the procedure. With a good explanation of the examination, and clear patient instructions such as cessation of breathing and movement for the duration of the exposure, voluntary motion can be reduced greatly or eliminated entirely. Using the shortest possible exposure time is also a helpful technique with both voluntary and involuntary motion, but the shortest exposure time will not always produce the best diagnostic information. In this case, the needs of the examination should be weighed against the physical limitations of the patient and the likelihood of cooperation.

3. The answer is (D). The radiographic density produced using an AED is based on predetermined known correct values. Therefore, no cell change is necessary for a thin patient; the unit will compensate. An exception to this situation occurs if the patient is so thin that the exposure required is less than the absolute minimum exposure time the machine is capable of. In this case, kVp may be reduced so that greater mAs is required to produce the exposure, or master density selections may be reduced to minus settings.

4. The answer is (B). The normal anatomic position is standing erect with palms up and thumb facing away from the midline. In this alignment, the patient is said to be in the AP position. Therefore, a PA view requires the patient to pronate the hand.

5. The answer is (C). Pneumocystosis is infection with the parasite *Pneumocystis carinii,* which is sometimes found in infants, but in recent years this microorganism has become one of the hallmark conditions associated with HIV and AIDS patients. The condition is well demonstrated on standard PA and lateral chest radiographs.

6. The answer is (A). The prime consideration in this clinical setting is reduction of motion on the part of the pediatric patient; therefore, although other combinations listed would yield better radiographic resolution, the fastest possible combination of screen/film speed and technique would be best.

II. SPECIFIC IMAGING PROCEDURES
A. Thoracic Studies

The cone-shaped bony thorax is narrow superiorly and broader inferiorly. It is wider than it is deep, and longer posteriorly than anteriorly. The thorax consists of the 12 thoracic vertebrae, 12 pairs of ribs, and the sternum, which function together to protect the heart and lungs. The thoracic cavity extends from the thoracic inlet, superiorly, at the level of the first pair of ribs, to the diaphragm inferiorly. The mediastinum is a potential space between the lungs that extends from the thoracic inlet to the diaphragm and contains the trachea, esophagus, thymus gland, heart, and great blood vessels.

The respiratory system consists of the larynx, trachea, bronchi, and two lungs. The trachea is a fibrous tube, situated on the midline anterior to the esophagus, with 16 to 20 cartilaginous C-shaped rings embedded in its walls to provide rigidity. It is approximately 2 cm in diameter and 11 cm in length. The trachea is slightly displaced to the right at the level of the aorta, and courses through the mediastinum from its laryngeal junction at the level of C6 inferiorly to the level of T4 to T5. At this level, the trachea bifurcates into right and left primary bronchi, which slant obliquely and inferiorly into each lung. The right bronchus is shorter, wider, and more vertically situated than the left, and hence, when foreign bodies are aspirated, they are more likely to pass into the right bronchus than the left. At the level of the hilum, the primary bronchus subdivides into main stem bronchi, supplying oxygen to each lobe of the lung. The right lung has three stem bronchi, and the left lung has two. The bronchi continue to subdivide and diminish in size, ending in much smaller tubes called terminal bronchioles, which are less than 0.5 mm in diameter. Terminal bronchioles communicate with alveolar ducts, which in turn end as densely clustered alveolar sacs. Alveolar sacs resemble bunches of grapes and are lined with alveoli, which are the microscopic chambers where the bulk of gas exchange occurs **(Figure 5-6)**.

The lungs are situated on each side of the thoracic cavity and extend from the rounded apices above the level of the clavicles to their base, where they are concave in shape, resting on the obliquely placed diaphragm. Because of the position of the liver, the right lung is approximately 1 inch shorter then the left lung, and is also broader because of the position of the heart. The lungs are enclosed by a double-layered membrane called the pleura; the inner layer is called the visceral or pulmonary pleura,

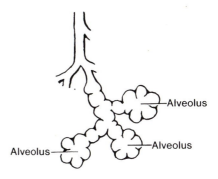

FIGURE 5-6.   A respiratory unit. Fifty to 100 of these make a tiny lobule. Bronchioles divide into alveolar ductules which open into alveolar saccules and alveoli. (Reproduced with permission from John V. Basmajian, MD, McMaster University, Hamilton, Ontario.)

and the outer layer is called the parietal pleura. The space between the two structures is called the pleural cavity. The pleura is moistened by serum to prevent friction between the lungs and chest walls during respiration. The right lung is divided into three lobes by two obliquely extending fissures, and the left lung contains two lobes, divided by a single oblique fissure **(Figure 5-7)**.

Anteriorly, the thorax is bounded at the midline by the sternum. The sternum is a narrow, flat bone, approximately 6 inches in length, that consists of three parts. The most superior part of the manubrium is the widest portion and contains the palpable manubrial (or jugular) notch on its superior medial aspect. The lateral aspect of the manubrium slants posterolaterally and contains an articular surface for the medial aspect of the clavicles, forming the sternoclavicular (SC) joints. The sternoclavicular joints are the only articulation between the upper extremity and the thorax, and are diathrotic (permitting limited movement) gliding type joints. The manubrium articulates with the longest portion of the sternum, the body or gladiolus, where it forms the palpable sternal angle. The smallest and most distal portion of the sternum is the xiphoid or ensiform process **(Figure 5-8)**, which lies approximately at the level of T10, is cartilaginous in early life, and ossifies with age.

The 12 pairs of ribs are numbered 1 to 12, beginning with the most superior first rib and increasing in number inferiorly. They are situated in an oblique plane, and extend from their posterior attachment to the thoracic vertebrae anteroinferiorly so that their anterior ends lie approximately 3 to 5 inches

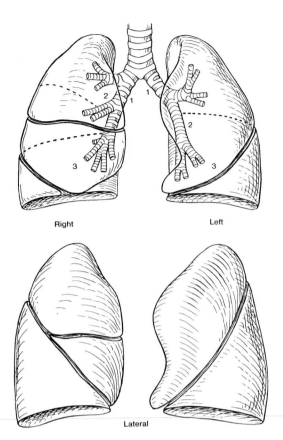

FIGURE 5-7. The right lung has three lobes and ten segments; the left lung has two lobes and eight segments *(broken lines),* each supplied by a tertiary bronchus. (Reproduced with permission from John V. Basmajian, MD, McMaster University, Hamilton, Ontario.)

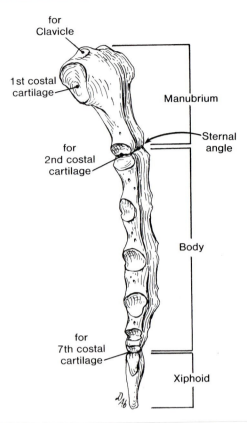

FIGURE 5-8. The sternum viewed from the right side. (Reproduced with permission from John V. Basmajian, MD, McMaster University, Hamilton, Ontario.)

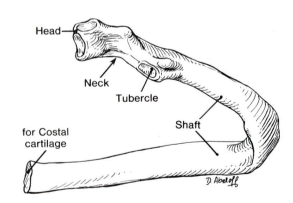

FIGURE 5-9. A typical right rib from behind (costal cartilage absent). (Reproduced with permission from John V. Basmajian, MD, McMaster University, Hamilton, Ontario.)

below the level of their vertebral ends. Ribs 1 to 7 attach directly to the sternum via costal cartilage, which are bars of hyaline cartilage, and are known as the true or vertebrosternal ribs. The remaining five pairs of ribs are called false ribs; ribs 8 to 10 attach to the sternum only indirectly, and ribs 11 and 12 lack anterior attachment altogether and are called floating or vertebral ribs. A typical rib is a bowed, flat bone, comprised of a head, neck, tubercle, and shaft **(Figure 5-9).**

The head of the rib contains two articulating facets; one joins the body of the same numbered thoracic vertebra, and the other articulates with the thoracic vertebra superior to it **(Figure 5-10).** The tubercle articulates with the transverse process of the same numbered thoracic vertebra. The first, eleventh, and twelfth ribs are atypical. The spaces between the ribs are known as intercostal spaces.

RADIOGRAPHIC PROCEDURES: THORACIC STUDIES

Chart 5-1 describes the procedures for imaging of the thorax.

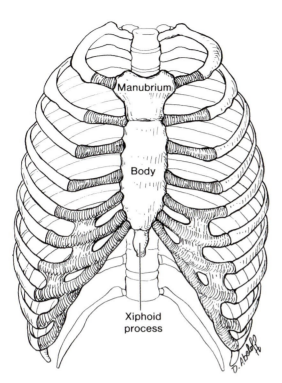

FIGURE 5-10. Thoracic cage. Costal cartilages are shaded. (Reproduced with permission from John V. Basmajian, MD, McMaster University, Hamilton, Ontario.)

▶ **CHART 5-1.** Procedures for Imaging of the Thorax

RAO STERNUM

Film Size and Centering. 10 × 12 LW bucky, centered to the midsternum.
Position. 15°–20° RAO, less oblique for larger patients, more oblique for thin patients. Shallow breathing technique may be used with low mA and long exposure time in order to blur pulmonary markings. Patients with large breasts should have the breasts drawn to the side and held in place with a wide bandage or tape.
Central Ray. Perpendicular to the midsternum.
Structures Visualized. PA oblique view of the sternum. Pulmonary markings will be blurred if breathing technique is applied.
Quality Control Criteria. The entire sternum will be visualized, with the sternum projected laterally into the cardiac shadow, free of superimposition of the thoracic vertebrae.

LATERAL STERNUM

Film Size and Centering. 10 × 12 LW bucky. The upper border is placed 1½″–2″ above the manubrial notch.

Position. Place the patient erect at the upright bucky, with hands joined behind the back in order to rotate the shoulders posteriorly. A 72-inch FFD may be used to decrease magnification. Have the patient suspend respiration on deep inspiration.
Central Ray. Perpendicular to the midsternum.
Structures Visualized. Lateral view of the entire sternum, superimposed SC joints, and media ends of the clavicles.
Quality Control Criteria. Entire sternum demonstrated; manubrium free of superimposition from the shoulders or ribs.

PA STERNOCLAVICULAR (SC) JOINTS

Film Size and Centering. 8 × 10 CW bucky. Centered to third thoracic (T3) spinous process, which is at the level of the jugular notch.
Position. Prone or erect, arms along sides, palms up. Bilateral examination is performed in the standard PA position. Unilateral examination may be performed; if so, turn the head toward the affected side, rotating the lower cervical (C) spine and upper thoracic (T) spine slightly. Exposure is made with suspended expiration.
Central Ray. Perpendicular to the T3 spinous process.
Structures Visualized. PA projection of the SC joints and the medial ends of the clavicles.
Quality Control Criteria. Both SC joints visualized, free of superimposition from thoracic vertebrae or ribs. No patient rotation is permissible on bilateral exam; slight rotation toward affected side on unilateral exam.

RAO AND LAO STERNOCLAVICULAR JOINTS—CR ANGULATION METHOD

Film Size and Centering. 8 × 10 CW screen or grid cassette. Using the bucky with this method would result in grid cutoff. Center at the level of the T3 spinous process.
Position. Prone or seated erect PA. Arms along patient's side, palms up. Head turned toward affected side.
Central Ray. From the side under examination, direct the central ray (CR) 15° toward the midsagittal plane (MSP) to the midpoint of the film. CR angulation projects SC joint nearest film away from overlapping structures.
Structures Visualized. Oblique projection of SC joint nearest film is demonstrated. Alternatively, one can oblique the patient 15° instead of the CR; however, in this case, the side up is demonstrated, resulting in more distortion and magnification.
Quality Control Criteria. SC joint should be projected onto the center of the radiograph, with the SC joint space open and free of superimposition. Manubrium and medial aspect of clavicle are included.

UPPER ANTERIOR RIBS—PA PROJECTION

Film Size and Centering. 14 × 17 LW bucky. Upper border of film 1½″ above the shoulders; MSP centered to grid.
Position. Patient should be erect if possible, in order to cause the diaphragm to move to its most inferior position. Shoulders are rolled forward to project scapulae away from the ribs. Respiration is suspended on inhalation, which also depresses the diaphragm.
Central Ray. Perpendicular to MSP at the level of T7.
Structures Visualized. Anterior ribs 1–9 in their entirety.
Quality Control Criteria. Anterior ribs 1–9 should be visualized above the diaphragm. Short scale of contrast is useful, using low kVp–high mAs technique, although this may be somewhat impractical with larger patients, because of extremely high dose.

POSTERIOR RIBS—AP PROJECTION

Film Size and Centering. 14 × 17 LW bucky. Upper border of film 1½″ above the shoulders. MSP centered to grid.
Position. Patient should be erect for ribs above the diaphragm, and supine for ribs below the diaphragm. For upper ribs, place the patient's hands resting behind his head. Respiration is suspended on inspiration to depress the diaphragm. For lower ribs, use a 14 × 17 cassette CW, and place the lower border at the iliac crest. Respiration is suspended on expiration to elevate the diaphragm.
Central Ray. Upper ribs are centered perpendicular to MSP at T7; lower ribs are centered at T12.
Structures Visualized. Posterior ribs above or below the diaphragm, as desired.
Quality Control Criteria. Posterior ribs 1–10 should be seen completely above the diaphragm, or posterior ribs 8–12 should be seen completely unobstructed by the diaphragm.

OBLIQUE RIBS

Film Size and Centering. 14 × 17 upright bucky for ribs above the diaphragm, table bucky for ribs below the diaphragm. Upper ribs centered 1½″ above the shoulders, lower ribs, place lower border of film 1½″ below the T12.
Position. For RPO and LPO (AP) projections, oblique the patient 45°, affected side toward the film. For RAO and LAO (PA) projections, oblique the patient 45°, affected side away from the film. Center on a sagittal plane midway between the MSP and the lateral-most surface of the body. Place the hand behind the patient's head, if possible. If the patient is supine, flex the elbow, and place the hand on the hip. Respiration is suspended on expira-

tion for ribs below the diaphragm, and on inspiration for ribs above the diaphragm.
Central Ray. CR at the level of T7 for upper ribs, and T12 for lower ribs, perpendicular to a sagittal plane midway between the MSP and the lateral-most surface of the body.
Structures Visualized. AP obliques demonstrate the axillary portion of the ribs closest to the film, whereas PA obliques demonstrate the axillary portion of the ribs away from the film.
Quality Control Criteria. Axillary portion of the ribs are elongated, demonstrated free of self-superimposition.

PA CHEST

Film Size and Centering. 14 × 17 LW or CW, depending on body habitus. Place the upper border of the film 1–1½″ above the level of the relaxed shoulders. A 72″ SID is used to reduce magnification of the heart.
Position. The patient is placed in the PA position at the upright bucky. The shoulders should be relaxed and rolled forward to project the scapulae away from the lung fields. The hands should be positioned with palms up to rotate the scapulae laterally, low on the hips, away from the lung bases. The chin should rest on top of the upright bucky. Patients with large breasts should be instructed to pull the breasts upward and laterally, and then hold them in place by leaning against the grid device. This method prevents underpenetration of the lung bases caused by dense breast tissue. Respiration is suspended on deep inspiration. Some authors advocate the use of a second deep breath to ensure full expansion of the lung fields.
Central Ray. Perpendicular to the MSP, centered at the level of T7.
Structures Visualized. Primary structures demonstrated include the costophrenic angles, diaphragm, heart and major vessels, aortic arch, air-filled lung fields, apical portion of the lungs, air-filled trachea, scapulae, and clavicles.
Quality Control Criteria. Both costophrenic angles must be included and adequately penetrated. The lung apices must be demonstrated. SC joints should be equidistant from T spine. Scapulae must be projected outside the lung fields. Ten posterior ribs should be demonstrated above the diaphragm.

AP SEATED ERECT (MODIFIED) CHEST

Film Size and Centering. 14 × 17 LW, or CW, depending on patient body habitus; 72″ SID. Upper border of film 1–2″ above upper border of shoulders. Compensatory caudal angulation may be necessary if examination is

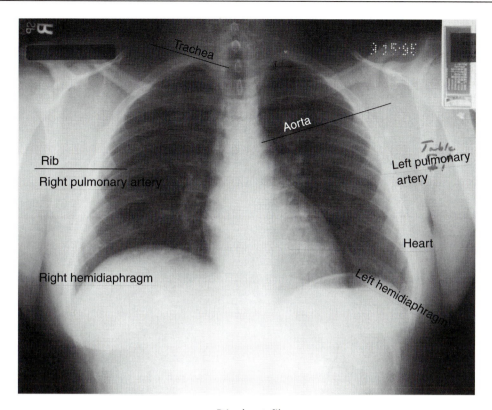

Trachea

Aorta

Rib

Right pulmonary artery

Left pulmonary artery

Heart

Right hemidiaphragm

Left hemidiaphragm

PA chest film

performed with the patient seated erect in a wheelchair or gurney.

Position. This modification is used when the patient is unable to stand erect, or for portable chest radiography. An erect film is generally preferred in order to demonstrate air/fluid levels, prevent engorgement of the pulmonary vessels, and move the diaphragm to its most inferior position.

Central Ray. Perpendicular to the plane of the film. A caudal angulation is usually employed, compensating for the more horizontal-appearing clavicles and freeing the apical portion from superimposition by the clavicles, and basal portion of the lung fields from superimposition of the anterior portion of the diaphragm.

Structures Visualized. The cardiac shadow and great vessels are more magnified than the PA projection because they are comparatively farther from the film. The lung fields also appear a bit shorter than on the PA, because the diaphragm is also magnified. Depending on angulation used, the clavicles are demonstrated somewhat more superiorly, and the ribs appear more horizontal.

Quality Control Criteria. Approximately equivocal to that of the PA projection, with the exceptions already mentioned.

LEFT LATERAL CHEST

Film Size and Centering. 14 × 17 LW bucky; upper border of film 1–1½″ above upper border of the shoulders; 72″ SID

Position. Patient is erect at the upright bucky, MSP perpendicular, with arms raised. Ideally, elbows should be flexed, with the patient's forearms resting on his head; this position allows maximum reduction of OFD by permitting the patient to stand flush against the upright grid. An IV pole may be employed for the patient to hold if he is unsteady. Respiration is suspended on full inspiration.

Central Ray. Perpendicular to the MSP and film at the level of T7.

Structures Visualized. The heart, aorta, and left pulmonary vasculature are demonstrated. Occasionally a right lateral is employed to demonstrate right pulmonary lesions. The lateral film aids in differentiation of lobes, demonstration of pulmonary fissures, and localization of lesions.

Quality Control Criteria. The ribs should be superimposed, and the apices free of superimposition of the arms. Sternum should be demonstrated in the lateral po-

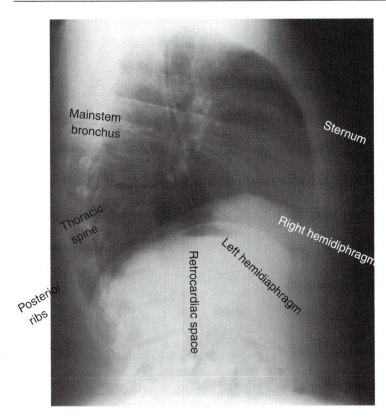

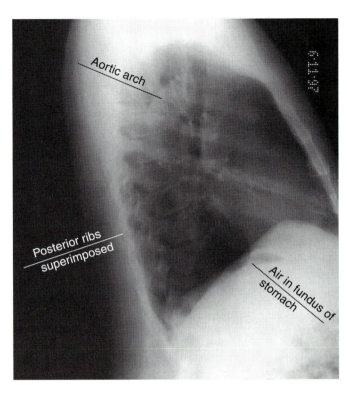

Lateral chest films

sition. Forward or backward leaning by the patient may obscure important structures. Thoracic vertebral spaces should be open, except with the presence of scoliosis.

QUESTIONS FOR THORACIC STUDIES

select the best answer

1. Which of the following are correct factors concerning the CR angulation method for an oblique projection of the SC joints?

   (A) Prone, 15 degrees cephalic
   (B) RAO, 15 degrees caudal
   (C) PA, 15 degrees toward the midpoint of MSP
   (D) RPO, 15 degrees toward the midpoint of MSP

2. An LPO projection of the ribs best demonstrates which of the following?

   (A) Posterior ribs
   (B) Anterior ribs
   (C) Left axillary portion
   (D) Right axillary portion

3. Which method of suspended respiration best demonstrates fully expanded lung fields?

   (A) Deep inspiration
   (B) Full expiration
   (C) Shallow breathing
   (D) Second breath inspiration

4. Compared with the left lung, the right lung is:

   (A) somewhat shorter and has an additional lobe.
   (B) broader and has only two lobes.
   (C) longer, but has an additional lobe.
   (D) broader and longer.

5. Which of the following best describes the term pneumothorax?

   (A) Air in the parietal pleura
   (B) Air in the visceral pleura
   (C) Air in the pleural cavity
   (D) Air in the mediastinum

6. How many pairs of ribs are considered true ribs?

   (A) 7
   (B) 10
   (C) 2
   (D) 12

▶▶ ANSWERS TO THORACIC STUDIES

1. The answer is (C). The CR angulation method for oblique SC joints demonstrates a slightly oblique projection of the SC joint with less distortion than that used when the body itself is placed in the oblique position, because comparatively less OFD occurs using this method. The patient is prone, and a 15-degree angulation toward the MSP is used in conjunction with a screen cassette in order to prevent grid cutoff.

2. The answer is (C). Oblique projections of the ribs are used routinely in order to demonstrate an elongated view of the axillary portion of the ribs. Anterior obliques best demonstrate the side away from the film, and posterior obliques best demonstrate the side toward the film.

3. The answer is (D). Particularly with hyperesthetic patients, more air is inhaled with less strain on the second inspiration than on the first. This method should be employed whenever possible; however, clinical restraints may require that the exposure be made as quickly as possible in order to prevent patient motion, in which case a single inspiratory effort is used.

4. The answer is (A). The right lung is divided into three lobes by two obliquely placed fissures. It is somewhat shorter than the left lung due to the position of the liver, and is somewhat broader because of the position of the heart.

5. The answer is (C). Each lung is contained by a double-walled, serous membrane called the pleura. The outer layer lines the cavity occupied by the lung and is called the parietal pleura, whereas the inner layer adheres to the surface of the lung, and is called the visceral pleura. The space between the two layers is called the pleural space or cavity. Pneumothorax is a collection of air in the pleural space that causes the lung to collapse. There are a number of conditions that may cause the condition, including an open chest wound, rupture of an emphysematous vesicle on the surface of the lung, severe coughing; or the condition may occur spontaneously. The lung is reinflated by insertion of a chest tube that expels the air via a water seal drainage system.

6. The answer is (A). Rib pairs 1 to 7 are considered true or vertebrosternal ribs because they attach via the costal cartilage directly to the sternum. Ribs 8 to10 are false ribs; they attach to the sternum via the costal cartilage superior to them; ribs 11 and 12 are also false ribs, but are referred to as floating ribs, because they have no anterior attachment at all.

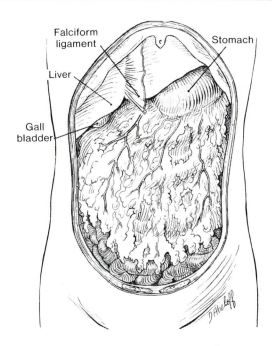

FIGURE 5-11. The greater omentum hangs like an apron from the greater curvature of the stomach. (Reproduced with permission from John V. Basmajian, MD, McMaster University, Hamilton, Ontario.)

B. Abdomen and GI Studies

The abdomen is bounded from its superior border at the diaphragm to its most inferior level at the symphysis pubis. Like the pleura in the thoracic cavity, the abdominopelvic cavity is lined by a double-walled seromembranous sac called the peritoneum. The outer portion of the peritoneum lining the body wall is known as the parietal peritoneum; that which covers the abdominal viscera, or organs, is known as the visceral peritoneum. The visceral layer forms folds called the mesentery and omentum, which aid in holding the organs in position **(Figure 5-11).**

Important visceral structures contained in the abdomen include the distal esophagus, stomach, small and large intestine, spleen, pancreas, liver, gallbladder, kidneys, ureters, and urinary bladder. Per the content specifications set out by the ARRT, the abdominal contents will be discussed according to systems, with the digestive system studied first, and the urinary system discussed in the following section.

GI Tract **(Figure 5-12)**

ESOPHAGUS

The esophagus is a collapsed, muscular tube lying posterior to the trachea, beginning at the level of C6. Total length is approximately 25 cm, with the upper

FIGURE 5-12. The digestive system. (Reprinted from Chung KW: *BRS Gross Anatomy,* 3rd ed. Baltimore, Williams & Wilkins, 1995, p 161.)

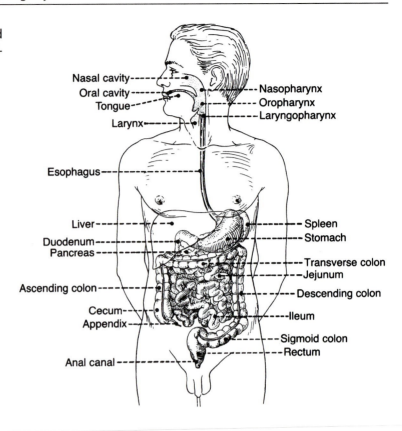

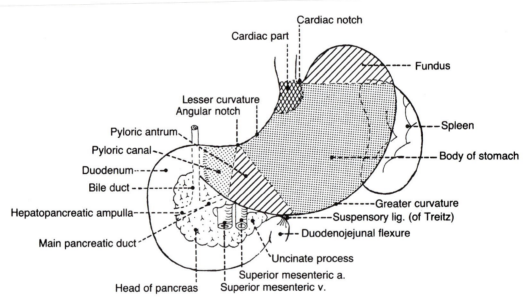

FIGURE 5-13. The stomach and duodenum. (Reprinted from Chung KW: *BRS Gross Anatomy,* 3rd ed. Baltimore, Williams & Wilkins, 1995, p 160.)

one fifth lying in the neck, and except for the most distal 2 to 3 cm, the remainder is located in the thorax. The distal esophagus turns slightly left, penetrating the diaphragm and descending 2 to 3 cm, where it joins the stomach at the cardiac orifice. Peristaltic contractions begin in the esophagus; food and water do not reach the stomach by gravity, but by muscular contraction.

STOMACH (Figure 5-13)

The roughly J-shaped stomach is the most dilated portion of the digestive tract, with an average capacity of approximately 1 liter. It is subject to great variation in size, shape, and location, according to body habitus. The stomach is marked by the lesser curvature, which descends nearly vertically from the cardiac orifice and forms its medial border. The lateral border is formed by the greater curvature, which varies in size and shape according to stomach contents. The most superior portion of the stomach is the upward ballooned recess superior to the cardiac orifice called the fundus. The fundus may be visualized on plain radiographs of the abdomen because it is frequently air-filled. The distal stomach becomes progressively narrower as it approaches the small intestine and is marked by its most inferior portion, the pyloric antrum, and then moves slightly superiorly and medially to form the pyloric canal, and the pyloric orifice, the exit of the stomach.

SMALL INTESTINE

The small intestine is divided into three portions. The first and shortest part is the horseshoe-shaped duodenum. The duodenum is approximately 25 cm (10 inches) in length, roughly the same length as the stomach and esophagus. The horseshoe, or C-shape of the duodenum, is formed by its proximal portion 2 to 3 cm to the right of the midline, and its distal portion approximately the same distance to the left. The two ends are approximately 5 cm apart. The duodenum surrounds the head of the pancreas and receives bile from the common bile duct and digestive enzymes from the pancreatic duct. The remainder of the small bowel measures approximately 20 feet and is subdivided into the proximal two fifths, called the jejunum, and the distal three fifths, called the ileum. The caliber of the small bowel varies according to its muscular activity, but in general decreases by half as it proceeds from duodenum to ileum.

LARGE INTESTINE (Figure 5-14)

The terminal ileum joins with the large intestine via a liplike portion of tissue called the ileocecal valve. The valve is a one-way passage into the cecum, a type of reservoir forming the first portion of the large intestine. Aside from the stomach, the lumen of the cecum possesses the largest caliber of any portion of the intestines. Attached to the posteromedial aspect of the cecum is the vermiform (meaning *wormlike*) appendix, the narrowest portion of the intestine, which measures approximately 2.5 × 3 inches.

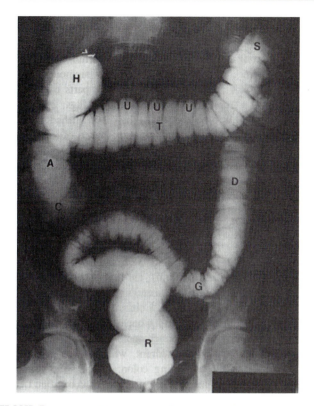

FIGURE 5-14. AP view, single-contrast barium enema. *C* = cecum; *A* = ascending colon; *H* = hepatic flexure; *T* = transverse colon; *S* = splenic flexure; *D* = descending colon; *G* = sigmoid colon; *R* = rectum; *U* = haustra. (Reproduced with permission from Moore KL: *Clinically Oriented Anatomy*, 3rd ed. Baltimore, Williams & Wilkins, 1992.)

The colon is first marked by its shortest portion—the ascending colon. The ascending colon rises through the retroperitoneum to the inferior surface of the liver, where it turns medially, forming a bend in the colon anterior to the right kidney, known as the hepatic or right colic flexure. The colon proceeds across the midline, forming the transverse colon. The transverse colon is approximately twice as long as the distance across the abdomen; its middle portion hangs downward to the level of the umbilicus when the patient is erect. At a point just anterior to the left kidney, the transverse colon bends inferiorly, forming the splenic or left colic flexure. From the splenic flexure, the colon proceeds inferiorly through the retroperitoneum until reaching the pelvic brim, where it becomes the sigmoid colon.

The sigmoid extends mediosuperiorly until reaching the rectum, which is approximately 6 inches in length. The rectum continues inferiorly, joining the anal canal and anus, which is the external orifice of

FIGURE 5-15. Anterior and visceral surfaces of the liver. (Reprinted from Dudek RW: *High-Yield Gross Anatomy.* Baltimore, Williams & Wilkins, 1997, p 163.)

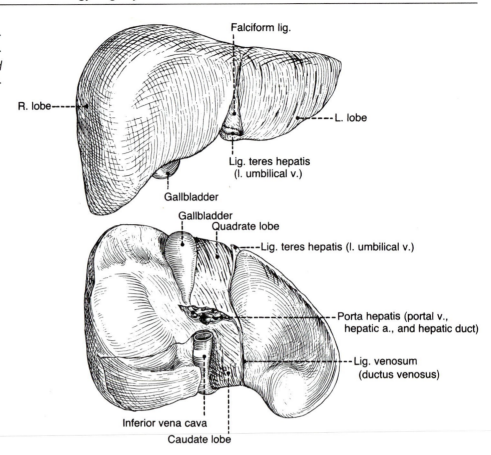

the intestine. Superior to the anal canal is a dilated portion of the rectum called the rectal ampulla.

A sagittal cross-section of the anal canal and rectum reveals two anteroposterior curves; the rectal ampulla almost forms a right angle with the anal canal, and following the sacrococcygeal curves superiorly, bends inferiorly before proceeding again in a superior direction. These two curves are significant to the radiographer from a clinical standpoint; they must be taken into account when inserting an enema tube.

Liver (Figure 5-15)

The liver is situated inferior to, and in contact with the right hemidiaphragm, and is protected in large measure by anterior ribs 8 to12. It is the largest gland in the body, comprising approximately one-fiftieth of total body weight.

The liver is marked by four lobes: (1) the largest right lobe; (2) a smaller left lobe; (3) the caudate lobe, which is located on the posterior surface of the right lobe; and (4) the quadrate lobe, which is found on the inferior surface of the right lobe.

The vascular supply of the liver is unique in that it receives blood from both the hepatic artery and the portal vein, which enter the hilum, or "door," of the

liver through a transverse slit between the caudate and quadrate lobes, known as the porta hepatis. The porta hepatis also carries the important right and left hepatic ducts, which leave the liver and form the common hepatic duct.

The physiologic functions of the liver are numerous and complex. Blood from the digestive tract, which is loaded with glucose derived from food, enters the liver via the portal vein. The liver converts the glucose to glycogen and stores it. When bodily activity demands an increase in glucose, glycogen is reconverted into glucose and circulated. The liver also metabolizes heparin, an important agent in the prevention of blood clotting. The organ produces and stores vitamin A, stores iron, helps to metabolize protein and fat, and acts as an important detoxifying agent. The liver secretes bile, which is the channel of elimination for dead red blood cells, and acts to emulsify and assimilate fat. Bile is carried to the gallbladder for storage purposes until poured into the duodenum via the common bile duct.

Biliary System

The biliary system, which is comprised of the gallbladder and bile ducts, acts as an excretory system for the

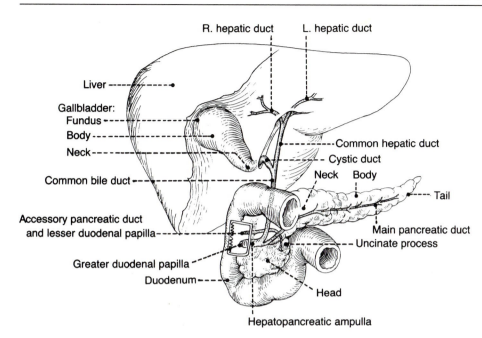

FIGURE 5-16. The biliary system. (Reprinted from Chung KW: *BRS Gross Anatomy,* 3rd ed. Baltimore, Williams & Wilkins, 1995, p 165.)

liver. The gallbladder has an elongated pear shape, measuring approximately 2.5 cm at its widest diameter and approximately 10 cm in length **(Figure 5-16).** It is located in a fossa on the inferior visceral surface of the right lobe of the liver, although it may become embedded in the liver or, alternatively, may hang free completely. It is comprised of thin-walled, musculomembranous tissue and has a capacity to store approximately 2 oz (50 cc) of bile. The gallbladder concentrates bile from the liver by absorbing the bile's water content; the gallbladder then stores the bile during interdigestive periods. Bile released from the gallbladder is up to 10 times as concentrated as bile entering it. An overconcentration of biliary salts may lead to the formation of gallstones. During digestion, a hormone called cholecystokinin is secreted by the duodenum, causing the gallbladder to contract and release bile into the biliary ductal system. The gallbladder is comprised of a rounded fundus, which projects beyond the liver and is in contact with the abdominal wall, and a constricted neck, which is continuous with the cystic duct (see Figure 5-16).

Emerging from the porta hepatis of the liver, the right and left hepatic ducts join to form the common hepatic duct. In turn, the common hepatic duct joins the cystic duct from the gallbladder to form the common bile duct. Bile enters the duodenum through the sphincter of Oddi, which is closed to protect the duodenum against the entry of bile and pancreatic juice until it is needed for digestion. During a meal, the gallbladder contracts, and the sphincter relaxes, al-

lowing passage of bile and pancreatic juice into the duodenum.

Pancreas

The pancreas is a soft, pink, roughly triangular accessory digestive organ associated with the small intestine (see Figure 5-16). It is the principal digestive-enzyme-producing organ of the digestive system. It extends transversely across the retroperitoneum from its tail, which is continuous with the spleen, to its 6-inch long body, which lies behind the greater curvature of the stomach, to its rounded head, which is encircled by the duodenum. The pancreas contains specialized cells called acini, which secrete pancreatic juice, an alkaline fluid containing a broad spectrum of enzymes. Pancreatic juice is drained by the pancreatic duct, which may unite with the common bile duct to form a single passage into the duodenum via the ampulla of Vater, but may also remain separate from the common bile duct until reaching the sphincter of Oddi at the duodenum.

Spleen

The spleen, situated in an oblique plane inferior to the diaphragm and posterior to the stomach (see Figure 5-12), is roughly the size of a fist. It is discussed in this section by virtue of its location, but it is not a digestive organ; rather it belongs to the lymphatic system. The spleen has three visceral surfaces that are named according to their contacts: renal, colic, and gastric. The

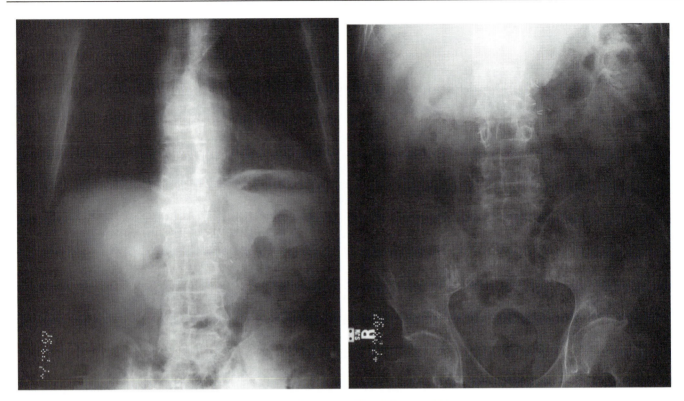

Flat (A) and upright (B) abdominal films.

spleen functions to produce lymphocytes and contains reticuloendothelial cells, which are the "scavenger" cells of the body. The spleen removes debris from disintegrated red blood cells, destroys worn out red blood cells, and filters bacteria. The spleen is a sort of built-in blood transfusion supply; it may add blood to the general circulation by contracting.

RADIOGRAPHIC PROCEDURES: ABDOMEN AND GI SYSTEM

Chart 5-2 describes the procedures for imaging of the abdomen and the GI system.

► CHART 5-2. Procedures for Abdomen and GI Studies

AP ABDOMEN—KIDNEYS, URETERS, AND BLADDER (KUB)

Film Size and Centering. 14 × 17 LW bucky.
Position. Patient is supine; a support may be placed under the knees to relieve back strain. MSP centered to midline of bucky. Cassette is centered roughly at the level of the iliac crest, although position varies according to body habitus. Symphysis pubis should be visualized at

the inferior border of the film. Respiration is suspended on expiration.
Central Ray. Perpendicular to the MSP at the level of the iliac crest.
Structures Visualized. A plain abdominal radiograph shows the size and shape of the kidneys, liver, and spleen. Abdominal gas and fecal material are visualized if present. The psoas muscles are appreciated.
Quality Control Criteria. Abdominal contents from upper abdomen to symphysis pubis are included. Lower thoracic and lumbar vertebrae should be seen in the center of the radiograph. Moderate long-scale contrast is appropriate; 70 kVp is considered optimal for visualization of calcified densities, although this may not be practical with obese patients.

ACUTE ABDOMINAL SERIES (FLAT AND UPRIGHT ABDOMEN, OR FLAT AND UPRIGHT WITH A PA CHEST)

Film Size and Centering. All films on 14 × 17 table or upright bucky, as appropriate, LW or CW according to body habitus. Extremely wide patients may require 2 CW exposures for the supine examination as well, to ensure the entire abdominal contents have been visualized.
Position. As per AP abdomen for the supine examination. Patient's MSP should be centered to the upright

bucky for the upright film. Respiration is suspended on inspiration for both PA chest and upright abdomen, and on expiration for the supine examination. A left lateral decubitus film of the abdomen to detect free air beneath the diaphragm may be substituted for the upright examination if the patient cannot stand.

Central Ray. Centered at a level 2″–3″ higher than the supine examination for the upright abdominal film to ensure diaphragm is visualized.

Structures Visualized. As previously discussed per the PA chest and KUB. Upright examination should demonstrate the diaphragm and should be marked with an upright marker. PA chest or upright radiograph may demonstrate free air under the diaphragm if present.

Quality Control Criteria. As previously discussed per PA chest and KUB; diaphragm should be demonstrated on upright examination. If lateral decubitus film is performed, the side down is of most importance when fluid is suspected, and the side up when the presence of free air is to be ruled out.

ESOPHAGUS

Routine exam includes AP or PA, RAO, and lateral views. Either single contrast examinations using 30%–50% wt/volume suspension of barium only, or double contrast, using low viscosity, high-density barium, and carbon dioxide–producing crystals, may be the routine, depending on the preference of the radiologist.

Film Size and Centering. 14 × 17 LW for overhead projections. Digital, 105 mm, or 9 × 9 spot films are generally obtained in the upright, or supine position, as indicated by the radiologist. Film is centered approximately at the level of T5–T6 in order to demonstrate the esophagus in its entirety.

Position. Unless the upright position is indicated, the patient is placed in the recumbent RAO, PA, and lateral positions, which demonstrate the esophagus more completely filled, by having the contrast flow against gravity. The recumbent position also demonstrates esophageal varices, as optimum filling of the varices occurs against gravity. The patient is instructed to hold a cupful of barium, placing a straw in the cup and in his mouth. He is instructed to drink continuously, and an exposure is made after several mouthfuls are ingested.

Central Ray. Perpendicular to the midpoint of the film at the level of T5–T6.

Structures Visualized. A contrast-filled esophagus is visualized from its proximal end at the level of C6 to the cardiac orifice. Single contrast is generally used for overhead projections; if double contrast is used, it is generally administered by the radiologist during fluoroscopy.

Quality Control Criteria. Exposure factors must include high kVp (110 or over) in order to adequately penetrate barium. If water-soluble contrast is used, lower kVp, in

the range of 70–80, is used instead. The esophagus should be demonstrated in the center of the film, between the cardiac outline and the thoracic vertebrae for the oblique views, and through the superimposed thoracic vertebrae on the AP/ PA views. The technologist must ensure the arms are raised enough to eliminate superimposition of structures over the proximal esophagus on the lateral projection.

UPPER GASTROINTESTINAL (UGI)

Single-contrast, double-contrast, or biphasic examinations may be performed, according to the diagnostic information desired, the limitations of the patient, and the clinical situation. Double-contrast exams are considered standard because of the superior visualization of the gastric and intestinal mucosa, but this requires comparatively more movement and ability to cooperate on the part of the patient than with single-contrast examinations. Single-contrast studies may not reveal small lesions. For biphasic examinations, the patient is examined with double contrast first, then with single contrast, combining the advantages of both approaches.

Film Size and Centering. Spot films are obtained by the radiologist during fluoroscopy. Preliminary scout view is a KUB on a 14 × 17. Esophagram is also taken on 14 × 17, usually in the RAO position. Stomach overheads are obtained in varying positions, on a 10 × 12, LW or CW, depending on body habitus. If small-bowel examination is also requested, the patient is given another cup of contrast following the UGI, and the progress of the contrast through the small intestine to the terminal ileum is monitored by obtaining sequential films, usually every 30 minutes.

Position. Routines may vary by facility, but generally include PA, AP, RAO, LPO, and right lateral views. The stomach is located in varying positions, but can almost always be demonstrated by placing the patient so that the bucky is centered to a sagittal plane midway between the midline and the left lateral border of the patient at the level of L2. For lateral projection, position the patient so that a coronal plane passes midway between the midaxillary line and the anterior border of the patient. Respiration is suspended on exhalation for all views.

Central Ray. Perpendicular to the midpoint of the film at the level of L2, slightly more superiorly for the PA projection.

Structures Visualized. PA projection demonstrates barium-filled stomach with air in the fundus. The prone position pushes the stomach superiorly 1″–4″; and slightly transversely, decreasing in length. It is best to observe the range of this movement during fluoroscopy if possible. RAO degree of rotation varies from 40°–70°, according to body habitus, and gives view of pyloric canal and duodenal bulb without superimposition of structures.

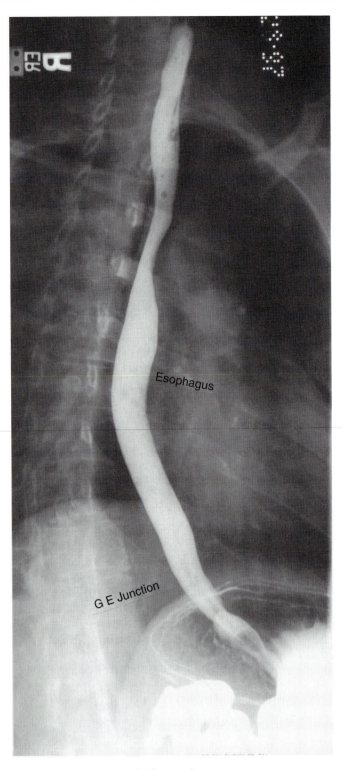

RAO esophagus

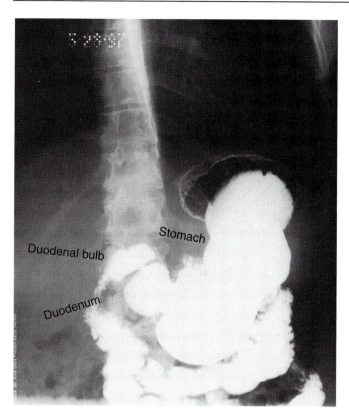

RAO stomach

LPO obliquity also varies; 30°–60° best demonstrates fundus of stomach. Right lateral projection best demonstrates right retrogastric space and duodenojejunal junction.

Quality Control Criteria.   Barium must be adequately penetrated. Entire stomach and duodenal loop should be demonstrated. Pylorus and duodenal bulb are not superimposed on oblique views.

SMALL BOWEL FOLLOW-THROUGH

The small intestine is most often examined in conjunction with a UGI series. When this method is employed, the examination consists of a timed series of exposures taken following completion of the UGI. Timing varies according to radiologist preference, but a film every 30 minutes is average. It is common to administer water-soluble oral contrast medium following the initial GI examination, in order to further stimulate peristalsis. Some radiologists prefer to give the patient ice water, coffee, or tea for the same purpose. When the standard follow-through method fails to reveal a satisfactory diagnosis, two other methods may be used. The small bowel may be examined by **reflux filling,** which is accomplished via large-volume barium enema. Another procedure, **enteroclysis, or small bowel enema,** employs direct contrast medium injection into the duodenum via an intestinal tube to visualize the small intestine.

Film Size and Centering.   14 × 17 LW bucky; centered at the level of the iliac crest. When timed film reveals contrast has reached the terminal portion of the ileum, the radiologist takes spot views for documentation.

Position.   AP supine. MSP plane centered to the bucky. Respiration suspended on expiration. When taking spot films, the radiologist may oblique the patient slightly to isolate the cecum and terminal ileum, and may employ a pneumatic-type compression paddle to displace small bowel overlying the area of interest. The technologist should ensure this device is readily available.

Central Ray.   Perpendicular to the MSP at the level of the iliac crest.

Structures Visualized.   Entire small bowel is visualized on large-film radiographs, with the stomach demonstrated on the initial film. Spot films demonstrate the terminal ileum without superimposition of structures.

Quality Control Criteria.   Barium adequately penetrated with high kVp technique. Patient in true AP alignment. Entire small bowel demonstrated, with stomach on initial follow-up film. Radiographs should demonstrate right or left radiopaque markers as well as markers indicating the time since initial ingestion of the barium.

SINGLE- AND DOUBLE-CONTRAST BARIUM ENEMA (BE)

Single-contrast examinations are performed using 2000–3000 mL of 12%–15% wt/volume suspension of barium suspension only, whereas double-contrast studies use high-density barium suspensions of 75%–95% wt/volume, but use much less barium (about 300 mL) and copious amounts of air. Opinion concerning temperature of the barium solution varies, but it is generally acknowledged that a cold solution of about 40°F produces less irritation, has a mild anesthetic effect on the colon, and induces the anal sphincter to tighten, aiding in retention of the enema. Preparation of the patient for BE examination is critical; the presence of fecal material in the colon may conceal or imitate lesions. It is vital that the technologist explain the procedure to the patient in step-by-step detail in order to gain cooperation. Few patients will be unable to retain the enema if they understand what is expected of them.

Film Size and Centering.   Spot films are taken during fluoroscopy using the available device. Overhead films consists largely of 14 × 17 LW bucky films, centered at the iliac crest; however, CW films may be required instead for hyperesthetic individuals in order that the entire colon may be visualized, in particular the hepatic and splenic flexures. The lateral rectum view is obtained using a 10 × 12 film. Some radiologists prefer a cross-table approach be used for the lateral rectum, in which case a

10 × 12 grid cassette or screen with 12-to-1 or higher ratio focused grid is used instead. Air-contrast enema examinations include bilateral decubitus views, obtained on 14 × 17 with grid or grid cassette.

Position. Prior to the examination, the patient is placed in the Sims position for insertion of the enema tip. To attain the Sims position, instruct the patient to turn on his left side, and gently position the right leg forward, flexing the knee. The enema tip is lubricated with a water soluble material, and the tip is inserted, pulling forward the right gluteal fold, and directing the tip first anteriorly 1″–1½″ and then slightly superiorly, following the curve of the rectum until the tip is inserted approximately 3″. The enema kit is equipped with a disposable enema retention tip that has a rubber balloon incorporated on the end. The balloon tip is inflated under fluoroscopic guidance by the radiologist and then clamped to maintain inflation. Double-contrast enema bags have a similar apparatus, but with a separate tubing for instilling air into the colon. Overhead routine for single-contrast enemas usually includes AP, PA, and both anterior 35°–45° obliques centered at the iliac crest. A prone or supine rectosigmoid view is taken with a tube angulation of 30°–40° caudally for the PA method, and cephalic for the AP method. CR passes through the midline at the level of the ASIS. A lateral rectum view is obtained with the CR passing through a midcoronal plane 1″ superior to the pubic symphysis. The lower border of the film is placed slightly below the inferiormost aspect of the gluteal fold. Decubitus views are obtained with the patient in the right or left lateral position, directing the CR through the anterior or posterior midline. The patient is elevated on a suitable sponge or pad; otherwise, the side down may not be entirely demonstrated.

Central Ray. Perpendicular to the MSP at the level of the iliac crest for the AP and PA, and decubitus views; perpendicular to a sagittal plane midway between the midline and lateral surface of the body for the oblique views; 35°–40° caudal for PA axial rectosigmoid view (cephalic for AP method) through the level of the ASIS. Perpendicular to the midcoronal plane 5–7 cm superior to the level of the symphysis pubis for the lateral rectum view.

Structures Visualized. Double-contrast decubitus views primarily demonstrate the air-filled up side, which is the splenic flexure to the rectum on the left lateral decubitus, and the hepatic flexure to the rectum on the right lateral decubitus. Double-contrast method is superior for visualization of intraluminal lesions such as polyps. Oblique views are primarily taken to evaluate flexures; side down is best demonstrated on anterior obliques and side up on posterior obliques. Lateral rectum view demonstrates entire rectosigmoid colon, as does 40° axial view.

Quality Control Criteria. Air-filled side up on decubitus views is of primary importance, and must not be over-

penetrated. Both single- and double-contrast methods require high kVp technique to ensure adequate penetration. Oblique views should demonstrate the hepatic and splenic flexures more open than the PA view. Hyperesthetic patients must have CW films taken to ensure entire colon is visualized. Angled rectosigmoid view should demonstrate this area with less superimposition when compared with AP and PA views. Radiologist must determine whether post-evacuation film demonstrates adequate emptying of the colon before the patient is permitted to leave the radiology department.

OPERATIVE CHOLANGIOGRAPHY

Water-soluble iodinated compounds such as those used with intravenous urography are used for direct injection methods of radiography of the biliary tract, or cholangiography. These studies include operative, T-tube, and percutaneous transhepatic cholangiography. Operative cholangiography is performed during biliary tract surgery. It may reveal the presence of calculi too minute to detect by palpation, and demonstrates biliary tract patency.

Film Size and Centering. The surgical tables employed with operative cholangiograms vary; however, most are equipped with an underlevel upon which the x-ray cassette is placed. A grid and screen cassette or grid cassette is used, and is placed with the aid of the surgical staff, centered to the RUQ of the patient before surgery. Depending upon preference of the surgeon and radiologist, a 10 × 12 film or 14 × 17 size is used. Before surgery, the portable x-ray unit should be thoroughly disinfected and the machine checked for functionality. A number of cassettes should be ready in case the surgeon requires more than one exposure.

Position. In order to prevent superimposition of the bile ducts, some surgeons may rotate the patient into the RPO position at the time of exposure; an AP projection may also be used. After exposing and draining the biliary tract, and sometimes after excision of the gallbladder, the surgeon injects the contrast media into the common bile duct using a needle or small catheter. If cholecystectomy is performed, an indwelling tube called a **T-tube** is used to inject. If the tube is present, the examination is more properly termed **operative T-tube cholangiography.** Contrast media may be introduced into the biliary tract in stages, with a film being taken after each injection. Because the patient is intubated and under general anesthesia, suspension of respiration is achieved by having the anesthesiologist give the patient a breath and holding it via the endotracheal tube.

Central Ray. Perpendicular to the level of the biliary tract. The level of the gallbladder and biliary tract varies according to body habitus, so centering levels may vary. Generally speaking, the gallbladder can be located at about the level of T12, which is roughly equivocal to the level of the elbow when the patient has his arms extended by his side.

Structures Visualized. Contrast-enhanced gallbladder, right and left hepatic ducts, hepatic duct, cystic duct, common bile duct, pancreatic duct, and proximal duodenum are seen.

Quality Control Criteria. Short-scale contrast using 70 kVp is optimal for visualization of iodinated contrast-enhanced biliary system. With larger patients, this kVp is impractical due to the long exposure times required to produce adequate density, particularly in conjunction with fixed mA portable radiography units.

POSTOPERATIVE OR T-TUBE CHOLANGIOGRAPHY

A T-shaped tube is left in place in the left common bile duct following cholecystectomy to permit postoperative drainage. Low-density water-soluble contrast media (25%–30% concentration) is used because higher density may obscure small biliary calculi.

Film Size and Centering. The patient is placed in the LPO position with the biliary tract centered to the midline of the table. The radiologist injects contrast material in small amounts, obtaining spot films as the biliary tract fills. The examination may also be performed without the aid of fluoroscopy, and 10 × 12 films substituted for the spot films. Some authors advocate the use of a lateral projection to demonstrate branching of the hepatic ducts.

Position. LPO and right lateral projections, or variations as indicated by the radiologist. The T-tube is clamped before the examination, permitting bile to fill the tube as a measure to prevent air bubbles from flowing into the tube, which may simulate pathology on the radiograph. The patient should be NPO.

Central Ray. Perpendicular to the level of the biliary tract.

Structures Visualized. Contrast-enhanced right and left hepatic ducts, hepatic duct, cystic duct, common bile duct and connecting T-tube, pancreatic duct, and proximal duodenum are seen. The study is most often performed to demonstrate the presence of residual calculi, the patency of the ducts, and the status of the ampulla of Vater.

Quality Control Criteria. Short-scale contrast using 70 kVp is optimal for visualization of iodinated contrast-enhanced biliary system. Unlike the operative procedure, this range of kVp can generally be used, as x ray output with three-phase generators is much higher than with mobile x-ray units.

ENDOSCOPIC RETROGRADE CHOLANGIOPANCREATOGRAPHY (ERCP)

The ERCP is generally performed in the GI lab, if one is available, with the assistance of radiology personnel. The primary task of the technologist is to perform fluoroscopy, allowing the gastroenterologist to insert a small cannula through the fiberoptic endoscope into the ampulla of Vater, where contrast media are injected and spot films are taken at the direction of the physician. Before ERCP, ultrasound of the abdomen is generally performed to rule out the presence of pancreatic pseudocysts, because contrast medium injected into pseudocysts may lead to severe inflammation (pancreatitis), or rupture of the pseudocysts.

Film Size and Centering. The fluoroscopy tower is centered to the area of interest, and spot films are taken at the direction of the physician.

Position. The patient is placed in the prone position during fluoroscopy, and may be turned into an anterior oblique position at differing intervals of the study to prevent superimposition of the bile ducts on the radiographs. The technologist may increase his usefulness by assisting the physician with positioning, as the patient is under twilight anesthesia and cannot usually respond to commands.

Central Ray. Perpendicular to the level of the biliary tract.

Structures Visualized. Contrast-enhanced right and left hepatic ducts, cystic duct, common bile duct, pancreatic duct, and proximal duodenum are seen.

Quality Control Criteria. Contrast material drains quickly from the biliary ducts; taking the exposure promptly when instructed to do so is vital. Fluoroscopic kVp should be set between 70 and 80. Some motion may be visible; the patient is usually not able to respond to commands.

QUESTIONS FOR ABDOMEN AND GI SYSTEM

select the best answer

1. Which of the following examinations would best demonstrate the presence of free air under the right hemidiaphragm?

   (A) KUB
   (B) UGI
   (C) Left lateral decubitus abdomen
   (D) Right lateral decubitus abdomen

2. During a double-contrast UGI procedure, which position will optimally demonstrate the duodenal bulb and pyloric canal?

   (A) AP
   (B) LPO
   (C) PA
   (D) Right lateral

3. A UGI examination is to be performed on an ICU patient. The patient is a frail 65-year-old

man who has profound epigastric pain, nausea, and vomiting. The condition of his skin is poor. He has two peripheral IV sites and a nasogastric tube in place. The most likely examination to be performed is a:

(A) double-contrast UGI examination.
(B) single-contrast, high-density barium UGI examination.
(C) single-contrast, low-density barium UGI examination.
(D) single-contrast, water-soluble contrast UGI examination.

4. Which of the following best describes the position of the esophagus?

(A) Midline, anterior to the trachea, joins the stomach at the cardiac orifice
(B) Slightly left of midline, anterior to trachea, joins the stomach at the pyloric orifice
(C) Midline, posterior to the trachea, joins the stomach at the cardiac orifice
(D) Midline, posterior to the trachea, joins the duodenum at the sphincter of Oddi

5. Which of the following correctly describes the anatomy that joins to form the common bile duct?

(A) Cystic duct and common hepatic duct
(B) Pancreatic duct and duct of Wirsung
(C) Right and left hepatic ducts and cystic ducts
(D) Sphincter of Oddi and pancreatic duct

6. In a single-contrast barium enema examination, which projection demonstrates the sigmoid colon with the least amount of self-superimposition?

(A) AP
(B) LPO
(C) RPO
(D) 30-degree caudal PA axial

7. In a double-contrast barium enema examination, the primary area of interest for a 45-degree RAO projection is the:

(A) rectum.
(B) splenic flexure.
(C) hepatic flexure.
(D) sigmoid colon.

8. The primary area of importance for a left lateral decubitus projection in a double-contrast BE examination is:

(A) air-filled right side up.
(B) barium-filled left side down.
(C) barium-filled right side up.
(D) air-filled left side down.

9. Which of the following organs can be found in the left upper quadrant (LUQ) of the abdomen?

(A) Liver and spleen
(B) Spleen and stomach
(C) Cecum and ascending colon
(D) Appendix and sigmoid colon

10. A fiberoptic scope is positioned down the esophagus, and a cannula placed in the hepatopancreatic ampulla for the purpose of contrast-enhanced examination of biliary ducts. This statement best describes:

(A) operative pancreatography.
(B) T-tube cholangiography.
(C) percutaneous transhepatic cholangiography (PTC).
(D) endoscopic retrograde cholangiopancreatography (ERCP).

▶▶ **ANSWERS TO ABDOMEN AND GI STUDIES**

1. The answer is (C). The lateral decubitus position is used to evaluate the presence of air-fluid levels. The side up best demonstrates air, and the side down best demonstrates fluid. Therefore, the left side down, or left lateral decubitus position, best demonstrates right-sided free air.

2. The answer is (B). With a double-contrast UGI examination, the LPO position demonstrates a barium-filled fundus; the duodenal bulb and pyloric canal are seen without superimposition of structures. The projection is important because the duodenum is frequently the site of peptic ulcer disease, typified by a sharply circumscribed area of mucous membrane loss. In the LPO position, gravity drains some of the barium from the pylorus and duodenum, yielding a double-contrast projection of the area. The PA projection demonstrates the size, shape, and contour of the barium-filled stomach, and the AP view shows a barium-coated, air-filled body and antrum. The retrogastric area of the duodenum and proximal jejunum can be seen through the air-filled stomach on this projection. Lateral views show a barium-filled duodenum and pyloric canal, and are obtained primarily to demonstrate the anterior and posterior surfaces of the stomach, and to further interrogate the retrogastric space.

3. The answer is (D). Standard UGI examinations on

such patients are difficult, and therefore not often performed in the standard fashion, because the patients are unlikely to be able to attain the required positions necessary for full studies. Generally speaking, if a UGI is required, then water-soluble iodinated contrast is administered through the nasogastric tube, and spot films are attained by the radiologist. If this limited approach reveals the information necessary to treat the patient, then further diagnostic imaging is not required. However, if the presence of subtle or underlying pathology is suspected, then the patient may be further examined with other modalities; CT and ultrasound studies are most commonly used.

4. The answer is (C). The esophagus is a collapsed, muscular tube beginning at the level of C6, with its upper one fifth in the neck, and lower four fifths in the thorax. It lies posterior to the trachea, and moves slightly to the left at its distal end, joining the stomach at the cardiac orifice.

5. The answer is (A). The cystic duct descends from the gallbladder to join the common hepatic duct, which in turn emanates from the right and left hepatic ducts from the liver, to form the common bile duct. The common bile duct later joins the pancreatic duct at the sphincter of Oddi, where it pours bile into the duodenum. The sphincter remains closed, forcing bile from the hepatic ducts to back up into the cystic duct and gallbladder until, during a meal, the gallbladder contracts, relaxing the sphincter, and allows bile into the duodenum.

6. The answer is (D). The axial projection of the rectosigmoid colon can be performed in either AP alignment, using cephalic angulation, or PA alignment, using caudal angulation. The 30- to 40-degree angled CR passes through the sigmoid approximately at the level of the ASIS, projecting it nearly free of overlapping structures.

7. The answer is (C). The anterior oblique position best demonstrates the side down flexure, in this case the right-sided hepatic flexure. Posterior obliques best demonstrate the side up, or opposite flexure: The LPO projection is taken to demonstrate the hepatic flexure, and the RPO demonstrates the splenic flexure.

8. The answer is (A). For decubitus projections, the side down gives the name to the projection; hence a left side down decubitus is a left lateral decubitus. In a double-contrast BE examination, barium sinks to the side down, and air rises to the side up. Decubitus views are taken primarily to demonstrate the air-filled side up and should demonstrate the area from the flexure to the rectum.

9. The answer is (B). The abdomen is divided into four primary areas called quadrants, which are defined by transverse and midsagittal planes that intersect at the umbilicus. The stomach and spleen are found in the LUQ; the liver is in the RUQ; the cecum and appendix are in the RLQ; and the ascending colon is found in both the RUQ and RLQ.

10. The answer is (D). ERCP is performed by passing a fiberoptic endoscope through the mouth to the duodenum with the aid of fluoroscopy, and injecting contrast into the common bile duct. Operative pancreatography is achieved in the operating room, by injecting contrast material into the pancreatic duct. T-tube cholangiography is primarily a postoperative investigation of the biliary system, with injection of contrast through an indwelling T-shaped drainage tube. PTC is a preoperative examination of the biliary tract for patients who have obstructive jaundice and dilated ducts as demonstrated either by CT or ultrasound. With PTC, a "skinny" needle is placed into the dilated biliary ducts under fluoroscopic control, and contrast is injected. PTC is often performed in conjunction with biliary drainage or stone extraction procedures.

C. Urologic Studies

The purpose of the urinary system is to maintain the chemical balance and alkalinity of the blood by removing waste products.

1. Kidneys

Removal of waste, which consists of a solution of excess water, glucose, and salts known as urine, is accomplished by the kidneys, two bean-shaped organs located in the retroperitoneum and embedded in adipose tissue; their superior border begins approximately at the level of T12 and extends to the transverse process of L3. The right kidney is located slightly more inferiorly than the left because of the large space occupied by the liver.

Kidneys vary somewhat in size, but average approximately 11.5 cm in length and 7 cm in width. Movement of the kidneys on respiration (respiratory excursion) is approximately 2.5 cm, and their movement from the erect to supine position is 2.5 to 5 cm.

A coronal section of a kidney reveals its major divisions: the cortex, medulla, and renal pelvis (**Figure**

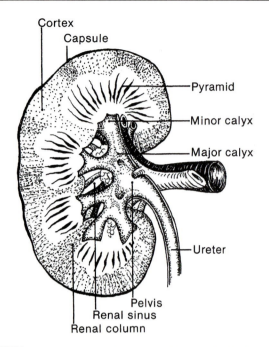

Cortex
Capsule
Pyramid
Minor calyx
Major calyx
Ureter
Pelvis
Renal sinus
Renal column

FIGURE 5-17. Coronal cross-section of the kidney. (Reprinted from April EW: *NMS Clinical Anatomy*, 3rd ed . Baltimore, Williams & Wilkins, 1997, p 386.)

5-17). The cortex is the outer area of the kidney, approximately 2 cm in thickness, and more pale in color than the medulla. The cortex has a granular appearance, whereas the medulla is longitudinally striated. The substance of the cortex is more compact than the rest of the kidney and extends from the periphery of the kidney to the bases of the medullary segments. The medulla is the inner, darker layer, consisting of 6 to 15 isolated triangular areas known as the renal pyramids. The cortex actually extends in between the pyramids, forming an area known as the renal columns. The medial border of each kidney is concave, giving way to a longitudinal slit called the hilum, into which the ureter, blood vessels, nerves, and lymphatic vessels pass. The proximal attachment of the ureter is expanded and funnel-shaped, forming a portion of the renal pelvis. The calyces arise from apical portions of the pyramids called the papillae. Each calyx (singular) encloses one or more papillae. Where they arise from the renal pyramids, the calyces are referred to as minor calyces, which vary in number from 4 to 14. Minor calyces unite to form two to three major calyces, which, along with the expanded portion of the ureter, form the renal pelvis (see Figure 5-17).

Microscopic evaluation of the kidneys clarifies the function of the anatomy. The functional unit of the kidney is an individual tubular unit called the nephron. The nephron is comprised of a proximal portion

called the glomerular (or Bowman's) capsule, which is invaginated to allow the presence of a cluster of specialized blood capillaries called the glomerulus.

The glomerulus is fed by a tiny branch of the renal artery called the afferent arteriole. Blood leaving the capsule exits by the efferent arteriole, which in turn feeds a capillary network communicating with the renal vein. It is the glomerulus that acts as a filtering system for the blood, allowing water, glucose, and salts to pass through the walls of the capillaries into Bowman's capsule. The filtered fluid is called glomerular filtrate. The glomerular filtrate is then absorbed by the epithelial lining of a specialized structure arising from the renal cortex called the renal tubule. The filtered blood passes through a capillary network to the renal tubules as well. The tubules travel a path through the cortex and medullary sections of the kidneys, and are divided into four important divisions, which are as follows: the proximal convoluted tubule, the descending loop of Henle, the ascending loop of Henle, and the distal convoluted tubule. Each portion of the tubule plays a specialized role in the filtering process. The distal tubule communicates with the origins of the collecting system (the renal pelvis), which passes urine down its various branchings to the ureter.

2. Ureters

The ureters convey urine from the renal pelves to the urinary bladder by means of peristalsis. Descending the peritoneum anterior to the psoas muscles and transverse processes of the lumbar spine, the ureters are approximately 10 to 12 inches in length and communicate with the posterolateral aspect of the bladder. Three normal constrictions of the ureter occur at the ureteropelvic junction (UPJ), the pelvic brim, and the ureterovesicular junction (UVJ). If the ureters are obstructed by calculus, a condition called hydronephrosis occurs. The urinary bladder is a reservoir for urine that is located superiorly and posteriorly to the symphysis pubis. The musculomembranous bladder is marked by three orifices, two on its posterior aspect through which the ureters pass, and the other, the internal urethral orifice, located on its most inferior portion, called the neck. The triangular area between the three orifices is called the trigone. The urethra, a slender musculomembranous canal arising from the internal urethral orifice, conveys urine outside the body. A sphincter type of muscle that controls the flow of urine is found at the base of the bladder. The urethra is relatively short in females, approximately 4 cm, and longer in males, measuring 17 to 20 cm.

RADIOGRAPHIC PROCEDURES: UROLOGICAL SYSTEM

Chart 5-3 describes the procedures for imaging of the urological system.

▶ CHART 5-3.   Procedures for Imaging of the Urological System

CYSTOGRAPHY, CYSTOURETHROGRAPHY, AND RETROGRADE URETHROGRAPHY

Radiography of the bladder (cystography) and urethra (cystourethrography) may be achieved either through intravenous injection or, more commonly, via a retrograde approach. Retrograde radiographic examinations of the bladder and urethra are performed under aseptic conditions. A catheter is passed into the urethra and iodinated contrast is injected, generally by drip infusion for cystography, and by contrast-loaded urethral syringe for cystourethrography. The contrast used is generally specially designed for cystourethrography, and is of a lower iodine concentration than that used for intravenous injection. A Foley catheter may also be used to occlude the vesicourethral orifice. Following introduction of the contrast agent, the catheter is clamped, and sometimes taped to the thigh to prevent displacement during positioning. Cystourethrography of the female patient is accomplished with the patient in the AP position, whereas a 35°–40° posterior oblique position is employed for the male patient.

Film Size and Centering.   10 × 12 CW bucky. Lower border of the film placed at the symphysis pubis. Larger films may be required if initial films demonstrate ureteral reflux.

Position.   AP, RPO, LPO, and lateral films are obtained. Films may be obtained during bladder filling and also during voiding, depending on radiologist's specification. If the voiding examination (commonly referred to as a voiding cystourethrogram, or VCUG) is to be performed, the radiographic table should be protected by placing a sheet or paper drape over it prior to the exam. The oblique cystograms employ a patient rotation of 40°–60°, with the pubic arch that is closest to the film adjusted to the midline of the bucky. The thigh away from the film should be abducted in order to prevent superimposition of the femur on the bladder. If an unobstructed view of the distal ureters is desired, the patient may be placed in the Trendelenburg position by lowering the head of the table 15°–20°. This position stretches the bladder superiorly, allowing the ureters to be seen without superimposition.

Central Ray.   A caudal angulation of 5°–15° is used with the AP projection of the bladder to project the pubis below the level of the bladder neck. Depending on body habitus, the caudal angulation may also be used with the posterior oblique positions.

Structures Visualized.   Urinary bladder, distal ureters, and urethra are visualized, depending on the area of interest. Physiologic examinations (voiding) are also routinely obtained.

Quality Control Criteria.   Area of interest should be seen without superimposition of structures. Hips are superimposed on lateral projection. For cystourethrography, the urethra should be filled with contrast and be visualized in its entirety.

INTRAVENOUS UROGRAPHY (IVU)

The patient is prepped the night before the exam, usually with a mild laxative, and is instructed to take nothing by mouth (NPO) after midnight. A scout film, usually a standard AP abdomen (KUB), is taken to evaluate the presence of stones and the efficacy of the patient preparation, or the presence of extrarenal lesions which may render the IVU unnecessary. If tomography is to be employed, a scout tomogram of the kidneys is obtained to check technique, position, and depth of the kidneys. Tomography greatly aids in examination of the kidneys, and in particular the renal parenchyma, by elimination of gas shadows and by increasing the clarity of small intrarenal lesions. A number of contrast injection methods may be employed, including the drip infusion method for nephrotomography; however, a bolus injection of 50–100 cc via the antecubital vein is most common.

Film Size and Centering.   Tomograms and stationary films of the kidneys and proximal ureters are obtained on 11 × 14 film CW, bucky, with the midline of the patient centered to the bucky, and the lowest portion of the cassette at the level of the iliac crest. Films of the kidneys, ureters, and bladder are taken using a 14 × 17 film LW, bucky, midline of the patient centered to the bucky and the lower border of the cassette placed at the symphysis pubis. If oblique views are required, a 30° rotation of the patient is employed. The prone position is recommended to aid in filling of the ureters. Bladder films are taken on a 10 × 12, CW, lower border of the film at the symphysis pubis.

Position.   Routine varies according to the diagnostic information desired; however, following bolus injection, a 30-second stationary film of the kidneys is obtained. This film demonstrates the renal parenchyma, and is sometimes referred to as a nephrogram. Films are taken at timed intervals following the 30-second film, with films at 1, 3, and 5 minutes being taken if the exam is being obtained to study hypertension. Generally speaking, tomograms of the kidneys are obtained at the 5-minute mark; usually three films 1 cm apart are taken through the center of the renal parenchyma. A full film on 14 × 17 may also taken at 5 minutes. Further radiographs are obtained at the direction of the radiologist, with a film every 5 minutes up to 30 minutes being common. At the end of the study, the patient is escorted to the restroom and instructed to void, and a postvoid film of the bladder is obtained to evaluate the presence of residual contrast in the bladder. If a renal calculus is suspected, the urine may need to be strained, because the patient may pass the stone with urination.

Central Ray. For full film, the CR is perpendicular to the MSP at the level of the iliac crest. Films of the kidneys and proximal ureters are centered at the level of the xiphoid process, and films of the bladder centered at the level of the greater trochanters.

Structures Visualized. Intravenous urography is a physiologic method of investigating the renal collecting (drainage) system. The kidneys, ureters, and bladder are demonstrated in various functional stages as timed images are obtained. Renal parenchyma is primarily visualized on the 30-second plain radiograph and on subsequent tomograms.

Quality Control Criteria. Entire renal parenchyma should be visualized on initial films; later films should include the entire bladder. Radiographs should possess the same degree of soft-tissue density as plain abdominal film; 70 kVp is considered optimum. A compression device may be applied over the distal ureters, centered approximately 2″ superior to the symphysis pubis, to slow the flow of opacified urine into the bladder and ensure adequate filling of the calyces. The oblique position should demonstrate the kidney away from the film without superimposition of the adjacent vertebral body. The prostate should be included on bladder radiographs of male patients. A time marker should be present on each radiograph. Postvoid radiographs should be labeled appropriately. Tomogram centimeter level should be indicated on tomographic films.

RETROGRADE UROGRAPHY

Unlike the physiologic method of contrast enhancement employed with intravenous urography, retrograde urography is an instrumental method of investigating the urinary tract. Contrast media is introduced via catheterization of the ureters for visualization of the upper urinary tract, and urethral catheterization for the lower portion. Cystoscopy, a procedure which directly visualizes the bladder by means of a cystoscope, is employed to locate the vesicoureteral orifices for placement of ureteral catheters. Once catheterized, the pelvicaliceal system is injected directly. As with any radiologic procedure requiring instrumentation, retrograde urography is classified as an operative procedure, and as such is carried out

under aseptic conditions. Therefore, the technologist must ensure that the radiographic equipment is disinfected and free of dust.

Film Size and Centering. Generally speaking, 14 × 17 films are used unless one is otherwise directed by the physician. The film is placed LW in the bucky tray and centering is at L3.

Position. The patient is placed supine on a specially designed cystoscopy table, in a modified lithotomy position, with the hips somewhat flexed and the knees flexed over the stirrups of the leg support. The examination is performed by a urologist with the assistance of a nurse and a radiologic technologist. Three films are generally performed. The first film is taken in order to demonstrate the ureteral catheters in position. Once catheter position is documented, a pyelogram and a ureterogram are performed. The patient may be placed 10°–15° Trendelenburg in order to more completely fill the renal pelves, and the head of the table may be elevated 30°–40° to more clearly delineate any tortuosity of the ureters. Respiration is suspended on exhalation if the patient is awake, or with the aid of the anesthesiologist if the patient is under general anesthesia.

Central Ray. Perpendicular to the MSP at the level of L3.

Structures Visualized. Compared with the intravenous method, a slightly more dilated projection of the kidneys and ureters is achieved on the retrograde examination.

QC Criteria. A short scale of contrast using 70 kVp is recommended. Kidneys and ureters are visualized in their entirety. If obliques are needed, 30° RPO and LPO positions are used, and should demonstrate the collecting system free of superimposition of the adjacent vertebral bodies.

QUESTIONS FOR UROLOGICAL STUDIES

select the best answer

1. The functional unit of the kidney is known as the:
   (A) nephron.
   (B) axon.
   (C) glomerulus.
   (D) renal tubule.

2. The contrast injection technique(s) used for voiding cystourethrography include(s):
   1. intravenous injection.
   2. percutaneous injection.
   3. injection through a catheter in urethral canal.
   (A) Choices 1 and 3 only
   (B) Choice 2 only

(C) Choices 2 and 3
(D) Choice 1 only

3. Which of the following conditions does NOT relate to the importance of obtaining a postvoid radiograph during an excretory urogram?

(A) Prostate hypertrophy
(B) Bladder neoplasm
(C) Residual urine
(D) Hydronephrosis

▶▶ ANSWERS TO UROLOGICAL STUDIES

1. The answer is (A). The nephron—consisting of Bowman's capsule, the glomerulus or renal corpuscle, the loop of Henle, and the proximal and distal renal tubules—is the unit that performs filtration by removal of water, glucose, and various salts from the blood. An axon is a portion of a nerve cell.

2. The answer is (A). Either method, whether intravenous injection in a bolus or drip infusion, or retrograde injection through a urethral catheter, may be used as a means of introducing contrast into the urinary bladder.

3. The answer is (D). Hydronephrosis is a condition whereby urine is backed up to the kidney tissue and exerting pressure on it. If untreated it may lead to necrosis and renal failure. Hydronephrosis may occur secondary to a number of conditions; renal calculus or a kink in the ureter secondary to renal ptosis are prominent among these conditions. The presence of residual urine on a post-micturition (postvoiding) radiograph may indicate the presence of a tumor (neoplasm) or prostatic enlargement (hypertrophy).

D. Extremity Studies

Classification of Joints

The joints of the body are classified according to structure or function. The structural category includes fibrous joints, which are immovable; synovial joints, which are freely movable; and cartilaginous joints, which may be either rigid or slightly movable. Functionally, joints are classified as synarthrodial, which are nonmovable joints; amphiarthrodial, which are semimovable joints; and diarthrodial, which are freely movable joints.

The limbs are composed predominantly of diarthrodial joints, and the axial skeleton, which is charged with the protection of vital organs, is composed of amphiarthrodial and synarthrodial joints.

The Lower Extremity

The lower extremity is grossly comprised of four primary parts: hip, thigh, leg, and foot. The bones and joints are constructed so that the activities of erect weight bearing and locomotion can be carried out.

THE FOOT (Figure 5-18)

The foot consists of 26 bones. Considered from anterior to posterior, the anterior half contains the 5 metatarsals, which are long bones, and 14 phalanges, or toes. The metatarsals and toes are numbered from 1 to 5 from medial to lateral so that the great toe is numbered 1, and the little toe is numbered 5. Except for the great toe, which contains two phalanges, each toe is individually comprised of three phalanges, which are named by their location as distal, middle, or proximal, accordingly. Each individual phalange is

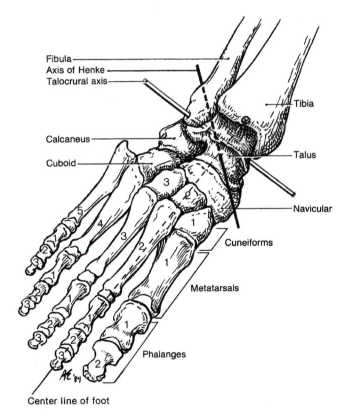

FIGURE 5-18. Bones of the distal leg, ankle, and foot. The talocrural axis and the axis of the subtarsal joint (of Henke) are shown. (Reprinted from April EW: *NMS Clinical Anatomy,* 3rd ed. Baltimore, Williams & Wilkins, 1997, p 202.)

called a phalanx. A phalanx consists of the longest middle portion, or shaft, and two expanded articular ends. The most distal portion of each toe contains a roughened segment of cancellous tissue for support of the toenail, called the ungual tuft.

The metatarsals, which are roughly comparable to the metacarpals of the hand, are longer and more slender, and the heads are less expanded than those of the hand. The first metatarsal rests on two pea-sized sesamoid bones that aid in transferring the weight of the body to the ground. The posterior half of the foot contains the seven tarsal bones. Of these, the talus and calcaneus are comparatively enlarged and geared toward weight bearing. The irregularly shaped talus is composed of a posterior body, a constricted neck, and an anterior head. The talus is the second largest tarsal bone and occupies the most superior position; its body rests on the middle superior surface of the calcaneus and occupies the socket of the ankle joint, which will be discussed later. The calcaneus, or heel, is the largest tarsal bone, and embodies three important articulating surfaces with the talus. The most significant of these, the sustentaculum tali, is a shelf of bone on the anteromedial aspect of the calcaneus that provides support for the head of the talus. Because of its attachment to the Achilles tendon, the calcaneus acts as a lever, whereby the muscles of the calf extend the ankle, permitting the body to be raised on tiptoes.

The cuboid bone is situated on the lateral aspect of the foot in between the fourth and fifth metatarsals and the anterior portion of the calcaneus. The navicular bone lies on the medial side of the foot between the talus and the three cuneiform bones. Each cuneiform articulates anteriorly with the same numbered metatarsal and posteriorly with the navicular. The third cuneiform articulates laterally with the cuboid. The foot contains three important arches consisting of bones, ligaments, and tendons that provide weight-bearing support. The arches give when weight is applied and spring back into position when weight is removed. The arches are named for their direction of travel; the lateral longitudinal arch, the longitudinal arch, and the transverse arch.

Radiographic Procedures: The Foot. **Chart 5-4** describes the procedures for imaging of the foot.

▶ CHART 5-4. Procedures for Imaging of the Foot

AP (Dorsoplantar) Oblique, and Lateral Toes

Film Size and Centering. 8 × 10 screen film. Cassette should be placed under the toes so that the midline of the cassette is parallel to the long axis of the foot on the AP and oblique positions, and parallel to the long axis of the toes in the lateral position. Collimation should be confined to the area of interest.

Position. The patient is seated on the x-ray table or is supine with the knee flexed for the AP and oblique views, and in the lateral recumbent position for the lateral projection. The unaffected lateral side is used if the great or second toe is the area of interest, and the affected lateral side for toes 3–5, because these positions will place the toes in closest proximity to the cassette. A true AP projection is achieved if a 15° cephalic tube angulation is used to compensate for the arch of the foot. A 15° wedge may be placed under the toes as a compensatory measure as well, if a vertical CR is desired instead. The patient is placed in the oblique projection by medially rotating the knee and foot so that the plantar surface forms a 45° angle with the surface of the film. In order to prevent superimposition of structures on the lateral projection, the toes should be isolated by taping or placing a gauze sponge between them.

Central Ray. The CR is angled 15° through the second metatarsophalangeal joint on the AP projection and directed vertically, perpendicular to the plane of the film, on the oblique and lateral views.

Structures Visualized. The 14 phalanges and distal metatarsals are seen in varying projections.

Quality Control Criteria. The AP view should demonstrate the phalanges free of rotation. The interphalangeal and metatarsophalangeal joints should be open. The toes should not overlie each other on the oblique projection and should be demonstrated individually in the true lateral projection.

AP, Oblique, and Lateral Foot

Film Size and Centering. Film size varies according to foot size. Generally, the AP and oblique are done two-on-one on a 10 × 12 or 11 × 14 cassette, and the lateral is done on a 10 × 12 or 11 × 14 cassette, placed so that its diagonal axis is parallel to the long axis of the foot, centered to the head of the third metatarsal.

Position. The patient is seated on the x-ray table or supine, with the knee flexed and the sole of the foot in contact with the x-ray cassette. Both medial and lateral oblique views may be obtained; the patient rotates the leg either medially or laterally so that the sole of the foot forms a 30° angle with the surface of the film. The preferred lateral projection is the lateromedial, with the medial aspect of the foot in contact with the cassette and the plantar surface of the film perpendicular to the cassette. This projection places the patient in a nearly exact lateral projection. This position is not always easy for the

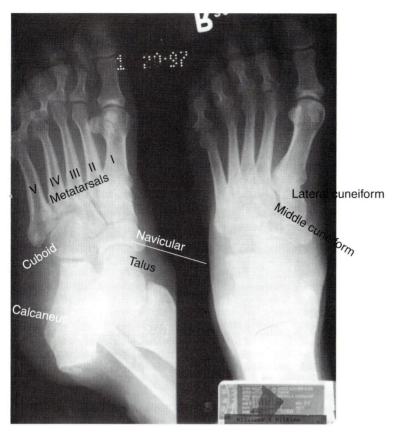

AP and medial oblique foot

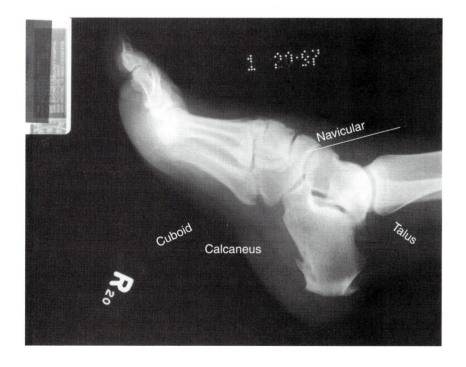

Lateral right foot

patient to achieve, however, so the mediolateral projection is often used instead.

Central Ray. The AP projection uses a 10° cephalic angulation directed through the base of the third metatarsal. The oblique and lateral projections use a vertical CR directed through the base of the third metatarsal.

Structures Visualized. The AP view demonstrates the phalanges, metatarsals, and tarsals anterior to the talus. The medial oblique view demonstrates the tarsometatarsal and intertarsal joints, and the bases of metatarsals 3–5 free of superimposition. The lateral oblique position is used to demonstrate the bases of the first and second metatarsals, as well as the interspace between the medial and intermediate cuneiforms. Lateral view demonstrates a profile view of the foot, including the distal tibia-fibula and ankle joint.

Quality Control Criteria. The technique used on the foot varies according to the area of interest, because the proxi-

mal aspect is more dense than the distal aspect. A wedge filter may be used to provide equivocal density throughout the radiograph. The lateral view should demonstrate the metatarsals overlapping each other, and the distal fibula should be shown overlapping the posterior distal aspect of the tibia. The lateral oblique position should demonstrate the bases of metatarsals 1 and 2, and the medial and intermediate cuneiform free of superimposition. The navicular should appear more elongated than on the AP or medial oblique projections. The medial oblique should demonstrate the bases of metatarsals 3–5 without superimposition. An equal amount of space between metatarsals 2–4 should be shown on the AP projection.

THE LEG

The leg is composed of two bones: the tibia and the fibula **(Figure 5-19).** The larger, medial tibia is the

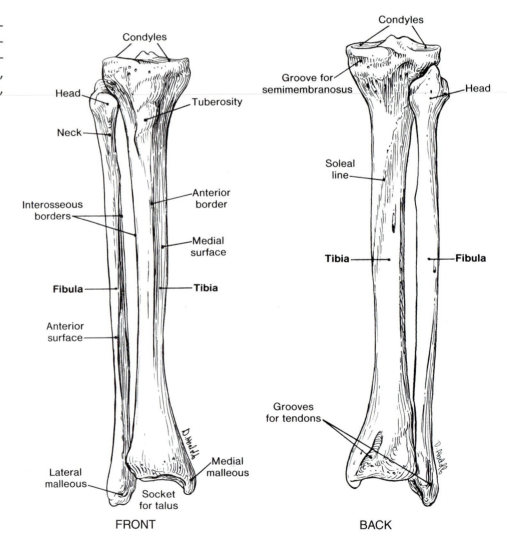

FIGURE 5-19. Right tibia and fibula from in front and from behind. (Reproduced with permission from John V. Basmajian, MD, McMaster University, Hamilton, Ontario.)

FRONT   BACK

The tibia itself embodies a shaft and two expanded ends. Proximally, the medial and lateral condyles articulate with the condyles of the femur above them. A sharp projection, formed by two peaklike projections and found in between the condyles, is called the intercondylar eminence, or tibial spine. The lateral condyle of the tibia forms a facet on its posterior surface that articulates with the fibular head. Inferior to the condyles on the anterior surface is a prominent process known as the tibial tuberosity, to which the extensor tendons of the knee are attached. The shaft of the tibia features a sharp ridge on its anterior surface, called the tibial crest. The shaft tapers as it approaches the ankle and then expands again, forming the large process known as the medial malleolus, which is the medial boundary for the ankle and an attachment point for several tendons.

The fibula is also comprised of a shaft and two expanded articular ends. Narrow in comparison to the tibia, its shape is influenced by its many muscle attachments. The proximal articular end is marked by an expanded head, on which a conical projection called the styloid process rests. The enlarged distal end of the fibula forms the triangular-shaped lateral malleolus, which is the lateral boundary of the ankle.

Radiographic Procedures: Ankle and Tibia-Fibula. **Chart 5-5** describes the procedures for imaging of the ankle and tibia-fibula.

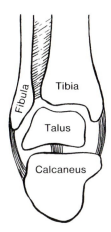

FIGURE 5-20. The ankle and talocalcanean joints in coronal section. (Reproduced with permission from John V. Basmajian, MD, McMaster University, Hamilton, Ontario.)

second largest bone in the body and bears the sole responsibility for weight transferred from the femur. The fibula is situated laterally and slightly more posteriorly than the tibia. The leg is an important component in two joints; together with the talus it forms the ankle distally **(Figure 5-20),** and with the distal femur and patella, the leg forms the knee proximally (see Figure 5-22).

Left ankle: Mortise (left) and AP (right) views

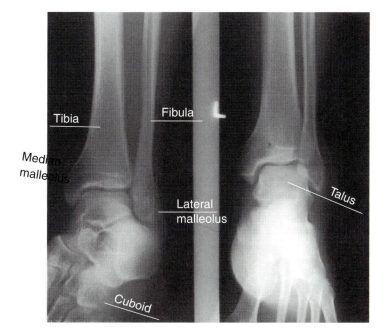

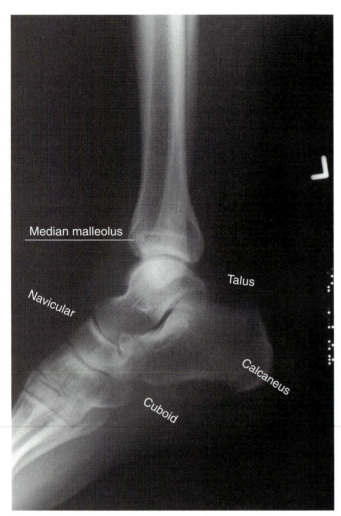

Median malleolus

Talus

Navicular

Calcaneus

Cuboid

Lateral left ankle

► CHART 5-5. Procedures for Imaging of the Ankle and Tibia-Fibula

AP, OBLIQUE (MORTISE VIEW) AND LATERAL ANKLE

Film Size and Centering. Film selection depends somewhat on radiologist preference. The examination may be performed on three individual 8 × 10 cassettes with the beam collimated to the area of interest, or may be done three-on-one on a 11 × 14 CW cassette, or also two-on-one on a 10 × 12, and the remaining view on a single 8 × 10 cassette. The ankle joint is centered to the center of the cassette for one-on-one views. For multiple projections on a single film, the cassette is divided into a number of sagittal planes and the part centered to the midpoint of the plane. As with all extremity radiography, the radiologist may prefer the initial examination be performed using a slow-speed, ultra-detail cassette, which demonstrates increased detail in comparison to standard

screens. Slow-speed screens require greater technical factors be used (see *Chapter 4, Image Projection and Evaluation*).

Position. The patient is supine on the x-ray table; a sponge may be placed under the affected-side knee to relieve stress. On the AP and oblique positions, adjust the patient so that the plantar surface of the foot is perpendicular to the surface of the film. The plantar surface is parallel to the film on the lateral projection, with the foot dorsiflexed (flexed upward); dorsiflexion of the foot is required in order to prevent rotation of the ankle on the lateral view. As with the foot, some authors suggest the lateromedial approach to the lateral position, because it places the relatively flat medial side in contact with the film, facilitating the production of a true lateral on the radiograph. If this method is used, turn the patient in a lateral recumbent position on the unaffected side.

The oblique ankle projection has always been a source of confusion for beginning technologists. It must be understood that in order to rotate the ankle, the leg must be rotated as well. Since the knee is a hinge-type joint, allowing only flexion and extension, rotation of the leg must emanate from the hip. Two medial oblique ankle projections are possible. If the mortise joint of the ankle is the area of interest, dorsiflex the foot and medially oblique the patient's ankle 15°–20°. This degree of rotation places both malleoli parallel to the cassette. (Some physicians, particularly orthopedic surgeons, may request a mortise view. If so, this is the position to which they are referring.) If the distal tibia-fibula is of more importance, a 45° medial oblique is performed instead.

Central Ray. The CR is directed vertically to a point midway between the lateral and medial malleoli. The CR should pass through the medial malleolus on the lateral projection.

Structures Visualized. The distal tibia, fibula, and talus are seen in their varying projections. Open mortise joint is best demonstrated on 15°–20° medial oblique position. Lateral view demonstrates the lower third of the tibia-fibula, with the fibula shown over the posterior half of the tibia. The tibiotalar joint is visualized, and the calcaneus and proximal tarsal bones are also seen.

Quality Control Criteria. The mortise view should demonstrate the mortise joint unobscured by the distal tibia and fibula. Lateral projection shows the fibula projected over the posterior portion of the tibia. Technique should be sufficient to ensure adequate penetration of all ankle constituents.

AP AND LATERAL TIBIA-FIBULA

Film Size and Centering. 14 × 17 LW, or diagonal axis of cassette parallel to the long axis of the film. Both the ankle and knee joints should be visualized; if the leg is longer than the cassette, then both proximal and distal

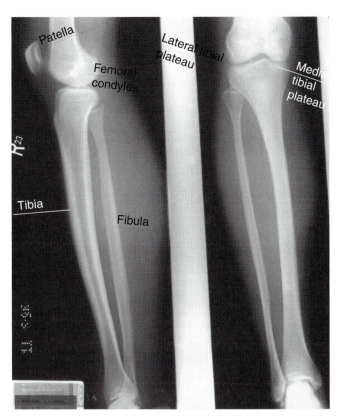

Patella

Femoral condyles

Lateral tibial plateau

Medial tibial plateau

Tibia

Fibula

AP and lateral right tibia-fibula

films are obtained. If the cassette is turned diagonally, then film coverage is not sufficient at 40″. Film coverage may be increased by increasing FFD 4″–6″, and compensating with a 4–6 kVp increase.

Position.   The pelvis should be free of rotation on the AP projection. The foot is inverted slightly, but the leg is not rotated. The patient is turned onto the affected side for the lateral projection, ensuring the patella is perpendicular to the plane of the film. Occasionally, oblique projections are requested; these are achieved with the patient in the supine position and rotating the leg 45° in either the lateral or medial direction, depending on the desired projection. The lateral oblique superimposes the fibula on the tibia, whereas the medial oblique opens the interosseous space between the tibia and fibula.

Central Ray.   Directed perpendicular to the plane of the cassette at the midpoint of the leg. FFD may be increased if increased film coverage in conjunction with a diagonally placed film cassette is desired.

Structures Visualized.   The tibia and fibula, along with their proximal and distal articulations, are demonstrated in their varying projections.

Quality Control Criteria.   Unless the examination is being performed in order to follow up on a known lesion, both joints must be demonstrated. The distal fibula overlies

the posterior half of the tibia on the lateral projection. Both ankle and knee should be demonstrated in the true AP projection on the AP examination.

THE FEMUR AND KNEE

The femur **(Figure 5-21)** is classified as a long bone, and in fact is the longest, strongest, and heaviest bone in the skeleton. Its articular ends are highly specialized for their role in the knee and hip joints, and its shaft, or diaphysis, is relatively simple in structure. The upper 10 cm of the femur traverses medially, forming a 125- to 140-degree angle with the shaft of the femur and a curved portion known as the neck. Due to osteoporosis, the neck is frequently the site of hip fractures, particularly in elderly persons (especially elderly women because of osteoporosis). The neck terminates in the articular portion known as the head, which is three quarters spherical and forms the ball of the ball-and-socket joint of the hip.

The hip is one of the most secure joints in the body. The head faces superomedially, and slightly anteriorly, where it articulates with the acetabulum of the pelvis. Two important prominences are seen along the femoral neck: the greater trochanter superiorly, and the lesser trochanter inferiorly (see Figure 5-21). The greater trochanter is the point of insertion for the gluteal muscles and is an important surface landmark for palpation. A large, roughened ridge that is the point of attachment for the vasti and adductor muscles runs superoinferiorly down the midline of the posterior aspect of the femoral shaft; this ridge is known as the linea aspera. The distal femur is broadened, and two prominent landmarks are seen: the medial and lateral condyles. Just superior to the condyles are two slight prominences, the medial and lateral epicondyles. The anterior surface between the condyles is a shallow, triangular, depressed area called the patellar surface. Posteriorly, the condyles are separated by a deep intracondylar notch or fossa.

The triangle-shaped patella is developed in the patellar tendon between the ages of 3 and 5; such bones, like the ones found in the first metatarsal, are called sesamoid bones. The patella is flat, relatively thick, and marked by its pointed apex, which is its most inferior aspect (see Figure 5-22). The apex of the patella lies slightly superior to the joint space of the knee and is attached to the tibial tuberosity via the patellar ligament. The primary purpose of the patella is to protect the anterior surface of the knee. When the knee joint is extended, the patella is freely movable and is easily palpated, lying as it is just deep to the skin. When the knee is flexed, however, the patella is locked in protective position.

FIGURE 5-21. Right femur from in front and from behind. (Reproduced with permission from John V. Basmajian, MD, McMaster University, Hamilton, Ontario.)

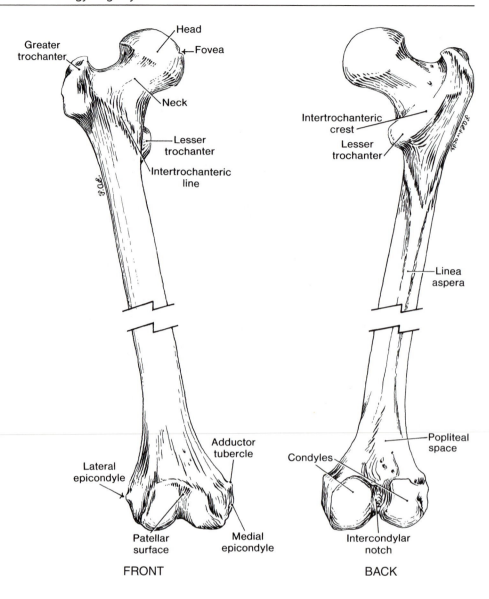

FRONT

BACK

The knee **(Figure 5-22)** is a modified hinge type of joint and is the largest and most complex joint in the body, allowing flexion, extension, and some rotation. The knee is actually three joints in one; consisting of the articulation between the patella and distal femur, as well as the medial and lateral articulations between the femoral condyles and the menisci of the tibia inferiorly. It is unique in that it is only partially enclosed by an articular capsule.

In between the articular surfaces of the femur and tibia are two important cartilaginous structures: the medial meniscus and lateral meniscus, or medial and lateral semilunar cartilage. The menisci act as shock absorbers and help control side-to-side motion of the femur on the tibia. A torn meniscus is a common sports injury that causes pain, edema, and decreased range of motion. Meniscal tears often require surgical intervention. Formerly, these procedures were necessarily accomplished by open surgical repair; however, they are now most commonly performed by arthroscopy. The menisci also increase the security of the joint by adjusting the two unmatched surfaces of the tibia and femur to each other.

The cruciate ligaments, thus named because they form an "X" in the intracondylar notch of the femur, are important structures in preventing displacement of the articular structures. The ligaments are named for their tibial attachment; the anterior cruciate ligament passes posterolaterally and superiorly from the intercondylar attachment on the tibia to the posteromedial surface of the lateral condyle of the femur. It is tight when the knee is in extension, and lax when the knee

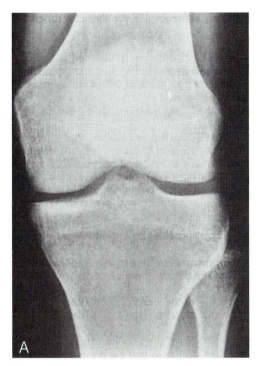

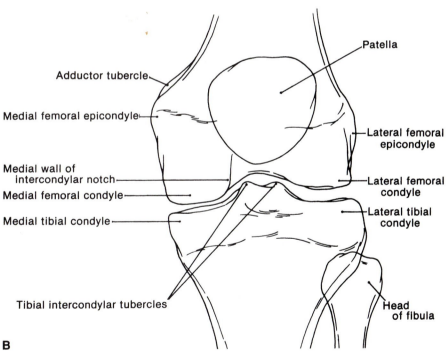

FIGURE 5-22. The knee. (A) Anteroposterior (AP) radiograph of the left knee. (B) Schematic representation. (Reproduced with permission from Slaby F, Jacobs ER: *Radiographic Anatomy.* Baltimore, Williams & Wilkins, 1990.)

is in flexion. The posterior cruciate ligament attaches to the posterior intercondylar surface of the tibia and moves anteromedially and superiorly to attach to the medial femoral condyle. This position allows the posterior cruciate ligament to prevent forward sliding of the femur and backward sliding of the tibia; thus it aids in prevention of hyperflexion of the knee.

Several other soft-tissue structures of the knee bear mention. The medial and lateral collateral ligaments aid in prevention of sideways displacement of the knee. There are many bursae (singular bursa) surrounding the anterior, posterolateral, and medial surfaces of the joint. Bursae are fibrous sacs lined with synovial membrane that contain synovial fluid, a substance that reduces friction between the structures. They are formed whenever a tendon rubs back and forth on a hard surface. A common condition known as housemaid's knee is an inflammation of the prepatellar bursa caused by prolonged pressure of the knee on a hard surface.

Radiographic Procedures: Femur and Knee. **Chart 5-6** describes the procedures for imaging of the femur and knee.

► CHART 5-6. Procedures for Imaging of the Femur and Knee

AP AND LATERAL FEMUR

Film Size and Centering. 14 × 17 or 7 × 17 LW, bucky.
Position. For AP projection, the patient is supine on the x-ray table with the affected-side toes inverted 15° in order to eliminate femoral neck anteversion. Generally, two projections must be obtained: one that includes the distal joint and one for the proximal joint. For the lateral view that includes the knee, turn the patient on the affected side with the pelvis in the lateral position. The unaffected knee is placed in front of the affected knee and flexed so that it is out of the x-ray field. For the lateral proximal femur, oblique the patient's pelvis into a 10°–15° posterior oblique position with the affected side down, and turn the affected leg laterally. Patients with suspected hip fractures should not have this projection because of the risk of further injury by rotation. Instead, a surgical hip view, which is discussed in the next section, is performed. Both the proximal and distal AP and lateral views should include approximately 2″ of the joint space.
Central Ray. Direct the CR perpendicular to the mid-thigh.
Structures Visualized. AP and lateral proximal views demonstrate the acetabulum, femoral head, femoral neck, greater and lesser trochanters, ischial tuberosity, and the

femoral shaft. Lateral view includes femoral shaft, femoral condyles, proximal tibia, and patella.
Quality Control Criteria. Femoral neck should be demonstrated without foreshortening. Patella should appear in profile on the distal lateral projection, and the patellofemoral joint should be open. Condyles should be free of rotation, and femoral condyles superimposed on lateral projection. When the patient is postoperative, any implanted hardware should be seen in its entirety.

AP, LATERAL, TUNNEL, AND SUNRISE KNEE

These four views represent a fairly standard routine knee series; however, as with all exams, routine may vary according to radiologist preference and information desired. Some commonly ordered variants of this routine are (1) standing AP or PA knees, which is performed to demonstrate the joint space in its weight-bearing position, and to ascertain the varus–valgus alignment of the knees preoperatively; and (2) medial and lateral oblique knee, which demonstrates the knee anatomy in the oblique projection.
Film Size and Centering. 10 × 12 LW for AP and lateral projections, screen or bucky. 8 × 10 CW for sunrise and tunnel views, bucky or screen, depending on method used. Some physicians prefer all views taken on 8 × 10.
Position. **AP:** MSP is centered to the center of the bucky or center of cassette, slightly inferior to the level of the patellar apex. The pelvis should not be rotated.
Lateral: The patient is turned onto the affected side with the nonaffected knee in front of the affected side and acutely flexed. Center slightly inferior to the level of the patellar apex. The affected knee is flexed 20°–30°.
Tunnel (intracondylar fossa): Many variants of this position exist. Perhaps the best known method is the Homblad position, which requires the patient to kneel on the table so that the femur forms a 70° angle with the surface of the table, centered at the level of the apex of the patella. If more comfortable for the patient, the position may also be performed with the patient standing. In this variation, the affected knee is placed on a stool and flexed, with the unaffected side firmly on the ground and the patient holding onto a step stool, IV pole, or other device as a means of support. The Camp-Coventry method for intracondylar fossa is also often performed. With this method, the patient is prone with the knee flexed 40°–50°, and the foot rests on a suitable support. The CR is directed caudally at the same angle used to flex the knee.
Sunrise view (tangential patella, Settegast method): Again, many variants of the basic position exist. The method described by Settegast is one popular method, whereby the patient is seated on the table with the knee acutely flexed. The patient holds the cassette

along the long axis of the femur so that the center of the cassette is at the level of the patellofemoral articulation. Ballinger warns against acutely flexing the knee too rapidly, causing the patient pain; this is sound advice. However, the knee need not be flexed as acutely as Settegast suggested in order to achieve the desired view. Experience has taught that knee flexion of 20°–30° is sufficient, providing the cassette is placed in proper tube part–film alignment and the CR is directed cephalic through the patellofemoral articulation.

Central Ray. A 5° cephalic angulation is used for the AP and lateral projections, directed through the patellar apex. CR angulation varies according to method used with intercondylar and tangential patellar views. With the methods described here, a 20°–25° tube angulation is sufficient for both tunnel and sunrise projections. The Camp-Coventry method for intracondylar fossa uses a 40°–50° caudal CR angulation, depending on the degree of knee flexion used.

Structures Visualized. AP view demonstrates the knee joint with patella projected superiorly, out of the joint space. Lateral view demonstrates a lateral projection of the joint space with the femoral condyles superimposed. Several methods described demonstrate the intracondy-lar fossa free of superimposition of the patella. Sunrise view is a tangential projection of the patellofemoral articulation.

Quality Control Criteria. Femorotibial joint should be open on both AP and lateral projections. Patella should be projected by CR angulation out of the joint space and superimposed on the femur on the AP view. Lateral view should demonstrate patella in profile and femoral condyles superimposed.

The Upper Extremity

The upper extremity is classified according to its four primary subdivisions, which are hand (including wrist), forearm, arm, and shoulder.

The hand, consisting of phalanges, metacarpals and carpals, is comprised of 27 bones **(Figure 5-23).** Except for the thumb, or first digit, which contains but two phalanges, the digits (fingers) consist of three phalanges, each of which is named by location as proximal, middle, and distal, and is numbered from lateral to medial. Each phalanx is a cylindrical shaft with slightly expanded articular ends. The phalanges are concave both anteriorly and at their bases to ac-

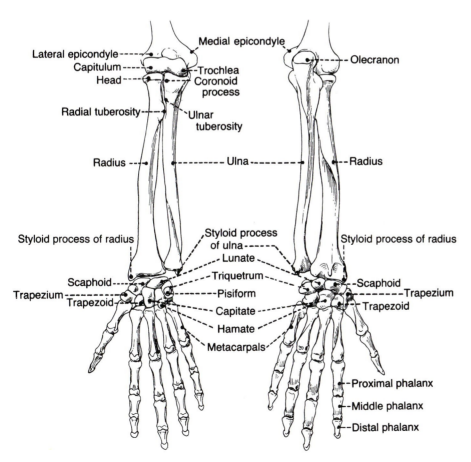

FIGURE 5-23. Bones of the forearm and hand. (Reprinted from Chung KW: *BRS Gross Anatomy*, 3rd ed. Baltimore, Williams & Wilkins, 1995, p 20.)

commodate the articular end of the metacarpals. The bones of the palm are known as metacarpals. They are classified as miniature long bones and as such consist of a cylindrical shaft and expanded extremities. The bases of the metacarpals are roughly square-shaped where they articulate with the distal carpals, forming a rounded head at the distal articulation with the proximal phalanges. The first metacarpal is also unique in that it forms a saddle-type joint at its base with the articular surface of the trapezium.

The eight bones of the wrist are known as carpals and are classified as short bones. They are arranged in two transverse rows of four and connected by interosseous ligaments. From lateral to medial, the bones of the distal row are known as trapezium (greater multangular), trapezoid (lesser multangular), capitate, and hamate; the bones of the proximal row are called navicular (scaphoid), lunate, triquetrum (triangular), and pisiform. The navicular is the most frequently fractured carpal bone, and the lunate is the most frequently dislocated bone. The two long bones of the forearm are the medially situated ulna and the laterally placed radius (see Figure 5-23). The two bones are connected along their entire length by the flexible interosseous membrane. Although both bones consist of a shaft and expanded articular extremities, the more significant bony structures of the ulna are proximal, whereas the distal aspect of the radius forms its more notable articulation. Therefore, the ulna is larger proximally, and the radius is larger distally.

The proximal aspect of the ulna forms two prominent processes and two concavities that are key structures of the elbow joint. The curved olecranon process is the more proximal of the two bony projections and forms the proximal portion of the semilunar, or trochlear, notch. The triangular-shaped coronoid process is more distal and shapes the distal portion of the semilunar notch. Together, these two processes grasp the trochlea of the humerus, forming a hinge-type joint at the elbow that permits flexion and extension. The olecranon process effectively locks into the olecranon fossa of the posterior aspect of the humerus, preventing hyperextension of the elbow. On the lateral aspect of the coronoid process is the remaining concave depression called the radial notch, which articulates laterally with the radial head. The shaft of the ulna is more or less triangular, tapering from its proximal end to a short bony projection at the wrist, known as the styloid process.

The proximal radius is marked by the disclike radial head, whose superior surface is concave in order to accommodate the articulation with the rounded capitulum of the humerus. Slightly inferior to the head is the smallest portion of the radius, the constricted neck, which gives way to a roughened projection called the radial tuberosity. The anteromedial tuberosity anchors the biceps muscle of the arm. The shaft, or diaphysis, of the radius is bowed quite laterally and is distinguished by the anterior oblique line, which runs obliquely from the radial tuberosity to the point of greatest convexity. At the wrist, the distal radius is nearly twice as large as it is at its proximal end and features a concave ulnar notch, with which a portion of the distal ulna called the ulnar head articulates, along with the bony projection called the radial styloid. The palpable radial styloid is somewhat larger than that of the ulnar styloid and projects farther distally.

In the normal anatomic position, with the hands supinated, the radius is positioned laterally and the ulna medially. However, when the hand is pronated, or turned so that the palms face backward, the radius crosses over the ulna, forming an "X." Notice that the head of the radius is at the elbow and the head of the ulna is at the wrist.

The humerus is the solitary bone in the upper arm; it articulates with the scapula proximally and the radius and ulna distally. It is the largest and longest bone of the upper extremity and bears the characteristics of a typical long bone. The humeral head forms the "ball" of the ball-and-socket joint at the shoulder. In actuality, the humeral head is not a complete sphere; rather, it is slightly more than one third of a sphere, carried atop the cylindrical humeral shaft. The humeral head faces superomedially and, covered in articular cartilage, is roughly three times the size of its articulating surface, the glenoid fossa of the scapula. Immediately inferior to the humeral head lies a constricted portion known as the anatomic neck. Slightly more inferiorly on the anterior surface are two bony projections called the greater and lesser tubercles. The greater tubercle is located laterally and the lesser tubercle medially; they are points of muscle attachment. The intertubercular, or bicipital, groove (sulcus) separates the two tubercles and guides the long head of the biceps tendon to its attachment point on the rim of the glenoid cavity. Still more inferiorly located on the proximal humerus is the surgical neck (see Figure 5-24), so-called because it is the frequent site of fractures that require surgical repair. The shaft of the humerus is cylindrical proximally; however, it becomes more triangular-shaped as it progresses inferiorly. The anterior aspect of the humeral shaft features the roughened deltoid tuberosity anteriorly, to which the deltoid muscle attaches, and the radial groove posteriorly, which marks the course of the radial nerve.

Radiographic Procedures: Upper Extremity.   **Chart 5-7** describes the procedures for imaging of the upper extremity.

▶ CHART 5-7.   Procedures for Imaging of the Upper Extremity

PA, LATERAL AND OBLIQUE DIGITS 2–5

Film Size and Centering.   Three views are easily obtained on one 8 × 10 cassette when collimation is confined to slightly beyond the lateral borders of each digit. The proximal interphalangeal (PIP) joint is centered to the midpoint of the cassette.

Position.   The patient is seated comfortably at the side or end of the x-ray table. The hand is placed on a screen cassette in the pronated position and the fingers are separated. The digit under examination is placed at the midline of the film and exposed. On all three views, the desired position can be easily demonstrated by using your own digit. For the lateral projection, the affected digit is extended and the rest of the hand closed into a fist. In order to minimize OFD, the patient is positioned with the radial surface closest to the film for lateral examinations of the second and third digit, while the ulnar surface is placed closest for examinations of digits 4 and 5. A 45° oblique angle is used for the prone oblique projection. Optimally, the patient's hand is placed on a 45° sponge so that the interphalangeal joints appear open when visualized.

Central Ray.   The CR is directed to a point perpendicular to the PIP joint of the affected digit on all three projections of the digits.

Structures Visualized.   A PA, oblique, and lateral image of the affected digit and distal metacarpal, along with adjoining soft-tissue structures, is seen.

Quality Control Criteria.   Technique should be short scale of contrast, demonstrating both soft tissue and bony detail. Joint spaces should appear open. Visualization of PIP and metacarpophalangeal (MCP) joints should not be obscured by adjoining digits. No rotation of the digit should appear on PA and lateral projections, as evidenced by open joint spaces and concavity of the affected phalanges' anterior surfaces.

AP, LATERAL, AND OBLIQUE THUMB (FIRST DIGIT)

Film Size and Centering.   Three views of the thumb are obtained on a CW 8 × 10 cassette, with the midline of each collimated area parallel to the long axis of the thumb at the MCP joint.

Position.   Show the patient how to obtain the desired position by demonstrating with your own thumb. The AP projection is accomplished by positioning the thumb in extreme internal rotation. The remaining digits are held out of the irradiated area with the unaffected hand or are otherwise immobilized using tape. The oblique position is quite simple, because the thumb is in a natural oblique position when the hand is pronated. Therefore, place the pronated hand in contact with the cassette and collimate to the area of interest. The lateral projection is also naturally achieved by placing the palmar surface of the hand in closest contact with the cassette and the rest of the hand in an arched position. With the hand arched, gently rotate the thumb until the lateral position is attained.

Central Ray.   Directed perpendicular to the first MCP.

Structures Visualized.   The thumb in AP, lateral, and oblique planes is visualized from the distal tip to the distal row of carpals.

Quality Control Criteria.   Technique should be appropriate for the part under examination, and the entire digit and distal carpal articulation demonstrated. Joint spaces should appear open on AP and lateral projections and rotated on oblique views. The saddle joint articulation of the proximal phalanx and trapezium is best seen on the AP or, alternately, on a PA projection.

PA, OBLIQUE, AND LATERAL HAND

Film Size and Centering.   8 × 10 LW one-on-one, or two views—10 × 12 and 8 × 10.

Position.   The patient is seated at the x-ray table with the palmar surface placed flat on the cassette for the PA projection. An AP projection may be substituted if the patient is unable to fully extend the fingers. The long axis of the hand is centered to the long axis of the film, and the fingers are spread slightly. A 45° oblique is performed optimally with the use of a foam wedge to prevent overlapping of the joint spaces. The lateral projection is performed with the ulnar surface of the hand in contact with the film, and the fingers aligned atop each other. The thumb is placed at a 45° angle relative to the hand. Alternatively, a "fan" lateral view may be performed, wherein the metacarpals are aligned but the fingers are positioned separately using a foam wedge to assist positioning. Less technique is required to penetrate the fingers individually than the metacarpals in the lateral position; therefore, technique varies according to the area of interest.

Central Ray.   Perpendicular to the third metacarpal head for all views.

Structures Visualized.   The entire hand is seen from the distalmost phalanges to the carpus in the various projections. Distal radius and ulna and carpals should also be demonstrated.

Quality Control Criteria.   No rotation of the joint spaces should be present on the PA view, and digits should demonstrate slight separation in order to prevent overlap of structures. Oblique view will demonstrate second and third metacarpals separated, and fourth and fifth metacarpals slightly overlapped if properly positioned. Lateral projection should demonstrate anatomy from the distal radius and ulna to the distal phalanges superimposed, with the exception of the fan lateral, which demonstrates the digits individually.

PA, Oblique, and Lateral Wrist

Film Size and Centering. Three views on one 10 × 12 cassette.
Position. The patient is seated at the x-ray table low enough to place the axilla in contact with it. This position allows the distal radius and ulna, elbow, and shoulder to occupy the same plane so that a true lateral view of the distal radius and ulna can be obtained. An AP projection may be substituted if the carpal interspaces or distal ulna is the area of interest, because the AP projection better demonstrates these areas. If the AP position is used, the fingers are slightly elevated using a sponge in order to place the wrist in closest contact with the cassette. The elbow is flexed at 90° for the true lateral wrist projection. A 45° oblique is used for the PA oblique projection, optimally using a 45° foam sponge under the elevated aspect of the wrist.
Central Ray. Perpendicular to the midcarpal area. If localized swelling makes determining the area of the carpus difficult, the patient is asked to flex the wrist and the CR directed to that point.
Structures Visualized. Distal radius, ulna, carpal bones, and proximal metacarpals are visualized in three planes. Oblique view best demonstrates bones on the lateral aspect of the wrist, the scaphoid in particular. Lateral projection view with palmar flexion is a variant view obtained to view "carpal boss," a bony outgrowth found on the dorsal surface of the carpometacarpal joint.
Quality Control Criteria. As with all extremity radiography, the technique used should be short-scale if the clinical situation permits. Thicker part-thickness view must be compensated for on lateral projections. Lateral projections should demonstrate superimposed distal radius and ulna, carpal bones, and proximal metacarpals.

AP and Lateral Forearm

Film Size and Centering. Two views on one cassette, 11 × 14 or 14 × 17 LW depending on length of the patient's forearm. The long axis of the patient's forearm is centered to the midpoint of a sagittal plane on each half of the cassette.
Position. As the with the wrist, the patient is seated at the x-ray table low enough to place the entire limb in

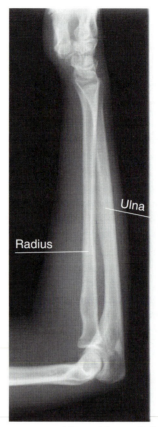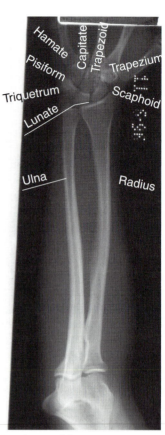

AP and lateral right wrist and forearm

the same plane. The AP view with the hand supinated is used, so that the radius crosses over the proximal third of the ulna in the normal PA position, producing an oblique view of the forearm. The elbow is flexed 90° and the forearm positioned so that the distal radius and ulna are superimposed for the lateral projection, with the ulnar surface of the forearm in contact with the film.
Central Ray. Directed perpendicular to the midpoint of the forearm.
Structures Visualized. An AP and lateral projection of the elbow, forearm, and proximal carpals is obtained.
Quality Control Criteria. Humeral epicondyles should be superimposed and the elbow flexed 90° on the lateral projection. The lateral view should demonstrate superimposition of the distal radius and ulna and the radial head and coronoid fossa. The AP view should demonstrate the elbow joint in an open position if the entire limb is placed in the same plane, and the radial head and neck will overlie a portion of the proximal ulna.

AP, Lateral, and Lateral Oblique Elbow

Film Size and Centering. AP and lateral performed, two views on one 10 × 12 cassette, lateral oblique view for radial head on 8 × 10.

Position. The patient is seated and positioned with the hand supinated for the AP projection and the elbow flexed to 90° for the lateral projection in the same manner as with the forearm. The lateral oblique projection requires that the elbow be positioned with the palm of the hand externally rotated so that the posterior surface of elbow forms a 40° angle with the cassette.

Central Ray. Perpendicular to the elbow.

Structures Visualized. The lateral oblique view demonstrates the radial head, neck, and tuberosity free of superimposition of the proximal ulna. If a medial oblique is performed, the coronoid process is seen in profile. The AP view demonstrates an open elbow joint, and the lateral view shows superimposed humeral epicondyles and the olecranon process in profile.

Quality Control Criteria. Radial tuberosity should face anteriorly on the lateral projection, with the humeral epicondyles superimposed. Oblique view should demonstrate radial head without superimposition from the proximal ulna. AP view should show the elbow joint open, and the humeral epicondyles parallel to the surface of the cassette.

AP AND LATERAL HUMERUS

Because of the painful nature of upper arm injuries, it is preferable to perform the examinations at the upright bucky. This technique allows positioning of the patient's body to achieve the desired projection with minimal risk of imparting further injury.

Film Size and Centering. 14 × 17 LW, upright bucky. The film is centered so that the upper border is 1½" above the humeral head.

Position. The patient is standing in the AP position with back to the upright bucky. For the AP projection, allow the arm to fall freely at the patient's side, with the hand supinated if tolerated by the patient. Because the arm will lie diagonally in relation to the film, collimation must be wide enough to permit visualization of the entire humerus. If the patient cannot achieve this position, gently palpate the affected humeral epicondyles and rotate the entire body until the epicondyles are parallel with the plane of the film for the AP projection, and form a 90° angle with the plane of the film on the lateral projection. For the lateral projection, place the hand of the affected arm on the same-side hip. This position abducts the shoulder and places the humeral shaft in a lateral position.

Central Ray. Perpendicular to the midpoint of the humeral diaphysis.

Structures Visualized. An AP and lateral view of the humerus from slightly above the humeral head to slightly below the humeral epicondyles is obtained with this method.

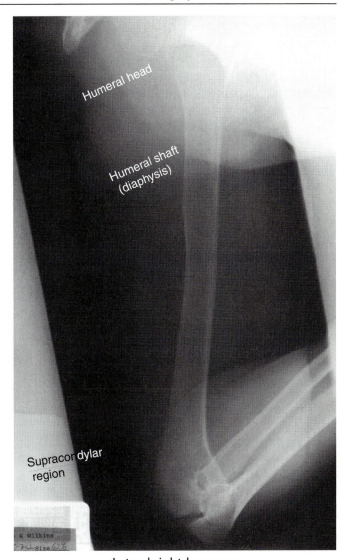

Lateral right humerus

Quality Control Criteria. The degree of correct positioning may be ascertained by the position of the epicondyles: they should appear without rotation on the AP projection and superimposed on the lateral projection. The elbow joint may lack the degree of openness seen on the AP elbow projection because of divergence of the x-ray beam. The humeral head appears in profile on the AP view. The lesser tubercle is seen in profile on the lateral projection.

TRANSTHORACIC VIEW OF THE PROXIMAL HUMERUS (LAWRENCE METHOD)

Film Size and Centering. 10 × 12 LW, upright bucky.

Position. This position is used to achieve a lateral projection of the humeral head and proximal humerus when abduction of the arm is not possible. The patient stands at the upright bucky in the lateral position, with the affected arm closest to the film. The unaffected arm is raised, and the affected side positioned so that the humeral head is centered, and the humeral epicondyles are parallel to the plane of the film. The film is taken on inspiration; the air-filled chest improves contrast and reduces the technique requirements. A low mA–long exposure time technique with the patient breathing may be used to blur the cardiac silhouette and lung parenchyma.

Central Ray. Perpendicular to the humeral head. Occasionally the patient may be unable to completely elevate the unaffected side; in such instances, a 10°–15° cephalic angulation may be used to avoid superimposition of the unaffected shoulder on the area of interest.

Structures Visualized. A lateral projection of the humeral head and proximal humerus through the lung parenchyma is seen.

Quality Control Criteria. The lesser tubercle is visualized in profile, whereas the greater tubercle is obscured by the humeral head. The humerus should be projected free

of the adjacent thoracic spine. If a breathing technique is used, the lungs and heart will be blurred but the humeral head and proximal humeral shaft will be demonstrated without motion artifact.

The Shoulder **(Figure 5-24)**

A distinction must be made between the shoulder joint and the shoulder, or pectoral girdle. The shoulder joint consists of the ball and socket, or diarthrodial, type articulation of the glenoid fossa of the scapula and the globular humeral head. The pectoral girdle is comprised anteriorly by the clavicle and its articulation with the sternum, the sternoclavicular (SC) joint, and posteriorly by the scapula. The SC joint is the sole articulation between the upper limb and the axial skeleton. The clavicle is united with the pectoral girdle at two other points. As the clavicle traverses posterolaterally from its sternal articulation, superior to the first rib, its lateral end forms an articulation with the acromion process, forming the acromioclavi-

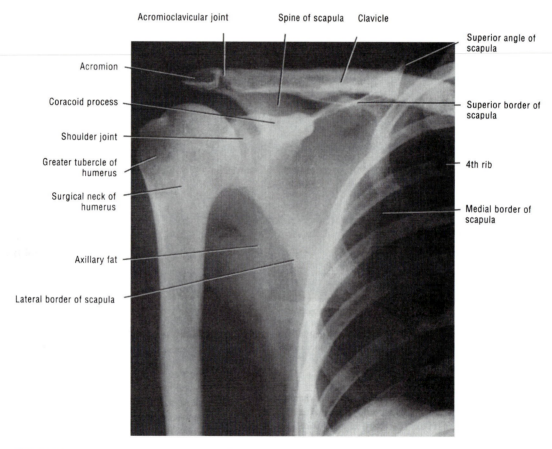

FIGURE 5-24. Anteroposterior radiograph of the right shoulder. (Reproduced with permission from Moore KL: Clinically Oriented Anatomy, 3rd ed. Baltimore, Williams & Wilkins, 1992.)

cular (AC) joint. The AC joint forges a sort of bony hood over the shoulder joint. Additionally, the strong coracoclavicular ligament serves to join the clavicle with the coracoid process of the scapula beneath it.

The shoulder joint is the most freely movable of all the joints; the joint capsule is extremely loose, permitting movement in every direction. This characteristic of the shoulder also renders it the most frequently dislocated joint.

Scapula. The triangular-shaped scapula is classified as a flat bone and forms the posterior portion of the pectoral girdle, covering ribs 2 through 7, and occasionally rib 8. The scapula has two surfaces, three borders, and three angles that are significant. The anterior surface of the scapula is marked by a broad concave area known as the subscapular fossa, to which the subscapularis muscle attaches. The posterior surface of the scapula is unequally subdivided by the scapular spine, an obliquely situated ridge of bone terminating in the acromion process, into the supraspinous fossa and infraspinous fossa. The borders of the scapula are named for their locations. The shortest, thinnest superior border extends from the superior angle to the coracoid process. The lateral or axillary border is the thickest portion of the three borders. It inclines from the inferior margin of the glenoid fossa in an oblique path to the inferior angle. The longest border is the medial or vertebral border, extending from the superior border to the inferior border. The superior border is formed by the junction of the superior and internal borders; the inferior angle by the union of the vertebral and axillary borders, and the lateral angle by the junction of the superior portion of the axillary border, where it forms the head of the scapula. The head presents a shallow articular surface called the glenoid fossa, which articulates with the humeral head.

Clavicle. The clavicle is a curved, long bone lying horizontally in the upper anterior thorax, superior to the first rib, forming the anterior portion of the shoulder girdle. Its two expanded ends articulate with the sternum medially and the acromion process laterally. The clavicle acts as a fulcrum for the pectoral girdle, allowing the arm to swing freely at the side by carrying the scapula laterally with it. A fracture of the clavicle results in the shoulder girdle collapsing in a medial direction. The superior surface of the clavicle is smooth, and its inferior surface is roughened to accommodate ligamentous attachments. The convex curvature medially and concavity laterally is more pronounced in men than in women.

Radiographic Procedures: Shoulder. **Chart 5-8** describes the procedures for imaging of the upper extremity.

► CHART 5-8.   Procedures for Imaging of the Shoulder

BILATERAL ACROMIOCLAVICULAR JOINTS (WITH AND WITHOUT WEIGHTS)

Because this exam is most often performed to rule out separation of the AC joints, it must be carried out in the upright position, because the recumbent position may produce an image that falsely demonstrates reduction of the affected joint. The exam uses two bilateral exposures: one with the patient holding sandbags or weights, and one without weights. If a dislocation is present, the weighted examination accentuates the widening of the joint on the affected side.

Film Size and Centering.   14 × 17 CW, upright bucky; the manubrial notch is centered to the cassette. If the patient is too large for the exam to be performed bilaterally, unilateral examinations may be substituted using 8 × 10 or 10 × 12 cassettes.

Position.   The patient is seated or standing in the AP position at the upright grid device. Center the patient so that the MSP is perpendicular to the cassette, and the shoulders lie in identical transverse planes. A 72″ FFD is employed. Collimation is restricted to a relatively thin transverse band across the AC joints. The patient's arms should hang freely at his sides. Instruct the patient to allow the muscles around the shoulder to relax. An exposure is made and the film marked with an appropriate marker indicating "without weights."

For the weighted examination, the patient is instructed to hold the sandbags in a way that allows the weights to pull freely on the joint. If the examination is performed correctly in the presence of a dislocation, the injured AC joint space will appear wider than the uninjured side. Respiration is suspended.

Central Ray.   Perpendicular to the jugular notch.

Structures Visualized.   A bilateral projection of the AC joints, distal clavicles, and both proximal humeri is produced using this method.

Quality Control Criteria.   The technique used should be somewhat less than what is conventionally used in conjunction with the shoulder, because the AC joints are less dense than the proximal humerus. Both AC joints should be demonstrated without rotation on one film, or separately in the case of a large patient. Films should include appropriate weight and right or left markers.

AP SHOULDER WITH INTERNAL, NEUTRAL, AND EXTERNAL ROTATION

Film Size and Centering.   10 × 12 CW, upright bucky.

Position.   The patient stands or is seated before the upright grid device, with the film centered at the coracoid process, which can be palpated slightly inferomedially to the AC joint. Three views are obtained sequentially. (1) For external rotation, turn the palm of the patient's hand up and laterally. (2) To obtain the neutral position, rest the patient's hand on his thigh. The epicondyles of the distal humerus should form a 45° angle with the plane of the film. (3) The internal rotation view is achieved by rotating the palm downward. Ask the patient to flex the elbow and rest the dorsal surface of the hand on the hip.

Central Ray. Perpendicular to the coracoid process

Structures Visualized. The external rotation position places the shoulder in the true AP position, demonstrating the glenohumeral relationship and the greater tubercle in profile. With the neutral position, the posterior portion of the supraspinatus insertion is seen, sometimes revealing calcifications not seen on other views. The internal rotation view demonstrates the humeral shaft in a true lateral position, with the region of the subdeltoid bursa visualized.

Quality Control Criteria. External rotation view should demonstrate greater tubercle in profile, and lesser tubercle is seen superimposed on the humeral head inferomedially to the greater tubercle. The neutral position demonstrates the greater tubercle superimposed on the humeral head. Internal rotation demonstrates lateral projection of the proximal humeral shaft; the lesser tubercle is seen in profile, pointing medially.

AXILLARY LATERAL SHOULDER, INFEROSUPERIOR PROJECTION (LAWRENCE METHOD)

A superoinferior modification of this position exists: the patient is seated and leaning laterally over the examining table with the arm abducted. A curved or conventional cassette is placed under the axillary portion of the arm and the CR directed 10°–15° laterally, toward the elbow. If the patient has a suspected subluxation or dislocation, it is prudent to consult the radiologist or referring physician as to the advisability of obtaining this view.

Film Size and Centering. 8 × 10 CW, screen. Film is placed in contact with the superior surface of the shoulder, firmly against the lateral aspect of the cervical spine.

Position. The patient is supine on the examining table, with the affected arm abducted. The shoulder and lateral aspect of the chest are elevated 3″–4″ because divergence of the beam may project the anatomy below the level of the film, causing "clipping" of the anatomy inferiorly. Respiration is suspended for the exposure.

Central Ray. If the patient is able to abduct the arm at a 90° angle with the thorax, the CR is directed horizontally. Otherwise, a medial angulation between 5°–30° is needed to maintain tube–part–film alignment.

Structures Visualized. A lateral projection of the glenohu-meral articulation is seen, along with the lateral aspect of the coracoid process and the AC joint.

Quality Control Criteria. The lesser tubercle should be seen in profile. The entire glenohumeral articulation should be visualized. The coracoid process should be included and facing anteriorly.

SCAPULAR Y VIEW

This position is often used as a substitute for the axillary position when the patient is unable to abduct the arm. The name is derived from the position of the scapula as it appears on the radiograph, with the scapular body forming the long axis of the Y, and the coracoid and acromion processes forming the upper extensions.

Film Size and Centering. 10 × 12 LW; upright bucky, centered to the glenohumeral articulation. The position may also be performed on the x-ray table; however, in most instances it is more comfortable for the patient to perform it upright.

Position. The patient is placed in either the prone or supine oblique position, so that the midcoronal plane of the body forms a 60° angle with the film. The PA oblique position is preferable if tolerated by the patient, because it places the part closer to the film, reducing OFD. Respiration is suspended for the exposure.

Central Ray. Perpendicular to the affected glenohumeral articulation.

Structures Visualized. The view demonstrates an oblique projection of the glenohumeral joint. It is used in determining anteroposterior dislocation of the humeral head. In the normal shoulder, the humeral head appears superimposed over the junction of the scapular Y. A posterior dislocation is demonstrated by the head projected over the acromion, and an anterior dislocation is shown by the head projected over the coracoid.

Quality Control Criteria. The scapular body and acromion process should be projected free of the thorax. The coracoid should be visualized, but superimposed on the thorax.

AP/PA AND AXIAL CLAVICLE

Film Size and Centering. 10 × 12 CW, upright or supine bucky centered at the level of the coracoid process.

Position. The exam may be performed in the upright or supine AP or PA position; the PA position is considered preferable because it places the part closer to the film. For both AP and axial views, the cassette is centered midway between the midline and the lateral border of the body at the level of the coracoid process. Respiration is suspended for the exposure.

Central Ray. The CR is directed perpendicular to the film on the AP/PA projections, and 25°–30° caudally for the PA, or 25°–30° cephalic for the AP projections.

Structures Visualized. The clavicle is projected superiorly and more horizontally on the axial projection, with only the medial end superimposed over the first and second ribs. The PA projection demonstrates the lateral half of the clavicle superior to the scapula and the medial half superimposed over the thorax.

Quality Control Criteria. The entire clavicle must be demonstrated on both views, with technique sufficient to penetrate the more dense medial aspect, but not overpenetrate the lateral aspect. Collimation should be confined to the area of interest.

AP and Lateral Scapula

Film Size and Centering. 10 × 12 LW. The AP position is centered to a point just medial to the axilla on the anterior surface of the thorax, and the lateral view is centered to the midpoint of the protruding medial border of the scapula.

Position. The exam may be performed in either the supine or erect position. For the AP position, the scapula is centered to the grid and the patient's arm is abducted at a 90° angle with the body in order to pull the scapula laterally, away from the thorax. The elbow is flexed and the forearm rests comfortably above it. The AP examination is performed with quiet respiration in order to blur the pulmonary markings. The lateral projection is performed in the upright position whenever possible. The patient stands or is seated before the upright bucky with the affected side in the anterior oblique position and rotated toward the film 50°–60°. The long axis of the humerus rests against the grid device, the elbow is flexed, and the hand is placed behind the patient's back; this position allows ready visualization of the medial border of the scapula. If the posterior oblique position is substituted, place the patient's hand across the chest and have the patient grasp the opposite shoulder. Respiration is suspended for this view.

Central Ray. Perpendicular to a point just medial to the axilla on the AP projection. Perpendicular through the medial border of the scapula with the humeral head centered to the film on the lateral projection.

Structures Visualized. AP and lateral projections of the scapula from the clavicle superiorly to a point just below the inferior angle.

Quality Control Criteria. The scapula should be pulled away from the thorax on the AP projection and should be free of superimposition from the thorax on the lateral projection. The humerus should not interfere with visualization of the scapular body. The scapula is more dense laterally, requiring technical adjustment.

Miscellaneous Related Extremity Studies

Occasionally radiographic studies of the extremities are needed that place emphasis on the soft-tissue structures adjacent to the affected extremity. Although other modalities such as CT, MRI, and ultrasound provide superior demonstration of virtually all soft-tissue abnormalities, there are occasions when a simple radiograph will suffice to provide the needed diagnostic information. When this is the case, a soft-tissue technique extremity examination is ordered. Clinical indications for soft-tissue studies vary, but include foreign body localization, diabetic gangrene, and evaluation of trauma-related edema. One commonly performed examination is the soft-tissue neck, which will be discussed later in this chapter. Compared with conventional extremity technique, the soft-tissue radiograph should demonstrate a long scale of contrast, with the bony structures appearing underpenetrated.

The bone age examination, consisting of a solitary PA left hand and wrist radiograph, is performed on pediatric patients whose developmental maturity is in question. The radiograph is centered at the third metacarpal head, with the fingers spread, and the thumb at a 30-degree angle relative to the second metacarpal, using a 30-inch SID. The finished radiograph is then measured against a known radiographic standard, using either the method described by Greulich and Pyle (1959) or the Tanner-Whitehouse method (Tanner et al., 1975).

Before the advent of more sophisticated imaging modalities, the bone survey examination was an integral part of metastatic disease assessment. But nuclear medicine, CT, MRI, and ultrasound have profoundly changed the manner in which oncologic evaluations are performed, rendering the bone survey nearly obsolete. Presently, the bone survey is used almost exclusively in conjunction with myeloma and plasma cell malignancy work-ups. When the examination is performed, it generally consists of the following protocol: lateral skull; AP and lateral cervical, thoracic, and lumbar spine; AP pelvis; and bilateral AP examinations of the shoulders, hips, ribs, femurs, and tibias.

A variety of disorders may cause clinical differences in leg length. Particularly with pediatric patients, surgical intervention may be required to correct the pathology. In this case, specialized radiographic measurements help determine the amount and type of surgical correction needed. The radiographic assessment of extremities to obtain long bone measurement, specifically the difference in leg length, is called scanography, or orthoroentgenography. The procedure uses a specialized metallic ruler in centimeter increments that is placed underneath the patient so that it is visualized on the radiograph. Orthoroentgenography minimizes beam divergence and associated leg length magnification by using three exposures on a single film. For bilateral examination, the scanogram ruler is placed along the MSP, and exposures made of both hips, knees, and ankles are obtained. The ruler has an approximate beam attenuation value of 8 to10 kVp; technical adjustment from the norm must be made. Additionally, the patient must be cautioned against even the slightest of movement between exposures, as any such action will invalidate the measurements. Because many of the patients requiring this examination are pediatric, it may be helpful to permit the parent to accompany the child into the exposure room for the examination; be sure to use prudent patient protection measures for both parent and child.

QUESTIONS FOR EXTREMITY STUDIES

select the best answer

1. Which of the following projections best demonstrates the articular surface of the radial head?
   (A) Lateral
   (B) AP
   (C) Medial oblique
   (D) Lateral oblique

2. In order to correctly center a PA view of the hand, the CR should be directed:
   (A) 5 degrees cephalic at the third metacarpal head
   (B) Perpendicular to the third metacarpal head
   (C) Parallel to the base of the third metacarpal
   (D) 5 degrees caudad at the third metacarpal head

3. The proximal ulna is marked to two prominent bony landmarks called the olecranon process and coronoid process. Which of the following correctly describes their articulations with the humerus?
   (A) Coronoid process with the olecranon fossa, posterior aspect of the humerus
   (B) Coronoid process with the coronoid fossa, posterior aspect of the humerus
   (C) Olecranon process with the olecranon fossa, posterior aspect of the humerus
   (D) Olecranon process with the coronoid fossa, posterior aspect of the humerus

4. The area between the anterior aspect of the calcaneus and the base of the fourth and fifth metatarsals is occupied by which bone?
   (A) Talus
   (B) First cuneiform
   (C) Cuboid
   (D) Navicular

5. A patient stands with the back to an upright grid device, with the supinated hand placed on the same-sided hip. The CR is directed to the midpoint of the humeral shaft. This description is called:
   (A) lateral humerus.
   (B) AP humerus.
   (C) oblique humerus.
   (D) transthoracic humerus.

6. Which of the following correctly describes the distal row of carpals from the radial to the ulnar side?
   (A) Navicular, lunate, triquetrum, pisiform
   (B) Trapezium, trapezoid, capitate, hamate
   (C) Scaphoid, lunate, os magnum, pisiform
   (D) Hamate, capitate, trapezoid, trapezium

7. A narrow, conical projection on the distal, posteromedial aspect of the ulna is known as the:
   (A) olecranon process.
   (B) coronoid process.
   (C) styloid process.
   (D) ulnar head.

8. Which of the following movements corrects the normal anatomic foreshortening of the scaphoid seen in a PA projection and opens the adjacent carpal interspaces?
   (A) Radial flexion
   (B) Palmar flexion
   (C) Dorsiflexion
   (D) Ulnar flexion

9. If a patient is supine on the x-ray table with the leg extended and the femoral condyles adjusted so they are parallel to the plane of the film, what orientation of the CR is used in order to best demonstrate the articulation between the proximal tibia and distal femur?
   (A) 5 degrees cephalic
   (B) 15 degrees cephalic
   (C) Horizontal CR
   (D) 15 degrees caudad

10. Which projection of the knee is a tangential projection of the patellofemoral articulation?

(A) Camp-Coventry
(B) Homblad
(C) Settegast
(D) Medial oblique

11. Which of the following bony lower extremity structures is easily palpated and often used as a bony landmark for positioning?
(A) Lesser trochanter
(B) Greater trochanter
(C) Acetabulum
(D) Femoral head

12. The lateral malleolus belongs to which of the following?
(A) Distal fibula
(B) Distal tibia
(C) Proximal fibula
(D) Proximal tibia

13. There are _____ bones in the foot.
(A) 23
(B) 25
(C) 26
(D) 27

14. Which of the following is the correct classification of the shoulder joint?
(A) Fibrous
(B) Amphiarthrodial
(C) Synarthrodial
(D) Diarthrodial

15. Of the following views, which can be used to obtain a lateral projection of the glenohumeral articulation when the patient is unable to abduct the arm?
(A) Axillary lateral
(B) Superoinferior lateral
(C) Inferosuperior lateral
(D) Transthoracic lateral

16. Which of the following views would be used to detect anteroposterior displacement of a fractured fifth digit of the hand?
(A) AP
(B) PA
(C) Lateral
(D) Oblique

▶▶ ANSWERS TO EXTREMITY STUDIES

1. The answer is (D). When the hand is externally rotated so that the posterior surface of the elbow forms an angle of approximately 40 degrees with the cassette, the result is an oblique view of the elbow, with the radial head projected free of superimposition of the ulna. The medial oblique view best demonstrates the coronoid process; the lateral view shows the humeral epicondyles superimposed and the olecranon process in profile; and the AP projection demonstrates the open elbow joint with the radial head, neck, and tuberosity superimposed over the proximal ulna.

2. The answer is (B). No tube angulation is required for the PA projection of the hand. The long axis of the fingers should be centered to the film cassette, and the CR should be directed perpendicular to the head of the third metacarpal. The fingers should be slightly apart to avoid possible superimposition of soft-tissue structures.

3. The answer is (C). The coronoid and olecranon processes join with the same named fossa of the humerus; the olecranon process articulates with the olecranon fossa on the posterior aspect of the humerus, and the coronoid process articulates with the coronoid fossa on the anterior aspect of the humerus. The two processes mark the borders of the deep trochlear notch, which grasps the trochlea of the humerus above it.

4. The answer is (C). The cuboid lies on the lateral aspect of the foot, occupying all of the space between the anterior calcaneus and the bases of the fourth and fifth metatarsals. The first cuneiform lies just medial to the cuboid, in the distal row of tarsals; the navicular lies on the medial aspect of the foot, and the talus lies medial, posterior, and somewhat superior to the cuboid.

5. The answer is (A). Placing the affected side hand on the same side hip abducts the shoulder and places the humeral epicondyles perpendicular to the film, with the humeral shaft in the lateral position. The humeral epicondyles are parallel to the film when the arm is in the AP position and tangential to the film in the oblique position. The transthoracic view of the humeral head is obtained with the patient in the affected-side lateral position, with the unaffected arm raised, and an exposure is made through the chest on suspended inspiration.

6. The answer is (B). The carpals are named from their radial, or thumb, side first. The distal row is trapezium (greater multangular), trapezoid (lesser multangular), capitate (os magnum), and hamate (unciform). The proximal row is navicular (scaphoid), lunate (semilunar), triquetrum (triangular), and pisiform.

7. The answer is (C). The styloid process of the ulna is a narrow bony projection that can be palpated on the distal aspect of the forearm. The ulnar

head is on the distal aspect of the forearm, but is not a bony projection. The olecranon and coronoid processes are found on the proximal aspect of the ulna and are important structures in the elbow.

8. The answer is (D). Ulnar flexion, or flexion toward the ulna and away from the radius, opens the lateral carpal interspaces and gives a view of the navicular bone (scaphoid) free of superimposition from the adjacent carpals. Radial flexion is used to view the medial carpal interspaces.

9. The answer is (A). The described position is an AP projection of the knee. A 5- to 7-degree cephalic angulation is used in order to project the patella superiorly out of the joint space. A horizontal CR may be used when the distal femur or the proximal tibia is the area of interest.

10. The answer is (C). The Settegast method, or sunrise view, is a tangential projection of the patellofemoral articulation that demonstrates the patella in profile and the articular surface of the femoral condyles. The Camp-Coventry and Homblad positions are obtained to demonstrate the intracondylar fossa. The medial oblique is sometimes used as a positioning variant and best demonstrates the lateral tibial plateau.

11. The answer is (B). The greater trochanter is an easily palpable, somewhat rectangular bony landmark that can be located on the body surface on the proximal lateral aspect of the thigh. It is particularly useful when other familiar landmarks such as the iliac crest or symphysis pubis cannot be easily located because of patient obesity. For example, using the greater trochanter as an orienting landmark, the technologist knows that the femoral head is slightly superior and medial to it, and that the symphysis pubis lies inferomedially approximately 1 to1.5 inches.

12. The answer is (A). The easily palpable, bony projection known as the lateral malleolus belongs to the fibula, which is the lateral bone of the leg. Its analogue is the medial malleolus; located on the distal aspect of the tibia. The malleoli should be parallel to the plane of the film on an AP ankle or tibia-fibula examination, and perpendicular to it on lateral projections.

13. The answer is (C). The bones that compose the foot are: 14 phalanges, 5 metatarsals, and 7 tarsals, which are the calcaneus, talus, navicular, cuboid, and first, second, and third cuneiforms.

14. The answer is (D). The shoulder is the most freely movable of all the joints in the body; therefore, it is classified as a diarthrodial, or synovial, type joint. The joints of the body are classified according to structure or function. The structural category includes fibrous joints, which are immovable; synovial joints, which are freely movable; and cartilaginous joints, which may be either rigid or slightly movable. Functionally, joints are classed as synarthrodial, which are nonmovable joints; amphiarthrodial, which are semimovable joints; and diarthrodial, which are freely movable joints. The limbs are composed predominately of diarthrodial joints, and the axial skeleton, which is charged with the protection of vital organs, is composed of amphiarthrodial and synarthrodial joints.

15. The answer is (D). The transthoracic view is used when arm abduction is not possible. The patient stands or is seated at the upright bucky with the unaffected arm raised. The CR is directed perpendicular to the midpoint of the film centered at the humeral head. The examination is performed on suspended respiration.

16. The answer is (C). AP or PA projections demonstrate mediolateral displacement of fractures, whereas lateral projections demonstrate anteroposterior displacement.

E. Spine and Pelvis Studies

1. THE VERTEBRAL COLUMN

The vertebral column is formed along the MSP by 26 irregular bones from the base of the skull to the pelvis, in a manner that results in a flexible curved structure. The spine functions to support the trunk and surround and protect the spinal cord, and also serves as an attachment point for the muscles of the back, the ribs, and via extension, the limbs. The vertebral column is held in place by an elaborate muscular support system. Two of the primary connecting ligaments are the anterior and posterior longitudinal ligaments **(Figure 5-25),** which are continuous bands of tissue extending from the cervical region to the sacrum. The anterior ligament is wide and forms a strong attachment to the vertebrae and intervertebral discs, whereas the posterior ligament is narrow and comparatively weak and attaches only to the discs.

The intervertebral discs lie between the vertebral bodies (see Figure 5-25) and are composed of two ring-shaped portions. The inner, gel-like nucleus pulposus lends the disc elasticity and the ability to compress, whereas the outer, tougher, annulus fibrosis contains the nucleus pulposus and holds successive vertebrae together. Sudden trauma to the disc may result in a common condition known as herniated nucleus pul-

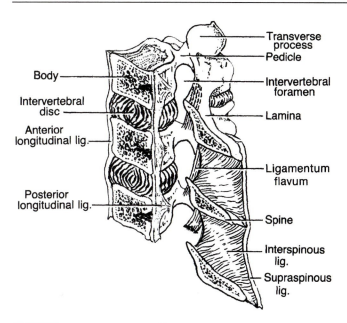

Body

Intervertebral disc

Anterior longitudinal lig.

Posterior longitudinal lig.

Transverse process

Pedicle

Intervertebral foramen

Lamina

Ligamentum flavum

Spine

Interspinous lig.

Supraspinous lig.

FIGURE 5-25. Principal ligaments of the vertebral column and intervertebral discs. (Reprinted from April EW: *NMS Clinical Anatomy*, 3rd ed. Baltimore, Williams & Wilkins, 1997, p 139.)

posus (HNP), which involves rupture of the annulus fibrosis and subsequent protrusion of the nucleus pulposus. HNP occurs most commonly in the lumbar or cervical region. When the nucleus pulposis impinges on a spinal nerve or on the spinal cord itself, severe pain in the neck, arm, lower back, or leg down the path innervated by the nerve results, depending on the location of the trauma. HNP is treated with bed rest, physical therapy, anti-inflammatory medicine, and analgesics. If conservative therapy is unsuccessful, surgery to remove the disc and vertebral lamina may be necessary.

The vertebral column has five major divisions and is approximately 70 cm in length in the average adult. The cervical spine consists of 7 vertebrae, lying in the region of the neck. Inferiorly, the thoracic, or dorsal, spine has 12 vertebrae, and the lumbar spine houses 5 vertebrae. Distal to the lumbar spine and articulating with pelvis is the sacrum. The sacrum articulates inferiorly with the terminus of the vertebral column, the coccyx.

Except for the coccyx, each section of the spine is curved, giving it a distinctive S shape when viewed laterally. The cervical and lumbar spine are convex anteriorly, and the thoracic and sacral spine are concave anteriorly. The spinal curvatures lend flexibility, strength, and resilience to the spine.

Several types of abnormal spinal curvatures are

significant to the radiographer. Scoliosis is an abnormal lateral curvature of the spine, occurring primarily in the thoracic region. The abnormality most commonly develops during late childhood, and is more prevalent among females than males. Kyphosis, also called hunchback, is an exaggeration of the dorsal spinal curvature, and is commonplace among elderly women; this condition occurs secondarily to osteoporosis. The familiar name for lordosis is swayback, an accentuation of the lumbar curvature. Lordosis may increase secondarily to weight gain as the obese or pregnant patient attempts to correct the center of gravity by shifting weight posteriorly.

All vertebrae share elements of a common structural design, but specific composition varies according to location. Each typical vertebra consists of an anterior body or centrum, and a vertebral arch posteriorly. The vertebral body and vertebral arch form the anterior and posterior boundaries of a rather large opening called the vertebral foramen, through which the spinal canal passes. As the vertebral foramina are stacked progressively on top of each other, they form the vertebral canal.

The vertebral arch is a complex structure whose boundaries are formed by the pedicles and the laminae. The pedicles are short, cylindrical, bony projections extending from the posterior vertebral body that form the sides of the neural arch. The laminae are located more posteriorly; they are flattened plates that fuse on the median plane and form the posterior portion of the neural arch. Seven processes extend from the vertebral arch. The spinous process is a single, posterior midline projection arising from the junction of the laminae. Two transverse processes project from the lateral aspect of the vertebral body. The four paired inferior and superior articular processes issue from the junction of the laminae and pedicles, and are covered with hyaline cartilage. The inferior process of a vertebral body articulates with the superior process of the vertebral body below it, forming the apophyseal joints. The pedicles contain notches on their superior and inferior surfaces that provide openings between adjacent pedicles called the intervertebral foramina. Nerves emanating from the spinal cord pass through these foramina.

Regional Vertebral Characteristics

Vertebral characteristics vary somewhat according to location and function **(Figure 5-26)**. For example, the transverse processes of the smallest, lightest cervical vertebrae contain foramina through which the vertebral arteries pass. Unlike the bodies of the thoracic and lumbar vertebrae, the body of the cervical

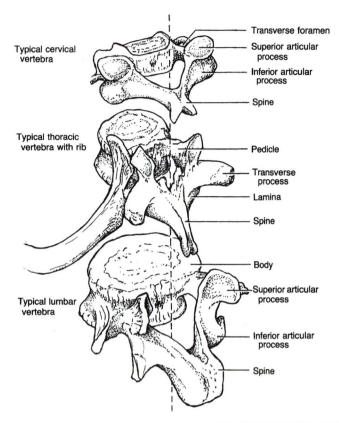

Typical cervical vertebra — Transverse foramen — Superior articular process — Inferior articular process — Spine

Typical thoracic vertebra with rib — Pedicle — Transverse process — Lamina — Spine

Typical lumbar vertebra — Body — Superior articular process — Inferior articular process — Spine

FIGURE 5-26. Typical cervical, thoracic, and lumbar vertebrae. The dashed line represents the center of the spinal canal. (Reprinted from April EW: *NMS Clinical Anatomy*, 3rd ed. Baltimore, Williams & Wilkins, 1997, p 135.)

spine is broader laterally than front to back, and except for C7, the spinous processes are bifid; that is, split at their tip. The spinous process of C7 is an important anatomic landmark; being easily palpated through the skin. C7 is sometimes referred to as vertebra prominens. C1 and C2, called the atlas and axis, respectively, are highly modified to accommodate for their specialized functions. C1 has no body or spinous process. It is a bony ring comprised of the anterior and posterior arches and lateral masses. The lateral masses have superior and inferior articular facets; the superior articular facets articulate with the occipital condyles of the skull, forming the atlanto-occipital joint; and the inferior articulating surface joins the superior articulating surface of C2. Arising from the body of the axis is a toothlike bony projection called the odontoid process, or dens **(Figure 5-27).** The dens forms a pivot point around which the body of C1 rotates. Thus, the C1 to C2 articulation is the joint that permits movement of the head to indicate "no,"

and the atlanto-occipital joint permits the movement of the head that indicates "yes."

The 12 thoracic vertebrae articulate with the ribs; their heart-shaped bodies bear two costal facets on their lateral aspects, which receive the head of the rib. With the exception of T1 and T12, the transverse processes present facets that articulate with the tubercles of the ribs. The thoracic vertebral foramen are nearly circular in comparison with the roughly triangular-shaped vertebral foramen of the cervical and lumbar spine. The spinous processes are long and project sharply downward.

The 5 lumbar vertebrae are quite sturdy; their structure is modified to accommodate their weight-bearing function. The lumbar pedicles and laminae are somewhat shorter and thicker than those of other vertebrae, and the spinous processes are short, flat, and project directly backward, an adaptation that facilitates attachment of the large muscles of the back. The facets of the lumbar articulating surfaces are modified in a fashion that locks the vertebrae together, supplying stability and preventing rotation.

The sacrum is a triangular-shaped bone formed by the fusion of 5 vertebrae, S1 to S5. It forms the posterior wall of the pelvis, strengthening and stabilizing it. The sacrum articulates superiorly, via its superior articulating surface, with the body of L5, and joins inferiorly with the body of the coccyx. The two alae of the sacrum are fused remnants of transverse processes that articulate laterally with the ilium of the pelvis, forming the sacroiliac (SI) joints. The weight of the body is transferred from the spine to the pelvis through the SI joints. The anterosuperior margin of S1 projects forward into the pelvic cavity, forming the sacral promontory. Directly posterior to the sacral body is the sacral canal, which is in essence a continuation of the vertebral canal contained within the bone of the sacrum. The sacral canal transmits the sacral nerves. The anterior and posterior aspects of the sacrum contain four pairs of foramina called the ventral and dorsal sacral foramina, which permit passage of the sacral nerves and blood vessels.

The triangular coccyx is a vestigial tailbone composed of three to five vertebrae diminishing in size from superior to inferior aspects, generally fusing into a single vertebra in adults. The name of the bone is derived from the Greek word that meant "cuckoo," because it was thought to resemble a bird's beak.

2. THE PELVIS **(FIGURE 5-28)**

The pelvic girdle attaches the lower extremity to the axial skeleton and supports the viscera of the pelvis.

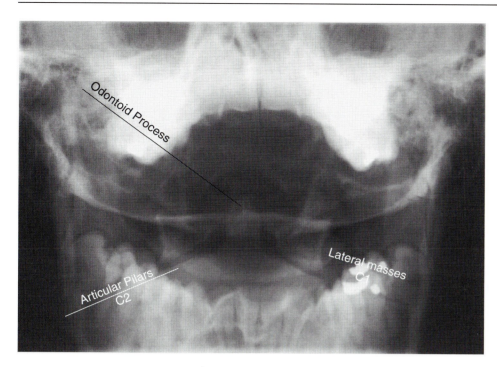

FIGURE   5-27.   Radiographic open-mouth view of the odontoid process.

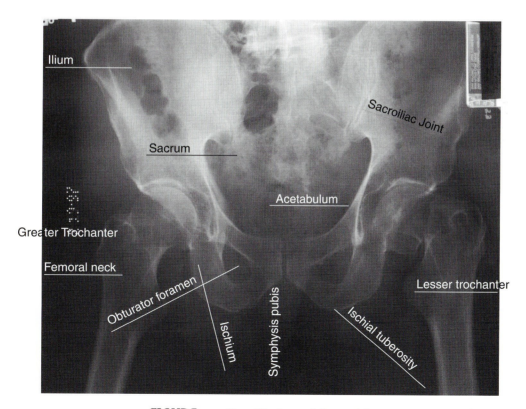

FIGURE   5-28.   AP view of the pelvis.

It comprises paired innominate (meaning *no name*) or coxal (meaning *hip*) bones, each of which unites with its partner anteriorly and with the sacrum posteriorly.

The term *pelvis* is derived from the Latin word for basin, which refers to the pelvic shape. It is formed by the joining of the sacrum, coccyx, and innominate bones. In childhood, the pelvis is made up of three distinct bones that later fuse; the names ilium, ischium, and pubis are retained in order to refer to their respective regions in the composite coxal bone. At the point of fusion of the three pelvic bones on the lateral aspect of the pelvis is a deep socket called the acetabulum, which articulates with the femoral head to form the hip.

The ilium represents the majority of the coxal bone and features several important anatomic landmarks. The flaring, winglike portion of the ilium is called the ala; the ala's thickened, superior border forms the iliac crests. When you instruct a patient to place hands on hips, the hands rest on the iliac crests. Inferior to the iliac crests are four bony projections that are also important landmarks, two located anteriorly and two posteriorly. The ASIS is the most easily palpable of these and can be visualized through the skin on a thin patient. Immediately inferior to the ASIS is the less prominent anterior inferior iliac spine (AIIS). The posterior superior iliac spine (PSIS) is difficult to palpate; however, its position can be approximated by a skin dimple caused by the attachment of the fascia to the PSIS at the level of S2. The posterior inferior iliac spine (PIIS) is located just inferior to the PSIS. Still further inferiorly, the ilium forms a deep indentation called the sciatic notch, through which the important sciatic nerve passes into the thigh.

The hip is one of the most secure joints in the body. Although it is a ball-and-socket joint like the shoulder, the range of motion permitted by the hip joint is much less than that of its upper extremity analogue. The femoral head faces superomedially, and slightly anteriorly, where it articulates with the acetabulum of the pelvis. The femoral head contains a small depression called the fovea capitis, to which an important ligament, the ligamentum teres attaches, extends to the acetabulum, and secures the femoral head in place. Two important prominences are seen along the femoral neck, which is the weakest part of the femur: the greater trochanter, superiorly, and the lesser trochanter, inferiorly. The greater trochanter is the point of insertion for the gluteal muscles and is an important surface landmark for palpation.

RADIOGRAPHIC PROCEDURES: SPINE AND PELVIS

Chart 5-9 describes the procedures for imaging of the spine and pelvis.

▶ CHART 5-9. Procedures for Imaging of the Spine and Pelvis

CERVICAL SPINE—AP, LATERAL, BOTH OBLIQUE, AND OPEN MOUTH ODONTOID (GEORGE) VIEWS

Film Size and Centering. 8 × 10 or 10 × 12 LW depending on the size of the patient; upright bucky for lateral and obliques; table bucky for AP 8 × 10 CW for odontoid view.
Position. For the lateral projection, the patient is placed before the upright grid device in the erect left lateral position, either seated or standing. The shoulders may be rotated either anteriorly or posteriorly, depending on body habitus, to avoid superimposition of the shoulders over the lower cervical vertebral bodies. Larger patients may hold sandbags or weights in either hand to further depress the shoulders. Another method to pull the shoulders away from C6 and C7 is to place a long, sturdy bandage under the feet so that the bandage forms a U, with an end in each of the patient's hands. Instruct the patient to pull downward to further depress the shoulders. The film is centered so that the upper border is approximately 1″ superior to the external auditory meatus. In order to position for the oblique projections, place the patient so that the entire body forms a 45° angle with the plane of the film, and the long axis of the cervical spine is parallel to the film. The chin should be elevated slightly to prevent the mandible from overlapping C1–C2. The CR is directed at a 15° caudal angle if PA obliques (RAO and LAO) are performed, and 15° cephalic if AP obliques are performed. The AP projection places the patient in the recumbent or erect AP position, with the chin slightly elevated, with the film centered at the thyroid cartilage. The open-mouth odontoid view is performed with the patient supine and the patient's mouth open at the time of exposure. Since the position is difficult to hold, technique should be set and tube part film alignment achieved prior to instructing the patient to open his mouth. Because of variations in skull formation, the positioning varies slightly from patient to patient. Generally speaking, the EAM should form an approximately 35° angle with the plane of the film. The patient is instructed to say "ah" during the exposure to position the tongue on the floor of the mouth, out of the way of the dens.
Central Ray. A 72″ FFD is used for the lateral and oblique projections. The CR is directed perpendicular to the level of C4 for the lateral projection, and angled 15° caudally for RAO and LAO obliques, and 15° cephalic for RPO and LPO projections through the level of C5. The CR is directed 15°–20° cephalic for the AP projection, through the level of the thyroid cartilage, and perpendicular to the midpoint of the open mouth for the odontoid projection. A 40″ FFD is used for the AP and open mouth views.
Structures Visualized. Open mouth view demonstrates AP

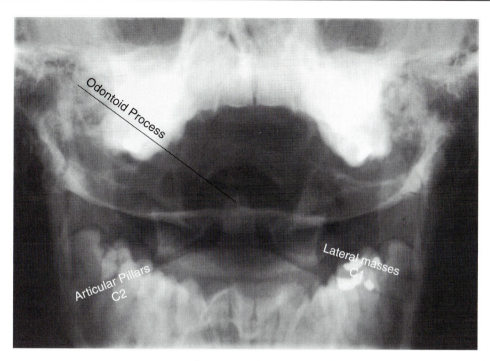

Open-mouth view of the odontoid process

projection of C1–C2 articulation through the open mouth. Visualized are the dens, the lateral masses and inferior articular facet of the atlas, and the body and spinous process of the axis. AP projection demonstrates C3–C7 and usually T1–T3. The interpediculate and intervertebral disc spaces are seen, and the spinous processes are seen on end. The lateral view demonstrates the vertebral bodies, inferior and superior articular facets of C3–C7, the intervertebral joint spaces, and the spinous processes of C1–C7. Oblique view primarily demonstrates pedicles and intervertebral foramina. The side closest to the film is demonstrated using PA obliques, and the side farthest from the film is demonstrated using the AP method. The AP projection demonstrates the five most inferior cervical vertebrae, along with T1–T3. The AP projection is also used to rule out the presence of a cervical rib.

Quality Control Criteria.   The dens should be unobscured by the teeth or occipital bone on the open-mouth view. AP view should minimally demonstrate C3–C7 without rotation, as determined by spinous processes being equidistant to the pedicles. The body and spinous processes of all seven cervical vertebrae should be demonstrated on the lateral projection. Intervertebral foramina should be open on oblique views. Chin should be slightly elevated to prevent superimposition of C1–C2 by the mandible on lateral and oblique projections. The area from C3–T2 must be included on AP projection, with disc spaces open and spinous processes equidistant to the pedicles.

THORACIC SPINE—AP, LATERAL, AND SWIMMER'S VIEW (TWINING) METHOD

Film Size and Centering.   14 × 17 or 7 × 17 LW, bucky, for AP and lateral views; 10 × 12 LW, bucky, for swimmer projection. Patient is placed in the upright or recumbent lateral position for the swimmer's view, with the midcoronal plane centered perpendicular to the film and centered to the cervicothoracic region. AP and lateral films are performed in their respective positions centered approximately at the level of T7, which can be located 3″ inferior to the sternal angle.

Position.   The patient is placed in the supine position for the AP projection, and in the left lateral recumbent position for the lateral projection. Dorsal kyphosis may be reduced in the AP position by having the patient flex the knees. Shallow breathing technique or respiration on full exhalation may be employed. Swimmer's view places the patient in the left lateral position with the shoulder closest to the film elevated and rotated posteriorly.

Central Ray.   The CR is directed to the level of T7 for the AP and lateral radiographs. The level can be located in a number of ways, the easiest being approximately ½″ superior to the level of the nipples, or 3–4 inches inferior to the jugular notch. The CR is directed perpendicular

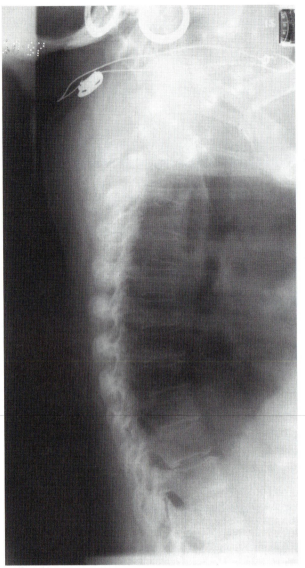

Lateral thoracic spine, breathing technique: blur lung and bone detail

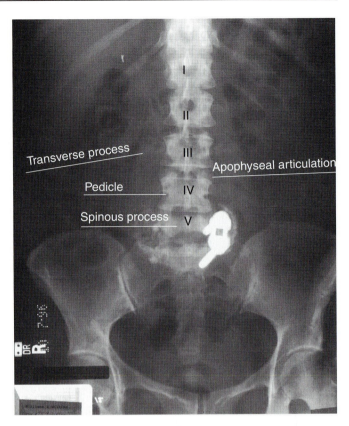

AP lumbar spine, post-laminectomy and fusion

radiograph. Twelve vertebrae included on AP projection. Lateral film includes L1; swimmer's view includes C5–T5. Collimation should be confined to the area of interest on all views.

LUMBAR SPINE—AP, BOTH POSTERIOR OBLIQUE, LATERAL, AND SPOT FILM L5–S1

Film Size and Centering. AP, LPO, RPO, and lateral films are obtained on 11 × 14 LW, bucky. Spot film of L5–S1 is obtained using 8 × 10 LW. AP film is centered so MSP is perpendicular to the midline of the grid device 1½″ above the iliac crest. Lateral film is centered at the same level along the midaxillary line. RPO and LPO films are centered at the same level also; however, the patient is adjusted so that a sagittal plane 2″ lateral to the midline is centered to the bucky. The film is centered 1½″ below the iliac crest for the spot film of L5–S1.

Position. Adjust the patient so that the MSP is perpendicular to the center of the grid for the AP projection. The patient's knees should be flexed and an appropriate support placed underneath them in order to reduce the lumbar lordosis and increase patient comfort. The most sensible sequence is to perform the oblique position next. A left lateral view is routine; therefore, perform the

to T2 for the swimmer's projection; a 5° caudal angulation may be used if the shoulder is difficult to depress.
Structures Visualized. AP view demonstrates the 12 thoracic vertebrae and interpediculate spaces. The intervertebral spaces are not well demonstrated because of beam divergence. The upper thoracic vertebrae are not generally visualized on the lateral projection; therefore, the film should include L1, because the absence of a rib at this level confirms the T12 vertebrae above it. Twining method demonstrates lateral projection of the area from C5–T5 between the shoulder images.
Quality Control Criteria. Anode heel effect may be used to advantage by placing thickest distal portion over cathode end of tube, providing more uniform density on the

RPO, followed by the LPO, followed by the lateral view in order to facilitate orderly positioning and reduce the amount the patient must move. Obliques are performed using a 45° angle of obliquity, with the side nearest the film being demonstrated. Adjust the patient so the CR enters a point 2″ lateral to the MSP 1½″ above the iliac crest. Rotate the patient into the left lateral position with the midaxillary line centered to the bucky. The patient remains in the same position for the spot lateral exposure of L5–S1, with the CR passing through a point 1½″ distal to the iliac crest. Respiration is suspended for the exposures.

A horizontal CR is used, directed through a point 1½″ superior to the iliac crest on all views, except for the spot film. In order to better demonstrate an open joint space on the spot film, the tube is angled 5°–8° caudally 1½″ inferior to the iliac crest.

Central Ray. AP projection demonstrates laminae, transverse processes, intervertebral disc spaces, the spinous processes on end, and the psoas shadow. Oblique projections are taken primarily to demonstrate the apophyseal articulations. Lateral view demonstrates the vertebral bodies, the spinous processes, and the superior four intervertebral foramina. Spot film demonstrates a lateral projection of the lumbosacral joint, the fifth lumbar vertebrae, and the superior portion of the sacrum.

AP film should be collimated to a width that permits visualization of the psoas shadows. SI joints should be equidistant from the midline. Lateral film must include spinous processes in their entirety, with the intervertebral disc spaces in an open position. L1–S1 joint space should be open on spot film and adequately penetrated. Typically, an 8–10 kVp adjustment from the technique used on the lateral view is employed. Apophyseal articulations, which when properly positioned appear somewhat like a "scotty dog" on the side nearest the film, should be demonstrated on the posterior oblique projections.

RPO and LPO Sacroiliac Joints

Film Size and Centering. 10 × 12 LW, bucky. Centered 1″ medial to the elevated iliac spine.
Position. From the AP position, elevate the SI joint under examination 25°–30°. Adjust the patient so that a sagittal plane 1″ medial to the elevated ASIS is perpendicular to the grid device. Respiration is suspended for the exposure.
Central Ray. Direct the CR 20°–25° cephalad through a point 1″ medial to the elevated ASIS.
Structures Visualized. A profile view of the elevated SI joint is seen. The joint should appear open, and both sides are examined.
Quality Control Criteria. An open joint space, or at least minimal overlap from the ilium and sacrum, should be demonstrated. The SI joint should be demonstrated in the center of the radiograph.

AP and Lateral Sacrum and Coccyx

Since the sacrum and coccyx are adjacent to the bladder and rectum, it is preferable to prepare the colon in a manner similar to that of a BE examination. The patient is instructed to void prior to the examination as well.
Film Size and Centering. 10 × 12 LW, bucky; 2″ superior to the symphysis pubis.
Position. The patient is positioned in the standard AP manner for both sacrum and coccyx, with the MSP perpendicular to the midline of the grid. The sacrum lies 3″ posterior to the midaxillary line in the lateral position, and the coccyx 5″ posterior; lateral centering should be adjusted accordingly. A lead rubber device should be placed behind the patient to absorb scatter and improve contrast on the lateral projections.
Central Ray. The CR is directed 15° cephalic for the AP sacrum passing 2″ superior to the symphysis pubis, and 10° caudally for the AP coccyx projection.
Structures Visualized. AP and lateral projections of the sacrum, SI joints, and coccyx are produced.
Quality Control Criteria. Correctly angled CR should produce a view of the sacrum and coccyx without foreshortening. Fecal material or a full bladder should not obstruct visualization of the part.

AP Pelvis

Film Size and Centering. 14 × 17 CW; upper border of the cassette 2″ superior to the iliac crest.
Position. The patient is placed on the examining table in the standard AP fashion. The feet should be inverted 15° to correct anteversion of the femoral neck, placing the long axis of the femur parallel to the cassette. Respiration is suspended for the exposure.
Central Ray. Perpendicular to the midpoint of the cassette, 2″ superior to the greater trochanter.
Structures Visualized. AP projection of the entire pelvic girdle is seen, along with the proximal third of the femur.
Quality Control Criteria. Entire pelvic girdle should be seen, including head, neck, and trochanters of the proximal femur. Ala of the ilium and obturator foramen will be symmetrical if positioning is correct. Ilia will be equidistant from the lateral borders of the radiograph if patient is centered correctly.

Frogleg Lateral of Hip—Modified Cleaves Method

This projection is not recommended for patients with suspected hip fracture, because positioning is extremely

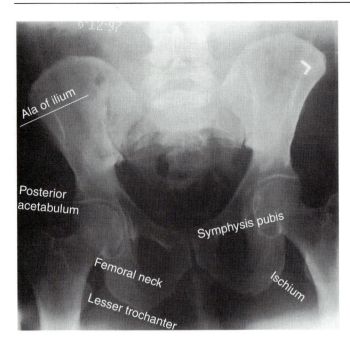

AP pelvis

painful for the patient and may make an existing injury worse.

Film Size and Centering. 14 × 17 CW for bilateral examination; 10 × 12 CW for unilateral examination. Center at the level of the symphysis pubis for bilateral exam and place the ASIS of the affected side at the midline of the cassette for unilateral exam.

Position. From the supine position, instruct the patient to flex the knees. Adjust the cassette and tube, and set technique before proceeding further. Abduct the thighs and brace the soles of the feet against each other for support. If unilateral exam is performed, turn the affected foot inward. The femoral neck(s) should form an angle of 40° with the plane of the table, placing the long axis of the femoral neck parallel to the table.

Central Ray. Perpendicular CR at the level of the symphysis pubis for bilateral examination and at the level of the affected ASIS for unilateral projection.

Structures Visualized. An axial projection of the femoral head, neck, and trochanter(s) is demonstrated.

Quality Control Criteria. Entire affected area should be demonstrated without rotation. If patient is postoperative following hip replacement or ORIF of the hip, entire prosthetic device must be visualized, sometimes requiring a larger film size. If previous films are available, the technologist should always consult them prior to performing the exam.

AP HIP

Film Size and Centering. 10 × 12 LW, bucky. Center the patient to a sagittal plane 2″ medial to the affected ASIS at the level of the greater trochanter.

Position. The patient is placed in the supine position with the foot internally rotated 15°. Respiration is suspended for exposure.

Central Ray. Perpendicular to a sagittal plane passing 2″ medial to the affected ASIS at the greater trochanter.

Structures Visualized. AP projection of the distal ilium, acetabulum, femoral head, neck, greater and lesser trochanters, and proximal portion of femur are seen.

Quality Control Criteria. Long axis of femoral neck seen in its entirety. Any orthopedic device must be completely visualized.

CROSS-TABLE SURGICAL LATERAL HIP—DANIELUS-MILLER METHOD

Film Size and Centering. 10 × 12 grid cassette, or cassette with fine-line stationary grid. The cassette is placed in an angled manner consistent with tube part film alignment so that its upper border is in contact with the body just superior to the iliac crest. The cassette is supported in place with sandbags, or the patient may support it by placing the hand on the rear of the cassette.

Position. From the supine position, the patient is elevated with a pad-type support or sheets, so that the trochanters are placed at the same level as the midpoint of the film. The knee and hip of the unaffected side are flexed and placed on a suitable support so as to permit unobstructed passage of the CR to the affected side.

Central Ray. The CR is directed in a cross-table manner so that it passes perpendicular to the long axis of the femur at the midpoint of the cassette.

Structures Visualized. An axiolateral projection of the acetabulum, femoral head, neck, and trochanters is seen.

Quality Control Criteria. The femoral neck should be seen without overlap from the greater trochanter; however, this is not always possible, because recent trauma may prevent the patient from attaining the needed degree of internal rotation of the foot. Entire length of orthopedic devices should be seen.

SCOLIOSIS SERIES—FERGUSON METHOD

This method is used in cases where scoliosis is present, specifically to distinguish the degree of deformity from the compensatory curve.

Film Size and Centering. 14 × 17 LW, bucky, PA erect; lower border of the film 1½″ below the iliac crests.

Position. The method uses a two-step procedure. (1) The first radiograph is obtained with patient in the PA position with the MSP centered to the grid device. Respiration is suspended on expiration. (2) For the second radiograph, elevate the foot on the convex side of the curvature roughly 3–4 inches. Ferguson states that, in order for the method to be reliable, the elevation must be sufficient to cause the patient to expend effort in holding the position correctly for the duration of the exam. *Central Ray.* Perpendicular to the midpoint of the film. *Structures Visualized.* PA projections of the thoracic and lumbar spine are demonstrated for the purpose of differentiating the primary, or deforming, curve from the compensatory curve.

Quality Control Criteria. Collimation to the area of interest should be in evidence, as should identifying markers. T and L spine should be demonstrated, including approximately 1″ of the iliac crests.

QUESTIONS FOR SPINE AND PELVIS STUDIES

select the best answer

1. Of the following, which type of vertebral foramen is (are) circular?

   (A) Thoracic
   (B) Cervical
   (C) Lumbar
   (D) Lumbar and thoracic

2. Of the following, which view (s) of the cervical spine will demonstrate the intervertebral foramina closest to the film?

   (A) Lateral
   (B) AP
   (C) RAO
   (D) LPO

3. A frail, 80-year-old female patient, having fallen out of bed on her right side, seeks evaluation in the emergency room. Her right hip is excruciatingly painful. She is unable to move her leg, and her toes are in the externally rotated position. The physician orders a right hip radiograph. Of the following, which is the most correct routine, considering the patient?

   (A) AP right hip, CXR
   (B) AP and frog leg lateral right hip
   (C) AP and surgical lateral right hip
   (D) AP pelvis, AP and surgical lateral right hip, CXR

4. Which of the following positions will most effectively demonstrate the left sacroiliac articulation?

   (A) PA with perpendicular CR
   (B) LAO with perpendicular CR
   (C) LAO with 25-degree caudal angulation
   (D) RAO with 25-degree angulation

5. The correct centering point used for a lateral view of the coccyx is:

   (A) the midcoronal plane, centered 2 inches below the ASIS.
   (B) 3 inches posterior to the midcoronal plane, with lower border of film at gluteal fold.
   (C) 5 inches posterior to the midcoronal plane, with lower border of film at gluteal fold.
   (D) 3 inches posterior to the midcoronal plane, centered 2 inches above the greater trochanter.

6. Which of the following projections is used to demonstrate the apophyseal articulations of the thoracic spine?

   (A) 70-degree anterior oblique
   (B) 45-degree anterior oblique
   (C) 45-degree posterior oblique
   (D) Lateral view

7. Which of the following projections is used to demonstrate the lateral C7 to T1 articulation when the standard Grandy method fails because of patient size or ability to cooperate?

   (A) Ottonello
   (B) Twining
   (C) Fuchs
   (D) Barsony

8. Which of the following is a single, midline bony projection arising from the pedicle–laminae junction?

   (A) Transverse process
   (B) Superior articular process
   (C) Inferior articular process
   (D) Spinous process

▶ ANSWERS FOR SPINE AND PELVIS STUDIES

1. The answer is (A). The thoracic vertebrae are the type that most closely resembles "typical" vertebrae. Their size increases as they descend inferiorly, with the upper vertebrae resembling the cervical spine, and the lower thoracic vertebrae resembling the lumbar spine. Their vertebral foramina are circular, whereas the vertebral foramina of the cervical and lumbar spine are approximately triangular.

2. The answer is (C). Oblique views of the cervical

spine are obtained primarily to demonstrate the pedicles and intervertebral foramina. Forty-five-degree PA obliques with a 15- to 20-degree caudal angulation (RAO and LAO) will demonstrate the foramina closest to the film, whereas AP obliques (RPO and LPO) with a 15- to 20-degree cephalic angulation will demonstrate the intervertebral foramina farthest from the film.

3. The answer is (D). A single view of the hip is insufficient, because there is no means of determining anterior or posterior displacement if a fracture is present. The frog leg hip view should never be used in conjunction with trauma; it may worsen a fracture or dislocation if one is present. The shoot-through, or surgical lateral view, is the desired projection with trauma cases, because it yields the desired information without further insult to the affected area. An AP chest radiograph is generally obtained for patients who have a fractured hip, because they are often taken to surgery quickly after their initial evaluation, and the chest radiograph is needed by the anesthesiologist to evaluate the patient's cardiac and respiratory status.

4. The answer is (C). In order to best demonstrate the sacroiliac articulation without overlap of the ilium and sacrum, the side down oblique, in this case the LAO projection, is used in conjunction with a 25-degree caudal angulation that exits the patient at the level of the ASIS.

5. The answer is (C). The coccyx lies approximately 5 inches posterior to the midcoronal plane. The lower border of the cassette is placed at the gluteal fold, and the patient is placed in a lateral position so that the CR is directed perpendicular to a coronal plane 5 inches posterior to the midcoronal plane. The technique used to visualize the coccyx should ideally be short scale, using tight collimation, with a leaded rubber absorber placed on the tabletop immediately behind the patient to absorb secondary and scatter-producing radiation. The exposure factors required are somewhat less than those necessary to expose the lateral view of the sacrum.

6. The answer is (A). The zygoapophyseal articulations of the thoracic spine are seen when the patient is rotated so that the coronal plane forms a 70-degree angle from the plane of the film. The lumbar apophyseal articulations are best seen using a 45-degree posterior (RPO and LPO) oblique position, although the degree of obliqueness varies among patients due to body habitus.

7. The answer is (B). The Twining method, commonly known as the swimmer's view, is used as a modification of the standard lateral when patient size makes appreciation of the lower cervical and upper thoracic spine difficult. The examination may be performed in the upright lateral or recumbent lateral position. The CR is directed through the level of T2 using a perpendicular beam or a 5-degree caudal angulation if depression of the shoulder cannot be achieved. The shoulder remote from the film is depressed as much as possible and rotated slightly posteriorly, while the shoulder closest to the film is raised and moved slightly anteriorly. It is common to find the Twining method as part of a routine protocol for radiographic examination of the dorsal spine, because the standard lateral method rarely demonstrates the upper 4 thoracic vertebrae.

8. The answer is (D). The vertebral arch is an aggregate structure formed by two pedicles and two laminae. Seven processes emerge from the vertebral arch. The spinous process is a single midline projection extending posteriorly from the pedicle laminae junction. The superior and inferior articular processes are paired processes that protrude superiorly and inferiorly from the pedicle–laminae junction. The two transverse processes project laterally from the sides of the vertebral arch.

F. Head and Neck Studies

The skull is formed by two sets of bones; the 8 cranial bones enclose and protect the brain and organs of hearing and equilibrium, whereas the 22 facial bones form the structure for the face, hold the eyes in anterior position, provide the cavities for the passage of air and food, secure the teeth, and provide muscle attachments for the muscles of the face (**Figures 5-29 and 5-30**). With the exception of the mandible, which is connected to the skull by the diarthrodial temporomandibular (TMJ) joint, the bones of the skull are joined by interlocking joints called sutures. The four major sutures consist of the coronal suture, which, as you might expect, divides the skull into anterior and posterior portions at the junction of the frontal and parietal bones; the squamous suture, which passes through the skull in an axial plane at the junction of the parietal bone superiorly and the temporal and sphenoid bones inferiorly; the lambdoid suture, which extends in a coronal plane between the occipital bone and parietal and temporal bones; and the sagittal suture, which divides the skull

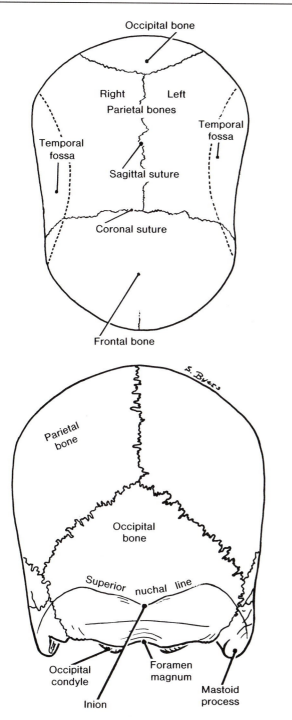

FIGURE 5-29. The cranium from above and behind. (Reproduced with permission from John V. Basmajian, MD, McMaster University, Hamilton, Ontario.)

into right and left portions at the junction of the two parietal bones.

The frontal bone forms the anterior portion of the cranium and the superior walls of the orbits. It is marked anteriorly by a region above the orbits with a thickened belt known as the supraorbital margins. The margins are pierced by the supraorbital foramen, which allows passage of the supraorbital artery and nerve. As the frontal bone extends posteriorly to its articulation with the paired parietal bones, it forms the anterior cranial fossa, which supports the frontal lobes of the brain. The glabella, which is an important surface landmark, is the smooth portion of the frontal bone between the orbits.

The occipital bone forms the walls of the posterior cranial fossa internally, and the base of the skull and posterior wall externally. At the base of the occipital bone is the foramen magnum, which is the crucial passageway between the vertebral and cranial cavities. On each lateral aspect of the foramen magnum are the occipital condyles, which articulate with C1. The external occipital protuberance is located just superior to the foramen magnum and is a bony landmark on the posterior aspect of the skull. The occipital bone articulates anteriorly with the parietal and temporal bones.

The paired temporal bones contain the organs of hearing and equilibrium. They lie inferior to the parietal bones; their junction is marked by the squamous suture. The temporal bones have a complex shape divided by four major regions. The squamous region abuts the squamous suture and features the jutting zygomatic process, which articulates with the zygoma anteriorly, forming the zygomatic arch. The inferior surface of the zygomatic process is remarkable for the mandibular fossa, which receives the mandibular condyle to form the TMJ. The tympanic region surrounds another important surface landmark, the external auditory meatus (EAM), through which sound enters the ear. Inferior to the EAM is the needlelike styloid process, an important muscle attachment point for the muscles of the neck and hyoid bone. The mastoid region contains the important mastoid air cells, which are crucial structures involved in equilibrium. Infection and inflammation of the mastoid air cells is a dangerous condition called mastoiditis. The condition is difficult to treat, and because the mastoids are separated from the brain only by a thin, bony plate, spread of the infection to the brain is likely if no treatment is instituted. Repeated bouts of mastoiditis are sometimes treated with surgical excision of the mastoid process. The petrous portion of the temporal bone houses the middle and inner ear cavities, which contain the sensory receptors for hearing and balance. This petrous portion is formed as a bony wedge between the occipital bone posteriorly and the sphenoid bone anteriorly. The petrous por-

FIGURE 5-30. The facial cranium. (Reprinted from April EW: *NMS Clinical Anatomy,* 3rd ed. Baltimore, Williams & Wilkins, 1997, p 587.)

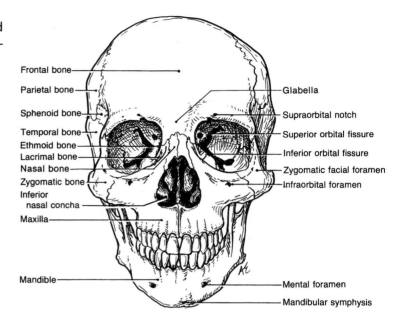

tion and the sphenoid bones together form the middle cranial fossa, which supports the temporal lobes of the brain. The jugular foramen penetrates the temporal bone at the junction of the occipital bone and petrous portion, allowing passage of the internal jugular vein and three of the cranial nerves. Anterior to the jugular foramen is the carotid canal, through which the internal carotid arteries pass. The internal carotids supply roughly 80% of the arterial blood supply to the cerebrum, and their proximity to the inner ear explains why, during excitement or exertion, we hear a "thundering" sound. Located slightly superior and lateral to the jugular foramen is the internal acoustic meatus, through which cranial nerves VII and VIII pass.

The bat-shaped sphenoid bone forms a central wedge with all other cranial bones. It consists of a central body and three pairs of processes. Within the sphenoid body are the paired sphenoid sinuses, and the saddle-shaped sella turcica, which contains the pituitary gland. Projecting laterally from the body are the greater wings, which form parts of the middle cranial fossa, the lateral walls of the orbits, and the external walls of the skull. The lesser wings form part of the anterior cranial fossa and the medial walls of the orbits. The pterygoid process extends inferiorly from the sphenoid body to form a portion of the lateral walls of the nasopharynx. The optic foramina are located anterior to the sella turcica and permit passage of the optic nerve and ophthalmic arteries. The superior orbital fissure is a long slit located between the greater and lesser wings through which the cranial

nerves pass. The superior orbital fissure is best seen on a PA or Caldwell view of the skull, the specifics of which will be discussed later in this chapter.

The ethmoid bone has an extremely complex shape, forming most of the area between the nasal passage and orbits. The superior surface of the ethmoid bone is distinguished by the horizontal plate, from which a triangular projection, the crista galli, emanates. The outermost covering of the brain, the dura mater, attaches to the crista galli. The bulk of the horizontal plate is formed by the cribriform plates, which are riddled with olfactory foramina. The olfactory nerves pass through the foramina. The perpendicular plate projects inferiorly from the center of the ethmoid, forming the superior portion of the nasal septum. The perpendicular plate is bordered on each lateral aspect by the lateral masses, which contain the ethmoid sinuses. The superior and middle nasal conchae, or turbinates, extend medially from the lateral masses into the nasal cavity. The lateral aspect of the lateral masses are known as the orbital plates, and form part of the medial wall of the orbit.

Except for the mandible and vomer, the 14 facial bones are paired, and include the palatine, inferior nasal conchae, zygoma, maxillae, nasal, and lacrimal bones.

The mandible is somewhat V-shaped and is the largest and strongest bone of the face. Its primary divisions are the jutting body, which forms the chin, and the upright rami, which are long, bony extensions that form part of the side of the face and terminate in the temporomandibular joint, the only freely movable joint in the skull. The rami are divided superiorly into an anterior and posterior process, partitioned by the mandibular notch. The anterior process is the coronoid process, which is the insertion point for the large chewing muscle, the temporalis. The posterior process is the mandibular condyle, which articulates with the mandibular fossa of the temporal bone, forming the TMJ. Inferiorly, the rami meet with the body of the mandible, forming the mandibular angle. The superior border of the mandible is known as the alveolar margin and contains sockets called alveoli in which the teeth are located. On the medial surface of each ramus is found the mandibular foramina, through which the nerves controlling teeth sensation pass. When working on the lower teeth, dentists anesthetize these nerves through the mandibular foramina.

The maxillary bones are fused centrally, forming the superior portion of the jaw and center portion of the face. Except for the mandible, all the facial bones articulate with the maxillae. Like the mandible, which carries the lower teeth, the maxillae hold the upper teeth in their alveolar margins. The palatine processes project posteriorly from the alveolar margins, fusing medially and forming two thirds of the hard palate, the roof of the mouth. Part of the lateral portion of the bridge of the nose is formed by the frontal processes, which extend from the superolateral aspect of the maxillae upward to the frontal bone of the skull. The largest of the paranasal sinuses, the maxillary sinus, is contained within the lateral portion of the maxillae. The zygomatic process of the maxilla articulates with the zygoma laterally.

The zygomas, or malar bones, are commonly referred to as the cheekbones. They articulate posteriorly with the zygomatic process of the temporal bone and anteriorly with the zygomatic process of the maxillae. The zygomas are important structures in forming the distinctive shape of the cheek and form a portion of the inferolateral aspect of the orbit.

The nasal bones are rectangular in shape. Their articulations include a superior articulation with the frontal bone, a lateral articulation with the maxillae, and a posterior articulation with the ethmoid bone. Inferiorly, the nasal bones form an attachment to the cartilage that forms the lower portion of the nose.

The tiny, fingernail-shaped lacrimal bones aid in forming the lateral portion of the orbital wall. The lacrimal sulcus is found in each lacrimal bone, permitting tears to flow from the surface of the eye into the nasal cavity. The articulations of the lacrimal bone are with the frontal bone superiorly, the ethmoid bone posteriorly, and the maxillae anteriorly.

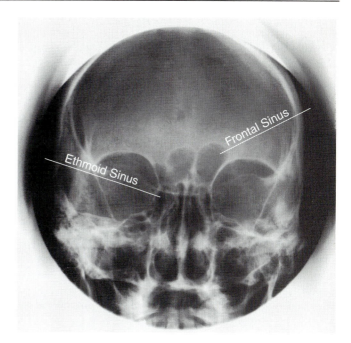

FIGURE 5-31. Frontal sinus, Caldwell view.

The palatine bones are approximately L-shaped. Their horizontal plates form the posterior one third of the hard palate. The diagonally oriented vertical plate invests part of the posterolateral portion of the nasal cavity and a small portion of the orbital wall.

Located within the nasal cavity, the vomer is thin and plow-shaped. It forms the inferior portion of the bony nasal septum. The nasal septum is the midline partition between the two nasal cavities.

The inferior nasal conchae (conchae = shell-like) are the largest of the three pairs of conchae. Like the superior and middle conchae, they invest the walls of the nasal cavity. The nasal septum and conchae are coated with mucus-secreting mucosa, which moistens, warms, and helps cleanse entering air. The shape of the conchae creates turbulence within the nasal cavity, which promotes bacteria and dust particles to adhere to the gluelike mucus.

Collectively known as the paranasal sinuses, the sphenoid, ethmoid, frontal, and maxillary sinuses are named for the bones that contain them **(Figure 5-31).** The sinuses connect with the nasal cavity, and like it are mucosa lined in order to warm and humidify inspired air. Air enters the sinuses from the nasal cavity, and mucosa from the sinuses drains into the nasal cavity, making the nasal passageways a kind of "two-way street." The sinuses lighten the skull and provide resonance to the voice.

RADIOGRAPHIC PROCEDURES: HEAD AND NECK

Chart 5-10 describes the procedures for imaging of the Head and Neck

▶ **CHART 5-10.** Procedures for Imaging of the Head and Neck

AP AND LATERAL SKULL

Film Size and Centering. 10 × 12 LW for PA projection, CW for lateral projection.

Position. For the PA projection, the patient is placed in the prone position, with nose and forehead resting against the table or upright grid device centered at the level of the nasion. Caldwell PA method uses 15° caudal angulation to demonstrate the petrous portion of the temporal bone in the lower third of the orbits. For the lateral projection, the patient is rotated slightly to the semiprone position with the elbow and knee flexed to provide support. The head is adjusted so that the interpupillary line (IPL) is perpendicular to the film, centered at a point 2″ superior to the external auditory meatus (EAM).

Central Ray. Perpendicular through the nasion for standard PA projection. Caldwell method uses 25° caudal angulation to project petrous ridge into lower third of the orbits and 25° angulation if petrous ridges are desired below the orbits. A perpendicular CR is used for the lateral projection, directed to a point 2″ superior to the EAM.

Structures Visualized. Lateral view demonstrates the superimposed halves of the cranium. Seen well in this projection are the sella turcica, clinoid processes, and dorsum sellae. Anatomy demonstrated on the PA radiograph is dependent on degree of caudal angulation. Frontal bone and portion of the parietal bones are seen. The crista galli and ethmoid sinuses are visualized.

Quality Control Criteria. Entire cranial vertex should be demonstrated. A larger film may be required in some instances. Skull demonstrated without rotation as evidenced by distance from the lateral border of the skull to the orbit. Lateral view is without rotation when TMJ joints, orbital roof, and both EAM are superimposed.

AP SEMIAXIAL CHAMBERLAIN-TOWNES VIEW

Film Size and Centering. 10 × 12 LW bucky.

Position. The patient is placed in the supine or seated erect position, MSP perpendicular to the midline of the grid device, with the orbitomeatal line (OML) perpendicular to the plane of the film. If the patient is unable to attain sufficient cervical flexion, increase angulation by 7°. The head is centered to the film so that the upper border of the cassette is slightly superior to the vertex of the skull.

Central Ray. The CR is directed caudally 30° to the orbitomeatal line or 37° to the infraorbital meatal line. If the foramen magnum is the area of interest, the CR angulation may be increased to a range from 40°–60°, depending on the degree of cervical flexion.

Structures Visualized. The posterior clinoid process and dorsum sellae are shown projected in the shadow of the foramen magnum. A symmetric view of the petrous ridges is seen. The occipital bone and the posterior portion of the parietal bone are also visualized.

Quality Control Criteria. The view is correctly positioned when the distances from the lateral borders of the foramen magnum to the lateral borders of the skull are equal. Technique should provide for adequate penetration of the occipital bone without overpenetration of the thinner lateral portion of the skull.

CALDWELL, LATERAL, WATERS, AND SUBMENTOVERTICAL (SMV) PROJECTIONS OF THE PARANASAL SINUSES

The Caldwell and lateral views have been previously described; centering and film size should reflect the area of interest. Sinus films are performed in the upright position in order to rule out the presence of air/fluid levels in the paranasal sinuses.

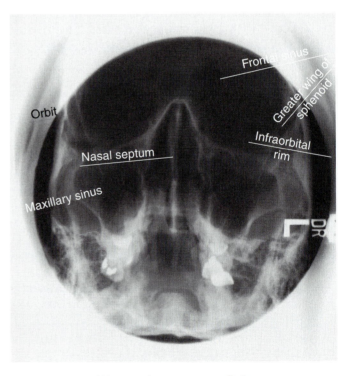

Waters view, paranasal sinus

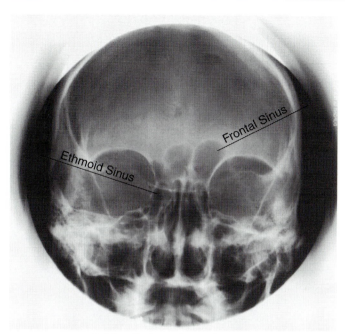

Caldwell view, frontal sinus.

Film Size and Centering. 8 × 10 upright bucky, or table tilted to the vertical position. Centering is at the level of the acanthion for the Waters projection, and the SMV is centered at the level of the sella turcica.

Position. In the Waters position, the patient is placed before the upright grid device, with the chin resting on its surface. The MSP is perpendicular with respect to the grid device, and the head is tilted with cervical flexion so that the OML forms a 37° angle to the plane of the film. The cassette is centered at the level of the acanthion. The patient is placed in the erect AP position for the SMV projection. A chair with a back support should be used if available. The patient is moved slightly away from the upright grid device and the head tilted backward by placing the cervical spine in complete extension, with the MSP perpendicular to the midline of the grid device. Because the position is difficult, centering of the film and setting technique should be accomplished prior to positioning the patient.

Central Ray. The CR is directed perpendicular through the level of the acanthion for the Waters projection. In order to perform the SMV, the tube is angled in a cephalic direction so that it is perpendicular to the infraorbital meatal line (IOML).

Structures Visualized. The Waters view demonstrates the maxillary and frontal sinuses. The view is also a standard projection in routine series of the orbit, zygomatic arches, and facial bones. When the SMV is performed for demonstration of the sinus, the examination reveals the sphenoid, ethmoid, and maxillary sinuses. However, the view is also used in conjunction with the facial bones

and the petrous portion of the temporal bones. When technique is decreased, the view is useful in demonstration of the zygomatic arches. The SMV view should demonstrate a basal view of the cranium, the petrous portion of the temporal bones, the internal auditory canals, and the mandible.

Quality Control Criteria. Waters view should demonstrate the orbits equidistant to the lateral borders of the skull, and the petrous portion should be projected below the level of the maxillae. Distance from the lateral border of the skull to the mandibular condyles should be equidistant on SMV projection. If correctly positioned, the mandibular symphysis is superimposed on the frontal bone. The petrous portion should appear symmetric.

ORBITOPARIETAL OBLIQUE OPTIC FORAMEN—RHESE VIEW

Film Size and Centering. 8 × 10 LW, bucky centered at the level of the orbit farthest from the film.

Position. Rotate the patient from the supine or prone position so that the MSP forms a 53° angle with the plane of the film. The acanthiomeatal line is perpendicular. Prone position is preferred, as it produces less dose to the lens of the eye and places the part closer to the film.

Central Ray. Perpendicular to the midpoint of the cassette.

Structures Visualized. The optic foramen is visualized in the inferior lateral quadrant of the orbit. The superior, inferior, lateral, and medial orbital margins are seen. The sphenoid ridge appears in the inferior third of the orbit.

Quality Control Criteria. Collimation should be confined to the area of interest. The optic canal should appear in the inferior lateral quadrant of the orbit, with the entire orbit visualized.

PA OBLIQUE AXIAL FACIAL BONES (ZYGOMA, ORBITAL WALL)—LAW METHOD

Film Size and Centering. 8 × 10 LW, table or upright bucky centered to the orbit closest to the film.

Position. With the patient in the PA position, rotate the head so the unaffected side is placed closest to the film, with the nose, cheek, and chin resting on the table or upright grid surface. Lift the chin so the neck is fully extended. Center the cassette to the orbit closest to the film.

Central Ray. The CR is directed 25°–30° cephalic, entering the patient slightly posterior to the mandibular angle.

Structures Visualized. All the facial bones are included. Ballinger notes that Law developed the view primarily to demonstrate the floor and posterior wall of the maxillary sinus, but the view is particularly useful for demonstration of the zygoma and external orbital wall as well.

Quality Control Criteria. All facial bones should be demonstrated. The side under examination should be seen without superimposition from the opposite side.

LATERAL NASAL BONES

Film Size and Centering. Two views on one 8 × 10 cassette centered to a level slightly distal to the nasion.
Position. The patient is placed in the lateral position on the x-ray table. A screen cassette is placed under the patient's facial area, with a side identification marker taped within the borders of collimation but out of the affected area. The MSP is perpendicular to the film and the IPL is perpendicular. Both sides are examined on a single cassette for comparison.
Central Ray. Perpendicular to a point slightly distal to the nasion.
Structures Visualized. A lateral view of the nasal bone and adjacent soft tissue structures, with the side nearest the film being demonstrated.
Quality Control Criteria. Technique should be appropriate for screen cassette, with factors that are approximate to that of a finger. A short scale of contrast is desirable. The nasal bones should be seen without rotation and the nasofrontal suture appreciated.

AP AXIAL VIEW OF ZYGOMA AND MANDIBLE

Film Size and Centering. 10 × 12 CW, bucky. Center at the level of the glabella.
Position. The patient is placed in the seated erect or supine AP position. MSP and OML perpendicular to the plane of the film. The chin and forehead may be immobilized with tape or other suitable immobilization device.
Central Ray. The CR is angled 30° caudad through the glabella.
Structures Visualized. An AP projection of the zygoma and mandibular rami free of superimposition is seen.
Quality Control Criteria. Zygoma must be seen without overlap from mandible; both structures must be free of rotation.

OBLIQUE MANDIBLE

The position can be altered slightly with technique and positioning to more clearly delineate the mandibular symphysis or ramus, if those areas are specifically of interest.
Film Size and Centering. 8 × 10 CW, slightly posterior to the mandibular angle.
Position. From the prone or erect PA position, adjust the patient's shoulders so that the horizontal axis of the mandible is parallel to the transverse axis of the cassette.
Central Ray. Twenty-five degrees cephalic through the area just posterior to the mandibular angle.
Structures Visualized. An axiolateral projection of the mandible from the mandibular angle to the region of the mandibular symphysis is seen.
Quality Control Criteria. The mandible should be free from superimposition from the opposite mandibular body. Entire area of interest should be included.

OPEN- AND CLOSED-MOUTH MODIFIED LATERAL VIEWS—TMJ

Film Size and Centering. 8 × 10 CW, table or upright bucky centered at the TMJ closest to the film.
Position. From the lateral position, rotate the patient's MSP toward the film. Adjust cervical flexion so that the acanthiomeatal line is perpendicular to the transverse axis of the cassette. After making an exposure with the patient's mouth closed, change cassettes; ensure that positioning has not changed and then, instructing the patient to open his mouth, make another exposure.
Central Ray. Fifteen degrees caudad through a point exiting at the TMJ closest to the grid device.
Structures Visualized. The relative position of the mandibular fossa and mandibular condyle is seen. Open-mouth view demonstrates the degree of inferior and anterior excursion of the condyle.
Quality Control Criteria. TMJ articulation clearly visualized. Normal closed-mouth radiographs demonstrate the mandibular condyle within the mandibular fossa. Open-mouth views demonstrate the condyle inferior to the fossa on a normal patient.

PA OBLIQUE FACIAL BONES

Film Size and Centering. 8 × 10 LW, bucky. Center through the infraorbital margin.
Position. From the semiprone or seated erect position, adjust the patient so that the nose, forehead, and cheek rest on the imaging surface. The MSP forms a 53° angle with the transverse plane of the film, with the acanthiomeatal line parallel to the transverse axis of the film.
Central Ray. Perpendicular to the infraorbital margin closest to the film.
Structures Visualized. An oblique image of the facial bones without overlap from the opposite side is seen. Both sides are routinely examined for comparison.
Quality Control Criteria. All facial bones should be included, without overlap from the opposite side.

SOFT TISSUE LATERAL NECK (INCLUDING SOFT PALATE, PHARYNX, AND LARYNX)

Occasionally, AP projections are obtained as well, depending on the pathology to be investigated.
Film Size and Centering. 10 × 12 LW, upright bucky. Center so that a coronal plane passes slightly anteriorly to the TMJ.
Position. The patient is placed in the standard lateral position, with the head slightly extended. Procedure may vary according to the area of interest. For example, the patient may be asked to phonate certain vowel sounds to demonstrate the vocal cords, or for cleft palate examination. The Valsalva maneuver is performed to distend the trachea with air.

Central Ray. Perpendicular to the level of the thyroid cartilage, although centering may vary slightly according to the area of interest.

Structures Visualized. The pharyngolaryngeal structures are identified.

Quality Control Criteria. Technical factors are adjusted so that soft tissue structures are clearly visualized. Shoulders are depressed to prevent overlap of the trachea, head, and neck.

QUESTIONS FOR HEAD AND NECK STUDIES

select the best answer

1. The anterior two thirds of the hard palate is formed by which bone(s)?

   (A) Maxillae
   (B) Palatine
   (C) Mandible
   (D) Vomer

2. The correct angulation for a routine view of the skull that demonstrates the dorsum sellae inside the foramen magnum is:

   (A) 15 degrees cephalic.
   (B) 5 degrees caudad.
   (C) 15 degrees caudad.
   (D) 37 degrees caudad.

3. With the patient in either the upright or supine lateral position, if the CR is directed to a point 1 inch anterior and 1 inch superior to the EAM, and a closely collimated 8 × 10 cassette is used, the primary anatomic structure(s) demonstrated will be the:

   (A) mastoid air cells.
   (B) sella turcica.
   (C) frontal sinus.
   (D) external occipital protuberance.

4. The correct number of bones that contain paranasal sinuses is:

   (A) three.
   (B) four.
   (C) five.
   (D) six.

5. A patient in the supine position is positioned so that the MSP forms a 53-degree angle with the plane of the film, and the acanthiomeatal line is perpendicular to the film. What view is performed when the CR is directed through the orbit farthest from the film?

   (A) Caldwell
   (B) Jones
   (C) Rhese
   (D) Waters'

6. Which view of the sinuses demonstrates all four sinuses?

   (A) Waters'
   (B) Caldwell
   (C) SMV
   (D) Lateral

7. The pterygoid process is a part of which bone?

   (A) Ethmoid
   (B) Vomer
   (C) Sphenoid
   (D) Lacrimal

►►ANSWERS FOR HEAD AND NECK STUDIES

1. The answer is (A). The anterior two thirds of the hard palate or roof of the oral cavity is formed by the palatine processes of the maxillae. The hard palate is completed posteriorly by the horizontal plates of the palatine bone.

2. The answer is (D). The routine view of the skull that demonstrates the dorsum sellae inside the foramen magnum is the Chamberlain-Townes view. Correct angulation of the view actually varies according to patient position and desired anatomic demonstration. The CR may be directed 30 degrees to the orbitomeatal line (OML), or 37 degrees to the infraorbital meatal line (IOML). Variants of the position include angulation of up to 60 degrees caudad.

3. The answer is (B). The position describes a lateral view of the sella turcica, in which the sella is placed in the center of the radiograph, and both the anterior and posterior clinoid processes are superimposed.

4. The answer is (C). The four paranasal sinuses are named for the bones that contain them: the sphenoid, ethmoid, frontal, and both maxillary bones.

5. The answer is (C). The described position is the oblique projection of the orbit and optic canal, or Rhese method. The optic foramen is demonstrated in the inferior lateral portion of the orbit using this method.

6. The answer is (D). Although the sphenoidal sinus is of primary concern, all four sinuses are demonstrated on the lateral view. The Waters' view demonstrates the maxillary and frontal sinuses; the Caldwell view demonstrates the frontal and eth-

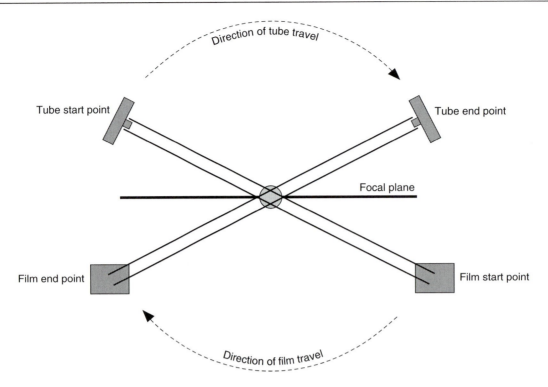

FIGURE 5-32. Basic priniciple of tomography.

moid sinuses; and the SMV chiefly demonstrates the sphenoid and ethmoid sinuses.

7. The answer is (C). The sphenoid bone somewhat resembles a bat with two sets of wings, the greater and lesser, projecting laterally from its body, and two processes, the pterygoid processes, extending inferiorly from the body. The sphenoid bone articulates with all the cranial bones, and its fragile appearing body is bound firmly together by them.

III. MISCELLANEOUS RADIOGRAPHIC PROCEDURES
A. Tomography

We have previously described techniques whereby superimposition of adjacent structures on the radiographic image can be partially or completely eliminated by the effect of motion. The breathing technique used in conjunction with the RAO view of the sternum and lateral thoracic spine is one such example of this kind of procedure. Tomography is a radiographic method that produces an in-focus image of a predetermined plane of the body, and structures above and below that plane are rendered as low-den-

sity blurs induced by motion. **Figure 5-32** illustrates the basic tomographic principle.

Remember that to produce a radiographic image, three basic elements—an x-ray source, an object, and a recording medium—are necessary. With tomography, a fourth element is added: the synchronous movement of the x-ray tube and film. Notice the horizontal line labeled focal plane. The focal plane is the fulcrum, or axis of rotation, around which the in-focus image is determined. Structures that are within the same level of the focal plane are demonstrated in focus, whereas those above it and below it are blurred. Thus, tomography is said to be a radiographic method of controlled blurring, that is, the focal plane structures are not enhanced in any way, they are simply less blurred than the surrounding structures.

With the advent of **computer assisted tomography (CAT scan),** plain film tomography is today used primarily in conjunction with excretory urography (nephrotomography) and occasionally to demonstrate fractures.

B. Arthrography

Arthrography is the radiographic examination of joints using either water-soluble iodinated contrast; gaseous medium, usually air; or both types of contrast

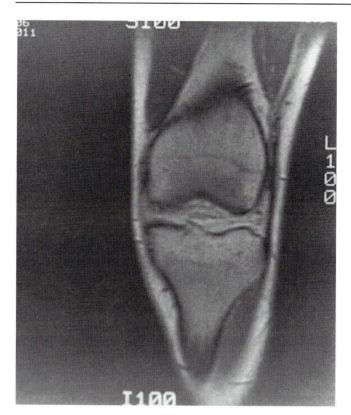

FIGURE 5-33. Coronal T1 view of the knee. (Reproduced with permission from Slaby F, Jacobs ER: *Radiographic Anatomy.* Baltimore, Williams & Wilkins, 1990.)

enhancement. Today, the examination has been largely replaced by noninvasive MRI examinations. The bulk of arthrography still performed uses the double-contrast approach. The joints most commonly investigated by arthrography are the hip, knee, shoulder, TMJ, and wrist **(Figure 5-33)**. The examination is performed under aseptic conditions, with the use of a sterile tray and local anesthetic. After aspiration of any joint effusion present, the contrast agent is injected under fluoroscopic control, and the joint is manipulated by the radiologist to ensure adequate dispersal of the contrast medium. Films are generally acquired by the radiologist using the available medium, usually digital 105-mm or 9 × 9 spot films. Overhead examinations are obtained as directed by the radiologist.

C. Myelography

Myelography is the radiographic examination of the central nervous system structures contained within the spinal canal, using water-soluble nonionic iodi-

nated contrast material, notably Iopamidol. Previously, non–water-soluble contrast-enhanced examinations using Pantopaque and gaseous contrast-enhanced examinations using air or oxygen were performed; however, these methods are now considered obsolete.

The radiographer prepares the examining room by ensuring cleanliness of the equipment, attaches the foot board and shoulder support, and selects fluoroscopic mode at the control panel. Some radiologists prefer to use an inflatable pillow placed under the patient's abdomen that can be filled to varying degrees by an oxygen tank in order to correct lumbar lordosis, which might otherwise prevent ready access to the subarachnoid space. A sterile myelogram tray is made ready for the radiologist's use as well as sterile gloves.

The patient is placed in the prone position on the x-ray table and prepped in the standard manner. Contrast material is introduced into the subarachnoid space by spinal puncture at the interspace level of L2 to L3, or L3 to L4. Because the spinal cord terminates at the conus medullaris at approximately the level of L1 in adults, there is no danger of puncturing the spinal cord using this method. A small amount of spinal fluid is generally withdrawn and sent to the laboratory for examination. Following introduction of the contrast, the table is angled upward or downward, and spot films are obtained, depending on the area of interest. The subarachnoid space is continuous with the ventricular system; therefore, if the cervical region is examined, care is taken to extend the head in order to prevent passage of contrast medium into the ventricles via the cisterna magna.

Spot films, generally in the PA and PA oblique positions, are taken by the radiologist. PA and cross-table lateral overhead films are performed by the technologist at the direction of the radiologist. Myelography is generally employed in order to demonstrate the size and extent of spinal cord lesions as well as posterior protrusion of herniated discs, which may encroach upon the spinal cord. CT myelography routinely follows standard myelography in order to demonstrate the size, position, and shape of the spinal cord and nerve roots.

Upper and lower extremity venograms are still performed on a limited basis; however, the examinations have been largely replaced by venous Doppler ultrasound, which is a noninvasive procedure. Both types of examinations are done to rule out the presence of deep venous thrombosis (DVT). The deep veins accompany an artery, and are usually wrapped in a sheath that encloses both the vein and associated artery. Thrombosis is an abnormal vascular condition, in which a thrombus, consisting of a collection of platelets and other cellular elements attached to the interior wall of a vein, forms. A thrombus may sometimes occlude the lumen of a vessel. With venography, an injection of water-soluble iodinated contrast is made via a needle or catheter directly into a superficial vein. In the case of the lower extremity, the foot is used, and with the upper extremity, the elbow or wrist is selected. Films for a lower limb venogram are obtained with the table placed at an angle of 45 degrees. Filming begins at the ankle, with the leg internally rotated 30 degrees. A tourniquet is placed proximal to the ankle and the knee to force filling of the deep veins. Filming continues superiorly, terminating at the inferior vena cava (IVC). Some radiologists prefer to perform a "dump" film of the IVC and iliac veins. This is accomplished by the radiologist raising the lower leg, draining the contrast into the thigh and pelvis, while simultaneously making an exposure of the IVC and iliacs. The radiographs are obtained 5 to 10 seconds apart, using a serial film changer, or bucky tray. Injections are accomplished by hand or using a volumetric injector set to deliver a 50- to 100-cc bolus at 1 to 2 mL/sec. The rate for the upper extremity is a 40- to 80-cc bolus at 1 to 4 mL/sec. The series obtained for upper film venography varies according to patient condition and area of interest. A tourniquet is applied proximal to the wrist and elbow to force deep vein filling.

D. Hysterosalpingography

Hysterosalpingography is the radiographic examination of the size, shape, and position of the uterus and fallopian tubes in nonpregnant females. The examination is carried out under aseptic conditions using a water-soluble iodinated contrast medium to investigate pathologic conditions of these areas. Investigation of fallopian tube patency in cases of sterility is one common reason the examination is performed.

Following emptying of the bladder and perineal cleansing, the patient is placed in the cystoscopic position on a standard radiographic table fitted with leg rests. A preliminary radiograph is performed to evaluate preparation of the intestinal tract. Uterine cannulation is performed, and contrast medium is introduced. The contrast flows through the uterus and uterine tubes and is allowed to spill into the peritoneal cavity. The contrast is absorbed and eliminated by the urinary system in approximately 2 hours. Filming for hysterosalpingography is exceedingly simple, sometimes consisting of a single 10 × 12 AP radiograph centered 2 inches superior to the symphysis pubis. Other radiographs are taken at the discretion of the physician.

QUESTIONS FOR MISCELLANEOUS RADIOGRAPHIC PROCEDURES

select the best answer

1. During upper extremity venography, where are tourniquets placed?
   (A) Distal to the wrist
   (B) Distal to the elbow
   (C) Proximal to the wrist
   (D) Proximal to the wrist and elbow

2. Which of the following examinations employs the use of a volumetric injector?
   (A) Hysterosalpingogram
   (B) Venogram
   (C) Arthrogram
   (D) Myelogram

3. Where are contrast media most commonly introduced during lumbar myelography?
   (A) Subarachnoid space at L3 to L4
   (B) Subdural space at L1 to L2
   (C) Epidural space at L3 to L4
   (D) Pia mater at L1 to L2

▶▶ ANSWERS FOR MISCELLANEOUS RADIOGRAPHIC PROCEDURES

1. The answer is (D). In order to facilitate filling of the deep venous system, including the basilic, cephalic, and subclavian veins, tourniquets are placed proximal to the wrist and elbow. AP projections, with the hand supinated, are most often employed.

2. The answer is (B). During venography, injection of the contrast medium is made by hand or with the use of a volumetric pressure injector, which delivers a bolus injection at a predetermined rate. Modern injectors can be programmed for multiple-phase injections that precisely deliver contrast to desired areas, which usually results in greater diagnostic accuracy and decreases the amount of contrast medium required.

3. The answer is (A). The subarachnoid space is continuous with the ventricular system and communicates with it via the foramen of Magendie and the foramina of Luschka, which are located between the cisterna magna and the fourth ventricle. Although the cisterna magna is sometimes used as a point of entry to the subarachnoid space, generally the L3 to L4 interspace, localized by fluoroscopy, is used for introduction of contrast media, because there is no danger of damage to the spinal cord, which terminates at the conus medullaris at the level of L1 to L2 in adults.

END-OF-CHAPTER EXAMINATION

▶▶ QUESTIONS

Select the best answer.

1. Which of the anatomic descriptions listed below is false concerning the spinal curvatures?
   (A) The cervical and lumbar curvatures are convex anteriorly.
   (B) The thoracic and sacral curvatures are convex anteriorly.
   (C) The cervical and lumbar curvatures are concave posteriorly.
   (D) The thoracic and sacral curvatures are convex posteriorly.

2. What bone houses the petrous region of the skull?
   (A) Occipital
   (B) Ethmoid
   (C) Temporal
   (D) Sphenoid

3. Which of the following bony landmarks can be described as a thin, sharp, bony projection located slightly inferior to the EAM?
   (A) Zygomatic arch
   (B) Styloid process
   (C) Mastoid process
   (D) Pterygoid process

4. Filming of the patient during micturition is a crucial view in which of the following examinations?
   (A) Cystography
   (B) Nephrotomography
   (C) Cystourethrography
   (D) Retrograde pyelography

5. A 15-degree caudal angulation directed through the OML demonstrates the petrous pyramids in the lower one third of the orbits. This position describes which of the following projections:
   (A) Caldwell
   (B) Waters'
   (C) Rhese
   (D) Arcelin

6. Which line must be perpendicular to the film for a true lateral projection of the skull?
   (A) OML
   (B) IOML (Reid's baseline)
   (C) Intrapupillary line (IPL)
   (D) Glabellomeatal

7. The vermiform appendix hangs from the inferior surface of which subdivision of the colon?
   (A) Rectum
   (B) Cecum
   (C) Ascending
   (D) Descending

8. Which of the following regions is the convex lateral surface of the stomach?
   (A) Greater curvature
   (B) Lesser curvature
   (C) Pylorus
   (D) Cardiac region

9. The common bile duct is formed by the fusion of the:
   (A) Pancreatic duct and common hepatic duct
   (B) Cystic duct and pancreatic duct
   (C) Right and left hepatic ducts
   (D) Cystic duct and common hepatic duct

10. Which of the following joints are synarthrotic?
    (A) Shoulder
    (B) Knee
    (C) Cranial sutures
    (D) Hip

11. Which of the following structures is (are) found in the left upper quadrant?
    1. Stomach
    2. Spleen
    3. Gallbladder
    (A) Choice 1 only
    (B) Choice 2 only
    (C) Choices 1 and 2
    (D) All of the aforementioned

(Continued)

12. Which of the following facial and skull landmarks describes the junction of the nose with the upper lip?

    (A) Glabella
    (B) Acanthion
    (C) Nasion
    (D) Outer canthus

13. The correct number of facial bones is:

    (A) 10
    (B) 12
    (C) 14
    (D) 16

14. Which of the following projections demonstrates the dorsum sellae within the foramen magnum?

    (A) AP axial
    (B) PA
    (C) Waters'
    (D) Rhese

15. Which of the following combinations of bones fuse in adults, resulting in the formation of the os coxae?

    (A) Ilium, ischium, pubis
    (B) Ilium, sacrum, coccyx
    (C) Coccyx, sacrum, pubis
    (D) Ischium, sacrum, pubis

16. Which of the following describes anatomic movement during respiratory expiration?

    (A) Elevated diaphragm, lowered ribs
    (B) Depressed diaphragm, elevated ribs
    (C) Elevated diaphragm, elevated ribs
    (D) Elevated diaphragm, elevated sternum

17. The base of the first metacarpal articulates inferiorly with which bone?

    (A) Navicular
    (B) Lunate
    (C) Trapezium
    (D) Trapezoid

18. Which one of the following anatomic locations corresponds to the region of the manubrial notch?

    (A) T5 to T6 interspace
    (B) T2 to T3 interspace
    (C) AC joint
    (D) Greater tuberosity of the humerus

19. Which of the following is not a criterion for quality control evaluation of a PA chest radiograph?

    (A) Scapula projected free of the lung fields
    (B) Clavicles above the lung apices
    (C) Pendulous breasts pulled upward and laterally
    (D) Costophrenic angles included

20. Which of the following would best demonstrate the presence of pleural fluid in the right lower lobe?

    (A) Apical lordotic
    (B) Erect lateral
    (C) Left lateral decubitus
    (D) Right lateral decubitus

21. The correct degree of flexion for a lateral view of the knee is:

    (A) 30 degrees
    (B) 45 degrees
    (C) 70 degrees
    (D) 90 degrees

22. A 55-year-old arthritic but otherwise healthy man undergoes preoperative radiographic evaluation for tibial osteotomy. Which of the following views is of most importance relative to pending surgery?

    (A) Settegast
    (B) Camp-Coventry
    (C) Bilateral weight-bearing AP
    (D) Lateral

23. The sustentaculum tali is found on what bone?

    (A) Calcaneus
    (B) Talus
    (C) Cuboid
    (D) Third cuneiform

24. Which of the following elements does not belong with the group describing a plantodorsal axial view of the os calcis?

    (A) Right-angle dorsiflexion
    (B) Weight bearing
    (C) 40-degree cephalic angulation
    (D) Exiting CR at the level of the ankle

(Continued)

25. The ankle mortise is best demonstrated on which of the following?

    (A) Weight-bearing AP
    (B) Lateral
    (C) 45-degree medial oblique
    (D) 20-degree medial oblique

26. Why are patients instructed to make a loose fist during a PA projection of the wrist?

    (A) The position makes the separation of the proximal and distal carpal rows more distinct.
    (B) The position is more comfortable for the patient.
    (C) The position reduces magnification.
    (D) The position defines the scaphoid free of superimposition from adjacent structures.

27. When performing an AP projection of the forearm, the hand must be:

    (A) supinated.
    (B) pronated.
    (C) flexed.
    (D) extended.

28. An AP projection of the cervical spine demonstrates:

    (A) C1 to C7
    (B) C2 to T2
    (C) C3 to T3
    (D) C1 to T4

29. An AP tangential view of the mastoid process involves which of the following?

    (A) Rotation of the head 30 degrees away from the area of interest
    (B) Rotation of the head 30 degrees toward the area of interest
    (C) Rotation of the head 55 degrees away from the area of interest
    (D) Rotation of the head 55 degrees toward the area of interest

30. Where is the renal hilum located?

    (A) Lateral border
    (B) Medial border
    (C) Superior pole
    (D) Inferior pole

31. A cervical and lumbar myelogram is performed using an L3 to L4 lumbar puncture. Which position fills the cervical nerve roots and prevents contrast agent flow into the ventricles?

    (A) Table angled down, head flexed
    (B) Table angled down, head extended
    (C) Table angled up, head flexed
    (D) Table angled up, head extended

32. Which of the following statements is false concerning tomography?

    (A) Objects in the focal plane are less blurred than those not in the focal plane
    (B) Section thickness is governed by exposure angle
    (C) The wider the exposure angle, the thinner the body section produced
    (D) The wider the exposure angle, the thicker the body section produced

33. Radiographic evaluation of the uterus and fallopian tubes by injection of iodinated contrast material via uterine cannulation is called:

    (A) Uterography
    (B) Pelvic pneumography
    (C) Hysterogram
    (D) Hysterosalpingography

34. The correct CR placement for the lateral nasal bones projection is:

    (A) 1 inch superior to the acanthion
    (B) 0.75 inch distal to the nasion
    (C) 1 inch superior and 1 inch anterior to the EAM
    (D) 1 inch posterior to the glabella

35. Which projection clearly delineates the olecranon process within the olecranon fossa?

    (A) Jones view
    (B) Lateral
    (C) Medial oblique
    (D) Lateral oblique

36. Which of the following structures contains a transverse foramen?

    (A) Sacral promontory
    (B) Thoracic transverse process
    (C) Cervical transverse process
    (D) Pedicle-laminae junction

(Continued)

37. A patient who has a suspected diagnosis of Crohn's disease would most likely undergo which of the following examinations?

    (A) Small bowel series
    (B) UGI
    (C) esophagram
    (D) Oral cholecystogram

38. An exposure is made with the patient in a 25- to 30-degree LPO position, with a 20- to 25-degree cephalic CR, entering the patient 1 inch medial and 1.5 inch distal to the right ASIS. What structure will be best demonstrated?

    (A) Right lumbar apophyseal articulation
    (B) Left lumbar apophyseal articulation
    (C) Right SI joint
    (D) Left SI joint

39. A true AP projection of the humerus requires which of the following?

    1. Supination of the hand
    2. Humeral epicondyles parallel to the image receptor
    3. 90-degree flexion of the elbow

    (A) Choices 1 and 2 only
    (B) Choice 3 only
    (C) Choice 2 only
    (D) Choices 1, 2, and 3

40. PA and lateral chest radiographs are performed with the CR directed perpendicular at the level of:

    (A) T5.
    (B) the SC joints.
    (C) the xiphoid process.
    (D) C7.

41. How many ribs attach directly to the sternum?

    (A) 7
    (B) 14
    (C) 10
    (D) 12

42. In order to obtain an elongated view of the right upper anterior ribs, which of the following shuld be used?

    (A) RAO with inspiration
    (B) RAO with expiration
    (C) LAO with inspiration
    (D) LAO with expiration

43. Which of the following is not a paired bone of the face?

    (A) Palatine
    (B) Vomer
    (C) Inferior nasal conchae
    (D) Maxillae

44. In a double-contrast–enhanced UGI series, which view demonstrates the air-filled duodenum in profile?

    (A) LPO
    (B) AP
    (C) Lateral
    (D) PA

45. The passage of an endoscopic tube down the esophagus through the stomach and duodenum, along with cannulation of the pancreatic duct in order to opacify the biliary system, describes which examination?

    (A) Percutaneous transhepatic cholangiography
    (B) Cholecystography
    (C) ERCP
    (D) IVC

46. A patient who has a diagnosis of dysphagia would most likely be scheduled for which of the following examinations?

    (A) UGI
    (B) BE
    (C) Barium swallow
    (D) IVP

47. A hysterosalpingogram (HSG) uses which type of contrast medium?

    (A) High-density barium
    (B) Iodized oils
    (C) Air
    (D) Water-soluble iodinated contrast

48. The distance between the fulcrum levels typically used during nephrotomography is:

    (A) 1 mm
    (B) 0.05 mm
    (C) 1 cm
    (D) 5 cm

(Continued)

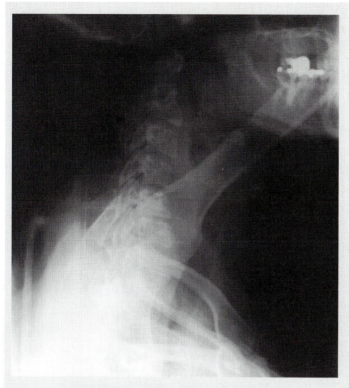

FIGURE 5-34.   **(Question 49)**

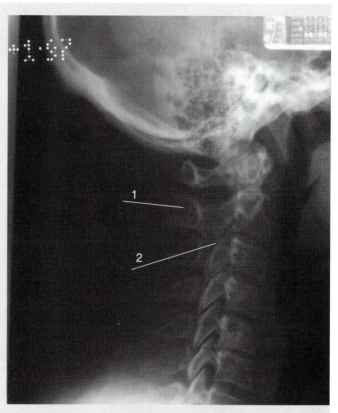

FIGURE 5-35.   **(Questions 50 and 51)**

49. The radiograph in **Figure 5-34** is an example of:

    (A) transthoracic humerus.
    (B) Twining, or swimmer's lateral.
    (C) AP axial oblique cervical spine.
    (D) oblique thoracic spine.

50. Look at the radiograph in **Figure 5-35.** The structure labeled *1* is the:

    (A) superior articular facet.
    (B) inferior articular facet.
    (C) spinous process.
    (D) transverse process.

51. Look again at the radiograph in Figure 5-35. The structure labeled *2* is the:

    (A) pedicle.
    (B) lamina.
    (C) transverse process.
    (D) superior articular facet.

52. Look at the radiograph in **Figure 5-36.** The structure labeled *1* is the:

    (A) transverse process.
    (B) pedicle.
    (C) lamina.
    (D) spinous process.

53. The structure labeled *2* in Figure 5-36 is the:

    (A) inferior articulating surface.
    (B) superior articulating surface.
    (C) pedicle.
    (D) lamina.

54. The radiograph in **Figure 5-37** demonstrates rounded areas of blastic metastatic disease overlying the ilium posteriorly. The area labeled *1* is the:

    (A) ilium.
    (B) ileum.
    (C) ischium.
    (D) pubis.

(Continued)

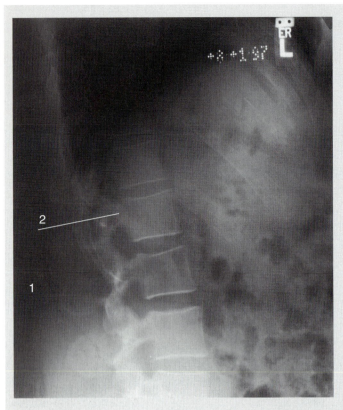

FIGURE 5-36. (Questions 52 and 53)

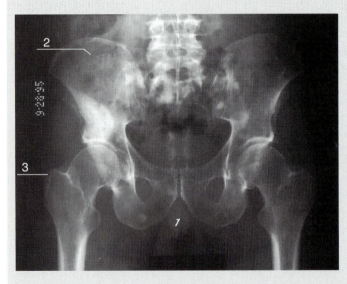

FIGURE 5-37. (Questions 54 and 56)

55. The area labeled *2* in Figure 5-37 is the:
    (A) symphysis pubis.
    (B) sciatic notch.
    (C) ala.
    (D) lesser sciatic notch.

56. The area labeled *3* in Figure 5-37 is the:
    (A) lesser trochanter.
    (B) greater trochanter.
    (C) linea aspera.
    (D) acetabulum.

57. Examine the PA chest radiograph shown in
    Figure 5-38. The structure labeled *1* is the:
    (A) left ventricle.
    (B) bicuspid valve.
    (C) aorta.
    (D) tricuspid valve.

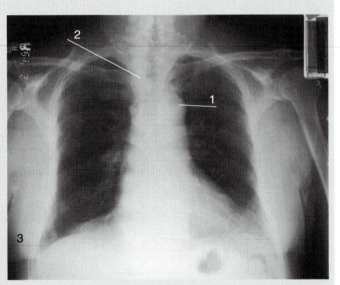

FIGURE 5-38. (Questions 57 and 59)

(Continued)

58. The structure labeled *2* in Figure 5-38 is the:

   (A) right sternoclavicular joint.
   (B) gladiolus.
   (C) xiphoid process.
   (D) sternal angle.

59. The structure labeled *3* in Figure 5-38 is the:

   (A) hilum.
   (B) mediastinum.
   (C) costophrenic angle.
   (D) diaphragm.

60. Concerning the paired radiographs in **Figure 5-39,** which of the following descriptions are true ?

   (A) View *A* is an AP lumbar spine film, and view *B* is an AP thoracic spine film.
   (B) View *A* is an upright abdominal film, and view *B* is a KUB.
   (C) View *A* is a KUB, and view *B* is an upright abdominal film.
   (D) Views *A* and *B* are both upright abdominal examinations.

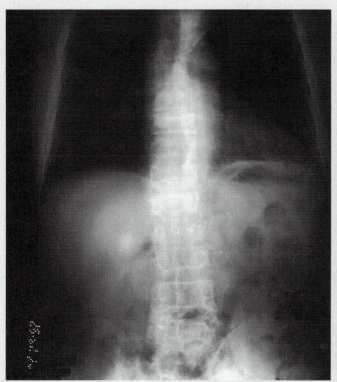 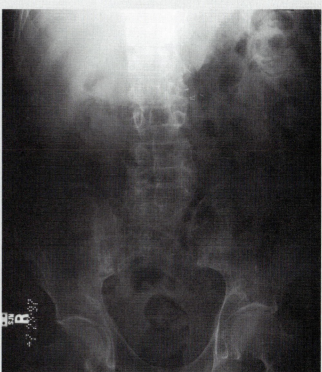

FIGURE 5-39. (Question 60)

▶▶ **ANSWERS TO END-OF-CHAPTER EXAMINATION**

1. The answer is (B). When viewed laterally, the four spinal curvatures give the spine its distinctive S shape, lending strength, resilience, and flexibility to the spine. The cervical and lumbar spine are convex anteriorly and concave posteriorly, whereas the thoracic and sacral spine are concave anteriorly and convex posteriorly.

2. The answer is (C). The petrous region of the temporal bone is seen as a dense wedge between the occipital bone posteriorly and the sphenoid bone anteriorly. The petrous portion houses the middle and inner ear cavities, which contain the sensory receptors for hearing and equilibrium.

(Continued)

3. The answer is (B). Located slightly inferior to the EAM on the inferior aspect of the temporal bone, the styloid process is a needlelike projection that forms an attachment point for the important stylohyoid muscles and ligaments that secure the hyoid bone.

4. The answer is (C). Micturition is the term for urination. Voiding cystourethrography demonstrates a contrast-filled bladder during micturition. Retrograde pyelography is an instrumental means of filling the ureters and renal pelvis. Cystography is a contrast-enhanced examination of the bladder, but does not require voiding. Nephrotomography is the tomographic evaluation of the kidneys following intravenous bolus injection of iodinated contrast.

5. The answer is (A). The Caldwell projection of the skull demonstrates the petrous portion of the temporal bone inferiorly through the lower one third of the orbits. When prescribed as a skull rather than sinus projection, Caldwell's projection primarily demonstrates the frontal, nasal, and ethmoid bones. The Waters' view chiefly demonstrates the maxillary sinus. The Rhese view is for demonstration of the optic foramen and optic canal, and the Arcelin projection is obtained for viewing mastoid air cells.

6. The answer is (C). The IPL must be perpendicular to the film in order to obtain a true lateral projection of the skull. The various anatomic baselines are descriptive of their path, for example, the IPL is formed by drawing a line between the two pupils; the orbitomeatal, or radiographic baseline, is formed by drawing a line from the orbit to the external auditory meatus, and so on.

7. The answer is (B). The cecum is a large-calibered, blind pouch lying below the ileocecal valve that forms the first part of the colon. Attached to its inferior surface is the vermiform (meaning wormlike) appendix, which is the narrowest portion of the digestive tract. The appendix is composed of lymphatic material similar to the tonsils. Like the tonsils, the appendix is a breeding ground for enteric bacteria; therefore, it frequently becomes infected and requires prompt surgical excision. If the appendix ruptures, it sprays bacteria over the abdominal contents, causing peritonitis, which is a potentially life-threatening condition.

8. The answer is (A). The large, convex lateral surface of the stomach is known as the greater curvature, whereas the smaller, concave medial surface is called the lesser curvature. The pylorus is the terminal portion of the stomach that is continuous with the duodenum and is marked by the pyloric sphincter, which controls emptying of the stomach contents. The cardiac region is the area surrounding the gastroesophageal junction.

9. The answer is (D). The cystic duct leaves the gallbladder and joins the common hepatic duct to form the common bile duct. The hepatic duct is a fusion of the right and left hepatic ducts. The pancreatic duct and common bile duct share a common entrance into the duodenal papillae, in the second portion of the duodenum. The sphincter of Oddi seals the common entrance to the duodenum, forcing bile from the liver up the cystic duct to the gallbladder, where it is stored and concentrated. During a meal, the gallbladder contracts and the sphincter of Oddi relaxes, which permits bile to enter the duodenum.

10. The answer is (C). Joints are classified according to structure as synovial, cartilaginous, or fibrous. Functional classification includes synarthrotic (nonmovable), amphiarthrotic (partially or somewhat movable), or diarthrotic (freely movable). The cranial sutures and the tibiofibular joint are examples of synarthroses. The shoulder, hip, and knee are all examples of diarthrodial joints.

11. The answer is (C). The stomach and spleen are both located in the left upper quadrant; the gallbladder is found on the inferior aspect of the liver, in the right upper quadrant.

12. The answer is (B). Landmarks of the skull and face are used as identifying points that aid in positioning. The acanthion is the point at the junction of the nose and upper lip. The glabella is the most superior landmark, located on the midline at the inferior portion of the frontal bone. The nasion is located inferior to the glabella at the junction of the nasal bones and the frontal bone. The outer canthus describes, from the lateral perspective, the junction of the upper and lower eyelids.

13. The answer is (C). With the exception of the vomer and the mandible, the bones of the face are paired, consisting of two of each of the following: maxillae, inferior nasal conchae, zygoma, lacrimals, palatines, and nasal bones.

(Continued)

14. The answer is (A). The AP axial, or Chamberlain-Townes view, demonstrates the dorsum sellae projected through the foramen magnum of the occipital bone. The patient is placed in the supine position with the OML perpendicular to the film, and the CR directed 30 degrees caudally, exiting at the foramen magnum.

15. The answer is (A). In children, the bones of the pelvis are distinct. Following fusion, the borders of the coxal bones are indistinguishable; however, the names ilium, ischium, and pubis are retained by convention.

16. The answer is (A). During respiration, the diaphragm moves inferiorly on inspiration and superiorly during expiration. The ribs and sternum move upward on inspiration and are returned to a lower position on exhalation.

17. The answer is (C). The first metacarpal is highly mobile due to the saddle-shaped articulation with the trapezium, or greater multangular. The trapezium articulates medially with the trapezoid, or lesser multangular. Both the navicular and lunate are in the proximal row of carpals; they do not articulate with the metacarpals.

18. The answer is (B). The sternal or manubrial notch is found at the level of the T2 to T3 interspace. The sternal angle is at the 5th thoracic vertebrae. The AC joint and greater tuberosity are both superior to the sternal notch.

19. The answer is (B). The shoulders should be depressed on a PA chest radiograph, in order to demonstrate 2 inches of the lung apex above the level of the clavicles. The shoulders are rolled forward to project the scapula away from the lung fields. Both costophrenic angles must be included in their entirety, because "clipping" may omit needed diagnostic information. The presence of pendulous breasts may lead to underpenetration of the central portion of the radiograph, so such patients should be asked to pull the breasts upward and laterally for the exposure.

20. The answer is (D). The affected side down recumbent lateral decubitus position best demonstrates the presence of fluid in the pleural cavity. The presence of free air is demonstrated on the affected side up decubitus view. Decubitus views are named according to the side down; thus, a right side down view is a right lateral decubitus.

21. The answer is (A). Flexion of 20 to 30 degrees is recommended for the lateral view of the knee because this position relaxes the surrounding musculature and demonstrates the maximum volume of the joint cavity. A 5-degree cephalic CR angulation is also recommended to prevent obscuring of the joint space by the somewhat magnified medial femoral condyle.

22. The answer is (C). Although all of the listed views aid in preoperative evaluation, the weight-bearing AP view may reveal joint space narrowing that appears normal on non–weight-bearing AP projections. Additionally, the view permits accurate preoperative evaluation of varus-valgus deformity corrected by osteotomy.

23. The answer is (A). The sustentaculum tali is a shelf of bone on the superior aspect of the calcaneus that supports the posterior aspect of the head of the talus. The anterior portion of the talar head has no bony support.

24. The answer is (B). Weight bearing is associated with the dorsoplantar (Kandel) method of imaging the calcaneus. Use of the dorsoplantar view is confined almost entirely to infant patients. To obtain the plantodorsal projection, the patient is placed supine with the leg fully extended and the foot maximally dorsiflexed. The CR is directed at an angle of 40 degrees cephalic, entering at the base of the fifth metatarsal and exiting at the level of the ankle joint.

25. The answer is (D). In order to best demonstrate the mortise joint of the ankle free of superimposition by the talus, tibia, or fibula, the leg is medially rotated 15 to 20 degrees so that the malleoli are parallel with the image receptor. A 45-degree oblique view demonstrates the distal tibia-fibula with superimposition over the talus. Both AP and lateral views primarily demonstrate the tibiotalar joint.

26. The answer is (C). The hand in extension places the wrist slightly farther away from the image receptor than when a fist is made. Because OFD is reduced by making a fist, magnification is also reduced.

27. The answer is (A). In order to view the radius and ulna without crossover of their proximal one third, the hand must be supinated. Flexion and extension of the hand have little impact on the position of the radius and ulna.

28. The answer is (C). The standard AP projection of the cervical spine does not demonstrate C1 or C2. Views exists for the atlas and axis; the most common being the open mouth, or George view. Generally speaking, the AP C-spine view also demonstrates the first 3 thoracic vertebrae.

(Continued)

29. The answer is (C). In the AP tangential view of the mastoid process described by Arcelin, the head is rotated away from the side of interest so that the MSP forms a 55-degree angle with the plane of the film. The CR is angled 15 degrees caudally, exiting at a point 1 inch inferior to the EAM.

30. The answer is (B). The hilum of an organ is a depression where vasculature, nerves, and other important structures enter and exit. The hilum of the kidney is located along its medial border, where the proximal ureter joins it.

31. The answer is (B). The table is angled downward for cervical myelography in order to permit contrast to flow into the cervical nerve roots. The head is extended to compress the cisterna magna sufficiently to prevent contrast agent from entering the ventricles. The cisterna magna is located posteriorly; flexion will not compress the cisternal cavity.

32. The answer is (D). The exposure angle is the angle described by the motion of the x-ray tube and film during exposure. The angle governs thickness of the section. The wider the angle, the thinner the section produced. Objects within the focal plane or fulcrum of the exposure are not enhanced; rather, they become less blurred as a result of controlled blurring of the structure above and below them, or not in the focal plane.

33. The answer is (D). Hysterosalpingography consists of radiographic delineation of the uterine cavity and the lumen of the tubal passages by introduction of room temperature iodinated organic compounds via uterine cannulation. Pelvic pneumography is the introduction of gaseous medium directly into the peritoneum in order to outline the external contours of the uterus, fallopian tubes, and ovaries. A hysterogram is confined to the delineation of the uterus.

34. The answer is (B). To obtain a lateral projection of the nasal bones, the patient is placed in the lateral position, and the CR is directed ¾ inch distal to the nasion. Routinely, both laterals are obtained: two views on one 8 × 10 cassette. A short scale of contrast is desirable.

35. The answer is (C). The lateral oblique projection demonstrates the radial head without superimposition of adjacent structures, and the lateral view demonstrates the olecranon in profile. The Jones view is obtained in complete flexion; the olecranon process is clearly seen, but the olecranon fossa is obscured. The medial oblique view demonstrates the olecranon process within the olecranon fossa and the coronoid process without superimposition of structures.

36. The answer is (C). The transverse processes of the cervical vertebrae contain transverse foramen through which the rather large vertebral arteries ascend to reach the brain. The transverse processes arise from the pedicle laminae junction. The thoracic transverse foramina are unique in that they include a facet for articulation with the rib. The sacral promontory is the most superior portion of the sacrum.

37. The answer is (A). Crohn's disease is a regional enteritis that affects the small bowel, usually at the terminal ileum.

38. The answer is (C). The sacroiliac joints are best demonstrated using a 25- to 30-degree posterior oblique position, and a 20- to 25-degree cephalic angulation, with the side remote from the film being demonstrated. This view should demonstrate the open sacroiliac joint space, without overlap from the ilium or sacrum.

39. The answer is (A). The AP of the humerus is generally performed in the upright position. In order to attain a true AP position, the hand should be supinated and the humeral epicondyles palpated to assure that they are parallel to the film.

40. The answer is (D). With the exception of lordotic views, chest radiography is performed with a perpendicular CR directed to the level of the 7th thoracic vertebrae. T7 may be localized by measuring approximately 7 inches inferior from C7 on female patients and 8 inches inferior on male patients.

41. The answer is (B). Seven pairs, or fourteen total ribs, attach to the manubrium and body (gladiolus) of the sternum directly, via the costal cartilage. Rib pairs 8 to 10 attach to the sternum indirectly, through the costal cartilage of the seventh rib. Rib pairs 11 and 12 are called floating ribs; they have no anterior attachment.

(Continued)

42. The answer is (C). The radiographer should always place the side of interest closest to the film, whenever possible. Therefore, anterior ribs are examined in the prone position and posterior ribs in the supine position. In this case, positioning would begin with a PA view. To obtain the oblique position that elongates the ribs, the radiographer must recall that the side up, or side away from the film, is the side demonstrated on the anterior oblique radiograph. Therefore, an LAO would best demonstrate the right axillary portion of the ribs. Upper ribs are best demonstrated on inspiration, because the diaphragm moves downward, and lower ribs are best seen using expiration as the diaphragm moves upward, out of the area of interest.

43. The answer is (B). Except for the vomer and the mandible, which is the only movable facial bone, all of the fourteen facial bones are paired. They include the pairs of maxillae, inferior nasal conchae, palatine, zygoma, nasal bones, and lacrimal bones.

44. The answer is (A). The LPO position demonstrates the barium-filled fundus of the stomach and the air-filled duodenum in profile. The AP and PA views are survey examinations. The right lateral position demonstrates the right retrogastric space and the C loop of the duodenum.

45. The answer is (C). Opacification and subsequent radiographic examination of the biliary system achieved via endoscopic means is called endoscopic retrograde cholangiopancreatography, or ERCP. Percutaneous transhepatic cholangiography is the passage of a long thin needle directly into the liver for the purposes of radiographic examination. Cholecystography is the generic name for a number of studies of the gallbladder and biliary system, and IVC stands for intravenous cholangiography, whereby opacification is achieved via the intravenous route.

46. The answer is (C). The term dysphagia means difficulty swallowing, which is commonly associated with obstructive or motor disorders. Patients who have obstructive disorders like esophageal neoplasms are unable to take solid food but can tolerate liquids, so they are good candidates for esophagography. Of the listed examinations, the barium swallow would be the study that most closely investigates the diagnosis.

46. The answer is (C). The term dysphagia means difficulty swallowing, which is commonly associated with obstructive or motor disorders. Patients who have obstructive disorders like esophageal neoplasms are unable to take solid food but can tolerate liquids, so they are good candidates for esophagography. Of the listed examinations, the barium swallow would be the study that most closely investigates the diagnosis.

47. The answer is (D). An HSG examination uses water-soluble iodine compounds that are readily absorbed by the body. Because the uterus and fallopian tubes are open-ended structures, when contrast material flows into the uterus, it spills into the peritoneum unless the tubes are obstructed. Therefore, the use of barium is ruled out because it would not be reabsorbed by the body and may cause peritonitis. Historically, the examination was performed using iodized oils; however, these materials were poorly reabsorbed and hence were replaced as better materials became available. An examination called pelvic pneumography was formerly performed using air as the contrast material; however, this examination has been largely replaced by diagnostic ultrasound examinations.

48. The answer is (C). Nephrotomography is tomographic evaluation of the kidney parenchyma in conjunction with excretory urography. Because the kidneys are approximately 3 cm thick, three cuts through the kidneys 1 cm apart are usually sufficient to demonstrate the area of interest. The kidneys lie in an oblique plane in the retroperitoneum, with the upper poles located more posteriorly than the lower poles.

49. The answer is (B). The Twining, or swimmer's lateral, is used when visualization of the C7 to T1 articulation is not possible, and as part of most routine thoracic spine series. The view demonstrates a lateral projection of the vertebrae from approximately the level of C5 to T5, projected between the shadows of the shoulder. An AP axial oblique of the cervical spine is a trauma modification of the standard oblique method, where the patient is placed supine on the table, and a screen cassette is placed under the cervical region. The central ray is directed 45 degrees medial and 15 to 20 degrees cephalic through the third cervical vertebrae.

50. The answer is (C). The structure labeled No. 1 is the most posterior structure on the vertebra, the spinous process. The specific vertebra is C7, also called vertebra prominens.

(Continued)

51. The answer is (D). The superior articular facet articulates with the inferior articular facet of the vertebra above it to form the zygoapophyseal articulation.

52. The answer is (D). The spinous process is the most posterior projection of the vertebrae, with the exception of C1, which has a posterior tubercle instead of a spinous process and is considered atypical. The spinous processes arise from the junction of the laminae. The cervical and thoracic spinous processes project posteriorly and caudally, and the lumbar spinous processes project posteriorly and horizontally.

53. The answer is (C). Typical vertebrae consist of two primary portions; the body or centrum is the disclike weight-bearing anterior portion, and the more complex posterior segment is the vertebral arch. The pedicles form the sides of the vertebral arch; they are short, bony cylinders projecting posteriorly from the vertebral bodies.

54. The answer is (C). The inferior portion of the pelvis that forms the posteroinferior part of the coxal bone consists of an upper thicker body and a thinner, more inferior ramus. The inferior surface of the ischium presents a roughened, thickened area called the ischial tuberosity. When we sit, our weight is borne entirely by this strongest portion of the os coxae.

55. The answer is (C). The superior, winglike portion of the ilium is known as the ala. The thickened upper portions of the ala are known as the iliac crests; they represent the place where you rest your hands on your hips. The sciatic notch is part of the ilium, and the lesser sciatic notch is part of the ischium. The symphysis pubis is the midline junction of the pubic bones.

56. The answer is (B). The greater trochanter is located laterally and is an important surface landmark. The labeled area is the lesser trochanter, which is a medial structure. Both trochanters are important muscle attachment points. The acetabulum is an inferior, hollow depression on the coxal bone that articulates with the femoral head. The linea aspera is a roughened area on the anterior aspect of the femur for muscle attachment.

57. The answer is (C). The aorta is seen as a rounded knoblike structure located just slightly to the left of the midline on a PA chest radiograph. The aorta arises from the heart and is guarded at its base by the aortic semilunar valve, which prevents backward flow of blood into the left ventricle. Differing portions of the aorta are named according to shape and location. The ascending aorta is the most proximal portion, persisting for only approximately 5 cm before becoming the aortic arch. The branches of the ascending aorta are the right and left coronary arteries. The aortic arch extends from the sternal angle at the level of T4 and has three major branches, which are the brachiocephalic, left common carotid, and left subclavian artery. These vessels are the arterial supply for the head, neck, and upper extremities.

58. The answer is (A). The lateral aspect of the manubrium slants posterolaterally and contains an articular surface for the medial aspect of the clavicles, forming the sternoclavicular joints. The sternoclavicular joints are the only articulation between the upper extremity and the thorax, and are diathrotic (permitting limited movement) gliding type joints. The manubrium articulates with the longest portion of the sternum, the body or gladiolus, where it forms the palpable sternal angle. The smallest and most distal portion of the sternum is the xiphoid or ensiform process, which lies approximately at the level of T10, and is cartilaginous in early life and ossifies with age.

59. The answer is (C). The area identified as *3* on the PA chest radiograph is the right costophrenic angle. The costophrenic angles are important radiographic structures; they are filled with fluid in the presence of pneumonia. A common reason for repeating the PA chest radiograph is exclusion or "clipping" of the angles, particularly in male patients who have large lungs.

60. The answer is (B). Views *A* and *B* are examples of a flat and upright abdominal examination. The upright film can be determined in a number of ways; the simplest is to look at the anatomy included on the film. Because view *A* includes the diaphragm and the lower portion of the lung fields, and because you know it is a paired examination in which the other radiograph includes the symphysis pubis, it is safe to assume that it is the upright examination. Note also the presence of air rising in the fundus of the stomach. One of the primary functions of an upright abdominal examination is to rule out the presence of free air under the diaphragm, or the presence of air–fluid levels.

CHAPTER 6

Simulated Full-Length Registry Examination

select the best answer

1. According to NCRP recommendations concerning patient protection, source-to-skin distance during conventional fluoroscopy using stationary equipment must be at least:
   (A) 40″.
   (B) 36″.
   (C) 12″.
   (D) 72″.

2. Which of the following are NOT included when calculating whole-body dose?
   (A) Lens of the eye
   (B) Spleen
   (C) Gonads
   (D) Hands

3. If the fluoroscopic portion of an upper GI examination is performed at 1.25 mA for 4 minutes, what is the approximate skin dose?
   (A) 10 rad
   (B) 5 rad
   (C) 25 rad
   (D) 2.5 rad

4. Which type of radiation monitoring device is a technologist most likely to use to calculate monthly occupational dose?
   (A) TLD
   (B) Film badge
   (C) Pocket dosimeter
   (D) Cutie pie

5. What unit of measurement is used to express occupational dose?
   (A) Sv
   (B) QF
   (C) LET
   (D) Roentgen

6. Which of the following are detectable effects of ionizing radiation?
   1. Luminescent effect
   2. Thermoluminescent effect
   3. Photographic effect

   (A) Choice 1 only
   (B) Choices 1 and 2
   (C) Choice 3 only
   (D) All of the above

7. Which type of x-ray interaction is responsible for most of the radiologic contrast on a routine radiograph?
   (A) Compton effect
   (B) Photoelectric effect
   (C) Pair production
   (D) Coherent scatter

8. To which of the following factors is exposure rate directly proportional, if all other factors are constant?

    (A) Tube current
    (B) Tube potential
    (C) Distance
    (D) Filtration

9. Which of the following is a true statement concerning the relationship between LET and RBE?

    (A) If LET increases, RBE increases
    (B) If LET increases, RBE decreases
    (C) LET and RBE are inversely proportional
    (D) LET and RBE are not related

10. Which of the following combinations of exposure factors will decrease patient dose if increased?

    (A) mA and time
    (B) kVp and FFD
    (C) mA and FFD
    (D) mA and kVp

11. The risk of congenital abnormalities resulting from fetal irradiation is greatest during:

    (A) third trimester.
    (B) second trimester.
    (C) first trimester after the first 2 weeks of development.
    (D) first 2 weeks of gestation after fertilization.

12. The primary difference between x-radiation and gamma radiation is:

    (A) mass.
    (B) ability to cause biologic change.
    (C) rate of travel in a vacuum.
    (D) source of origin.

13. The 10-day rule pertains to which of the following?

    (A) The last 10 days of the menstrual cycle
    (B) The 10 days after cessation of the menses
    (C) The 10 days before the onset of menses
    (D) The 10 days after the onset of menses

14. The effect of filtration on the primary beam can be described by the statement:

    (A) filtration decreases the overall energy of the primary beam.
    (B) filtration increases the overall energy of the primary beam.
    (C) filtration has no effect on the primary beam; it decreases scatter radiation.
    (D) filtration has no effect on the primary beam; it decreases secondary radiation.

15. Which one of the following produces the most significant amount of scatter radiation?

    (A) The patient
    (B) The x-ray table
    (C) The bucky
    (D) The film

16. The unit of measurement used to express the amount of radiation measured by an ionization chamber is:

    (A) rem.
    (B) rad.
    (C) roentgen.
    (D) gray.

17. In which of the following energy ranges will Compton type interactions predominate?

    (A) Less than 40 kVp
    (B) Between 40 and 50 kVp
    (C) Between 50 and 60 kVp
    (D) Greater than 70 kVp

18. Acute radiation syndromes may occur as a result of exposure to which of the following ranges of exposure?

    (A) 10 to 25 R acute whole-body exposure
    (B) 25 to 50 R acute whole-body exposure
    (C) 50 to 75 R lifetime whole-body exposure
    (D) Greater than 100 R acute whole-body exposure

19. Which of the following is not a factor affecting patient dose?

    (A) FFD
    (B) OFD
    (C) Inherent filtration
    (D) Added filtration

20. If an elderly patient is too frail to comply with needed positioning requirements, who among the following would be the best choice to hold the patient in the event that mechanical restraints prove inadequate?

    (A) Mammography technologist
    (B) QC technologist
    (C) Family member
    (D) Nurse

21. According to the laws of Bergonie and Tribondeau, which of the following cell types would be least radiosensitive?

    (A) Muscle cells
    (B) Gonadal cells
    (C) Eye cells
    (D) Bone marrow cells

22. Cell division of germ type cells in humans is called:

    (A) anaphase.
    (B) telophase.
    (C) meiosis.
    (D) mitosis.

23. Which of the following groups of exposure factors will deliver the lowest absorbed dose?

    (A) 20 mA, 80 kVp
    (B) 30 mA, 70 kVp
    (C) 20 mA, 60 kVp
    (D) 30 mA, 80 kVp

24. The optimum type of shielding for use during a lumbar myelogram is:

    (A) contour.
    (B) contact.
    (C) shadow.
    (D) half-apron.

25. According to NCRP guidelines, at least how much filtration is required of an exposure room used primarily for examinations of the gastrointestinal (GI) tract?

    (A) 2.5 mm Al
    (B) 0.0025 mm Al
    (C) 1.5 mm Mo
    (D) 0.5 mm Al

26. Radiation emanating from the tube housing in a different direction from the useful beam is considered:

    (A) Compton scatter.
    (B) photoelectric effect.
    (C) leakage radiation.
    (D) secondary radiation.

27. Which of the following techniques or devices protects the patient from unnecessary radiation exposure?

    (A) High mA, fast screens
    (B) Focused grids, detail screens
    (C) Greatest SID, nonscreen film
    (D) Immobilization devices, added filtration

28. A certain radiology department issues its technologists one film badge for radiation monitoring. Where should the technologist wear the badge when performing a thoracic spine examination?

    (A) On the wrist
    (B) On the collar
    (C) At the waist
    (D) At the most practical location, depending on attire

29. If the known dose for a given exposure is 50 mrem at a distance of 40 inches, what will the exposure be at 80 inches?

    (A) 100 mrem
    (B) 200 mrem
    (C) 25 mrem
    (D) 12.5 mrem

30. NCRP regulations require that lead aprons have Pb equivalents of:

    (A) > 0.50 mm Pb equivalent.
    (B) ~ 0.50 mm Pb equivalent.
    (C) = 0.50 mm Pb equivalent.
    (D) < 0.50 mm Pb equivalent.

31. Which process produces electrons in the x-ray tube?

    (A) Rectification
    (B) Mutual induction
    (C) Thermionic emission
    (D) Photoemission

32. Of the following exposure factor combinations, which will permit the greatest heat loading capacity?

    (A) 1-mm actual focal spot, 10° target angle
    (B) 0.5-mm actual focal spot, 10° target angle
    (C) 1-mm actual focal spot, 20° target angle
    (D) 0.5-mm actual focal spot, 20° target angle

33. Which of the following devices is responsible for kVp selection?

    (A) Rheostat
    (B) Capacitor
    (C) Autotransformer
    (D) Resistor

34. A double-focus x-ray tube has two:

    (A) filters.
    (B) windows.
    (C) filaments.
    (D) rectifiers.

35. An alternate means of expressing 500 mA and 80 kVp is:

    (A) 5 amps, 800 volts.
    (B) 0.5 amp, 80,000 volts.
    (C) 50 amps, 80,000 volts.
    (D) 0.5 amp, 8000 volts.

36. The star pattern test is used to measure:

    (A) focal spot resolution.
    (B) half-wave rectification.
    (C) incoming line voltage.
    (D) tube cooling properties.

37. Which of the following types of exposure timers is most accurate?

    (A) Phototimer
    (B) Electronic timer
    (C) Synchronous timer
    (D) Reciprocating timer

38. Which of the following waveforms has the least voltage ripple?

    (A) Single phase, half-wave rectified
    (B) Single phase, full-wave rectified
    (C) Three phase, six pulse
    (D) Three phase, 12 pulse

39. The principle that allows the primary side of the high-voltage (step-up) transformer to generate voltage in the secondary side is called:

    (A) self-induction.
    (B) mutual induction.
    (C) copper loss.
    (D) hysteresis loss.

40. Which device maintains electron flow from cathode to anode?

    (A) Stator
    (B) Rotor
    (C) High-frequency generator
    (D) Diode rectifier

41. The mA range used to record a fluoroscopic image is:

    (A) 200–400 mA.
    (B) 20–50 mA.
    (C) 10–20 mA.
    (D) 1–5 mA.

42. The function of the beam splitter in a conventional fluoroscopic imaging system is:

    (A) to divide x-ray beam between input and output phosphor.
    (B) to divide image between photocathode and output phosphor.
    (C) to split image data between TV monitor and photospot film camera.
    (D) to split electrons between input phosphor and photocathode.

43. A given image intensification system has an input phosphor measuring 10″ and an output phosphor measuring 1″. If the flux gain is 60, what is the brightness gain?

    (A) 6000
    (B) 7000
    (C) 7200
    (D) 8700

44. Which exposure factor, if decreased, would cause an undesirable decrease in density when using an AED?

    (A) mA
    (B) kVp
    (C) Screen speed
    (D) Patient thickness

45. A Franklin head unit is an example of which type of radiographic machinery?

    (A) Fixed
    (B) Dedicated
    (C) Mobile
    (D) Fluoroscopy

46. Suppose an exposure made using 500 mA, 0.02 second, and 70 kVp yields an exposure output of 250 mR. What is the mR/mA?

    (A) 50
    (B) 25
    (C) 12.5
    (D) 75

47. According to NCRP Report 102, an x-ray unit collimator must prevent the light field from exceeding:

    (A) ±2% FFD.
    (B) ±3% FFD.
    (C) ±2% FFD².
    (D) ±3% FFD².

48. Poor screen / film contact is tested by:

    (A) Wisconsin cassette.
    (B) spin top test.
    (C) wire mesh test.
    (D) star pattern test.

49. Which of the following formulas would be used to find current on the secondary side of a step-up transformer?

(A) $\dfrac{V_S}{V_p} = \dfrac{N_S}{N_p}$

(B) $\dfrac{V_S}{V_p} = \dfrac{N_p}{N_S}$

(C) $\dfrac{V_p}{V_S} = \dfrac{N_S}{N_p}$

(D) $\dfrac{N_S}{N_p} = \dfrac{I_p}{I_S}$

50. Which of the following formulas is used to determine HU output of a three-phase, six-pulse radiographic unit?

(A) HU = mA × s × kVp
(B) HU = mA × s × kVp × 1.35
(C) HU = mA × s × kVp × 1.41
(D) $\dfrac{I_1}{I_2} = \dfrac{D_2^2}{D_1^2}$

51. Which of the following components determines focal spot size?

(A) Rectifier
(B) Autotransformer
(C) Target material
(D) Filament size

52. Refer to the anode cooling chart in **Figure 6-1.** Suppose you are midway through a lengthy series of films on a large patient; the machine notifies you of a technic overload. Assuming you have reached the capacity for this machine, how long would you have to wait before continuing with a series of films that would generate 140,000 HU?

(A) Less than 1 minute
(B) 2 minutes
(C) 3 minutes
(D) 4 minutes

53. Four typical x-ray tube configurations are listed below. Which permits the greatest tube loading capacity?

(A) 15° target, 1-mm actual focal spot
(B) 15° target, 0.8-mm actual focal spot
(C) 10° target, 1-mm actual focal spot
(D) 10° target, 0.8-mm actual focal spot

54. Which of the following target angles will produce the most noticeable anode heel affect?

(A) 10°
(B) 12°
(C) 15°
(D) 20°

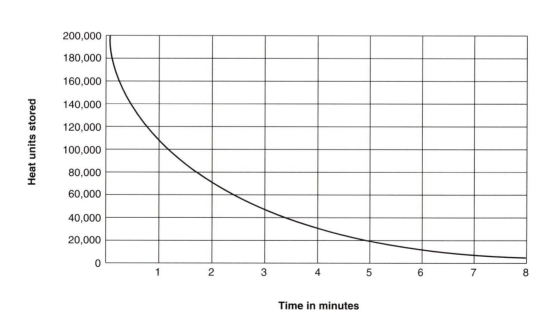

FIGURE 6-1.   Anode cooling chart.

55. All of the following relate to the x-ray cathode except:

(A) space charge.
(B) thermionic emission.
(C) filament current.
(D) focal track.

56. Where in the x-ray circuit is the step-down transformer located?

(A) Anode
(B) Filament circuit
(C) High-voltage side
(D) Rectification system

57. Which of the following describes most correctly the effect of collimation on image quality?

(A) Focuses the primary beam
(B) Ensures proper tube-part film alignment
(C) Hardens the beam
(D) Decreases Compton interactions

58. Roughening of the anode track and localized melting due to exceeding safe heat exposure limitations results in:

(A) overall increase in output.
(B) overall decrease in output.
(C) mA linearity out of calibration.
(D) filament burnout.

59. When using an AEC, what happens to a radiograph when the needed exposure is less than the minimum exposure time of the AEC?

(A) Overexposed film
(B) Underexposed film
(C) Blank film
(D) Film demonstrates grid lines

60. Which of the following are ways in which poor screen film contact can occur?

1. cracked cassette frame
2. bent or broken latches
3. exposure to excessive humidity

(A) 1 only
(B) 2 only
(C) 1 and 2
(D) All of the above

61. The following exposures are made to a certain cold anode. Which one represents the LEAST hazard?

(A) 10 mA, 80 kVp, small focal spot
(B) 10 mA, 80 kVp, large focal spot
(C) 20 mA, 75 kVp, small focal spot
(D) 20 mA, 75 kVp, large focal spot

62. In comparison with the first half-value layer (HVL), the second HVL of a given x-ray beam must be:

(A) equal to the first.
(B) equal to or greater than the first.
(C) equal to or less than the first.
(D) greater than the first.

63. Sodium carbonate is a commonly used chemical in automatic processing; it may be found in the _____ tank, where it performs its function of _____ .

(A) Fixer, reducing agent
(B) Developer, activator
(C) Fixer, restrainer
(D) Developer, preservative

64. A given exposure of the lateral cervical spine is made at 40", using 10 mA and 70 kVp. To decrease magnification, the exposure is repeated at 72". What is the new technique?

(A) 32 mA, 70 kVp
(B) 3.2 mA, 70 kVp
(C) 320 mA, 70 kVp
(D) 10 mA, 80 kVp

65. Which artifact is likely to occur when film boxes are improperly stored?

(A) Static artifact
(B) Tree artifact
(C) Pressure artifact
(D) Fingernail artifact

66. Which of the following is associated with grid radius?

(A) Focused grid
(B) Unfocused grid
(C) Parallel grid
(D) Cross-hatch grid

67. If a radiology department switches from a 200-speed system to a 400-speed system, what technical adjustment is required to maintain the same density on the produced radiographs?

(A) 2 × increase in mA
(B) ½ original mA
(C) 4 × increase in mA
(D) ¼ original mA

68. All of the following are undesirable characteristics pertaining to intensifying screens EXCEPT:

(A) luminescence.
(B) phosphorescence.
(C) screen lag.
(D) crossover.

69. A densitometer reading on the unexposed portion of a collimated, processed radiograph of the knee should produce a reading of no more than:
    (A) 0.2.
    (B) 2.0.
    (C) 20.0.
    (D) 0.002.

70. Gradient screens are likely to be used in which of the following examinations?
    (A) Lumbar spine
    (B) Cervical spine
    (C) Scoliosis survey
    (D) Lateral sacrum/coccyx

71. Of the following, which are characteristics unique to a focused grid?
    1. canting
    2. radius of infinity
    3. grid radius
    4. grid ratio

    (A) 2 and 3
    (B) All of the above
    (C) 1 and 3
    (D) 1 and 4

72. Compared with an 6:1 grid, a 12:1 grid exhibits which of the following characteristics?
    (A) Greater cleanup, less positioning latitude
    (B) Less cleanup, greater positioning latitude
    (C) Greater patient dose, greater positioning latitude
    (D) Greater selectivity, less patient dose

73. An AP tabletop knee examination is performed using 5 mA, 70 kVp, and 40″ SID. The patient is large, and a significant amount of image-degrading scatter is produced at this technique. To clean up scatter, a 10:1 bucky examination is performed instead. If all other factors remain consistent, what new technique should be used to reduce scatter and maintain density?
    (A) 10 mA
    (B) 15 mA
    (C) 20 mA
    (D) 25 mA

74. Which of the following is NOT used to control the production of scatter radiation?
    (A) Grids
    (B) Filtration
    (C) Optimum kVp
    (D) Collimation

75. A decrease in exposure factors is required during radiography of patients with which of the following conditions?
    (A) Osteoarthritis
    (B) Osteochondritis
    (C) Osteoporosis
    (D) Osteoblastoma

76. Which of the following conditions requires an increase in exposure factors in order to maintain correct radiographic density?
    (A) Emphysema
    (B) Congestive heart failure
    (C) Cardiomegaly
    (D) Mitral valve stenosis

77. Using the bucky factor, adjust the technique of an exposure of 75 mA, 75 kVp, 10:1 grid to nongrid tabletop technique. The new correct factors will be:
    (A) 15 mA, 85 kVp.
    (B) 15 mA, 75 kVp.
    (C) 25 mA, 75 kVp.
    (D) 75 mA, 75 kVp.

78. An examination of the abdomen is performed using a 16:1 fine-line bucky with the tube placed 2″ off center toward the right side of the patient. The resulting radiograph will demonstrate:
    (A) overall loss of density.
    (B) unilateral right-sided loss of density.
    (C) unilateral left-sided loss of density.
    (D) loss of density on the anode side of the tube.

79. The AED accounts for all of the following exposure factor variables EXCEPT:
    (A) distance.
    (B) part thickness.
    (C) pathology.
    (D) positioning.

80. Silver recovery is accomplished by which of the following methods?
    1. from used film
    2. from metallic cartridge
    3. from electrolytic plating unit

    (A) All of the above
    (B) None of the above
    (C) 2 only
    (D) 1 and 2

81. All other exposure factors remaining constant, which of the following factors is most important concerning recorded detail?
    (A) Grid ratio
    (B) Exposure time
    (C) Screen speed
    (D) kVp

82. The single best method the technologist can use to decrease voluntary motion is:
    (A) short exposure times.
    (B) long exposure times.
    (C) good communication.
    (D) fast screens.

83. What type of image misrepresentation, if any, occurs if a wedge-shaped object is tilted relative to the film and the central ray is angled so it is perpendicular to the long axis of the object?
    (A) Blurring
    (B) Elongation
    (C) Foreshortening
    (D) No geometric unsharpness will occur

84. Two radiographs of the chest on a small patient are made. Radiograph #1 is collimated to 14 × 17. Radiograph #2 is collimated so that it demonstrates a 2″ border around the edge of the film. Which of the following statements are true concerning the comparison between the two radiographs?
    (A) Radiograph #1 demonstrates higher contrast than radiograph #2
    (B) Radiograph #2 demonstrates higher contrast than radiograph #1
    (C) The two radiographs will produce equal scales of contrast
    (D) Not enough information is provided to answer the question

85. The differing absorption properties of various anatomic tissue types result in which radiographic property?
    (A) Density
    (B) Scale of contrast
    (C) Distortion
    (D) Magnification

86. Which factor controls the amount of film replenishment?
    (A) Emulsion thickness
    (B) Film size
    (C) Solution temperature
    (D) Dryer temperature

87. Which type of technique chart is based on changes in quality of radiation delivered to the patient?
    (A) Fixed mA
    (B) Fixed kVp
    (C) Caliper method
    (D) Point system

88. Which of the following is NOT a rare earth material?
    (A) Gadolinium oxysulfide
    (B) Calcium tungstate
    (C) Lanthanum oxysulfide
    (D) Lanthanum oxybromide

89. The effect of FFD on recorded detail can be best described by the statement:
    (A) FFD has no effect on detail.
    (B) increased FFD increases detail.
    (C) decreased FFD increases detail.
    (D) 40″ FFD is the optimum distance for diagnostic radiography.

90. A fractional x-ray tube achieves an improvement in recorded detail by:
    (A) increasing the anode angle.
    (B) decreasing the anode angle.
    (C) increasing the heel effect.
    (D) using fractional exposure times.

91. Which of the following is most likely to result in radiographic elongation?
    (A) Improper FFD
    (B) Excessive OFD
    (C) Grid cutoff
    (D) Tube angulation

92. The term "base plus fog" describes:
    (A) unwanted exposure of film to light.
    (B) unwanted exposure of film from scatter radiation.
    (C) inherent manufacturing and processing density.
    (D) contributing environmental exposure factors, such as radon.

93. Increasing screen speed is accomplished by:
    (A) using light-restricting dyes.
    (B) decreasing crystal size.
    (C) decreasing phosphor thickness.
    (D) increasing phosphor thickness.

94. Quantum mottle is most likely to appear with which of the following system speeds?
    (A) 100
    (B) 200
    (C) 400
    (D) 800

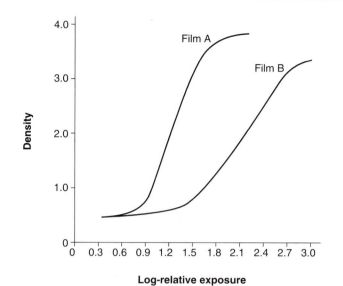

FIGURE 6-2.

QUESTIONS 95-97

Using the characteristic curve shown in Figure 6-2, answer the following:

95. In comparison with film A, film B:
    (A) is faster and has less latitude
    (B) is slower and has greater latitude.
    (C) is faster and has greater contrast.
    (D) is slower and has less contrast.

96. In comparison with film B, film A:
    (A) is higher contrast, shorter scale.
    (B) is higher contrast, longer scale.
    (C) is longer contrast, longer scale.
    (D) is longer contrast, shorter scale.

97. Approximately how much faster is film A than film B?
    (A) 2 ×
    (B) 3 ×
    (C) 4 ×
    (D) 5 ×

QUESTIONS 98-200

select the best answer

98. Portions of the characteristic curve that represent densities outside the useful density range include:
    (A) straight line and toe.
    (B) toe and shoulder.
    (C) straight line and shoulder.
    (D) there are no densities on the curve that are outside the range.

99. An examination of the abdomen is performed using a 12:1 oscillating bucky with the tube placed 2″ off center toward the right side of the patient. The resulting radiograph will demonstrate:
    (A) overall loss of density.
    (B) unilateral right-sided loss of density.
    (C) unilateral left-sided loss of density.
    (D) loss of density on the anode side of the tube.

100. Which of the following sets of exposure factors would be most appropriate for use for an RAO projection of the esophagus?
    (A) 10 mA, 110 kVp
    (B) 50 mA, 70 kVp
    (C) 25 mA, 80 kVp
    (D) 100 mA, 65 kVp

101 Which of the following combinations will produce the most density on a radiograph if film and screen speed remain constant?
    (A) 70 mA, 70 kVp, 40″ FFD, 10:1 grid
    (B) 35 mA, 80 kVp, 40″ FFD, 8:1 grid
    (C) 40 mA, 70 kVp, 72″ FFD, 8:1 grid
    (D) 70 mA, 70 kVp, 72″ FFD, 10:1 grid

102. Which of the following technique combinations would be appropriate for a PA projection of the hand, using rare earth screens and fast film?
    (A) 10 mA , 60 kVp
    (B) 5 mA, 70 kVp
    (C) 1 mA, 50 kVp
    (D) 10 mA, 80 kVp

103. Which of the following combinations would produce the longest scale of contrast on a 72″ PA chest radiograph if the same film type is used for all exposures?
    (A) 10 mA, 80 kVp, 12:1 grid
    (B) 5 mA, 92 kVp, 12:1 grid
    (C) 2.5 mA, 106 kVp, 12:1 grid
    (D) 1.25 mA, 122 kVp, 12:1 grid

104. Of the following factors, which is the most effective control of involuntary motion?
    (A) mA
    (B) kVp
    (C) Patient instructions
    (D) Distance

105. Of the following colors emitted by radiologic accessories, the color LEAST likely to fog orthochromatic film would be:

    (A) amber.
    (B) green.
    (C) blue-violet.
    (D) red.

106. All of the following are possible darkroom-related causes of film fog EXCEPT:

    (A) white light leak.
    (B) film illumination by safelight over 1 minute.
    (C) humidity under 40%.
    (D) Wratten 6B filter used with rare earth screen film system.

107. A pinhole-type artifact is the result of which type of improper cassette handling?

    (A) Humidity over 80%
    (B) Dust and lint on the intensifying screen
    (C) Defective manufacturing of film
    (D) Dropping the cassette

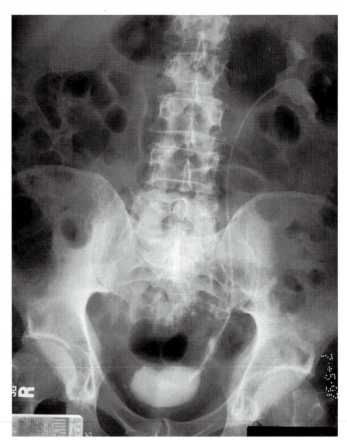

FIGURE 6-4.

108. Examine the radiograph in **Figure 6-3.** The most likely cause of underexposure is:

    (A) incorrect positioning.
    (B) incorrect patient instruction.
    (C) insufficient mA.
    (D) insufficient distance.

109. Which of the following techniques is most appropriate for the radiograph in **Figure 6-4?**

    (A) 20 mA, 70 kVp, 40″ FFD
    (B) 40 mA, 70 kVp, 72″ FFD
    (C) 20 mA, 90 kVp, 40″ FFD
    (D) 10 mA, 100 kVp, 48″ FFD

110. Why did the radiograph in **Figure 6-5** have to be repeated?

    (A) Technique, too dark
    (B) Positioning
    (C) Technique, too light
    (D) Artifact

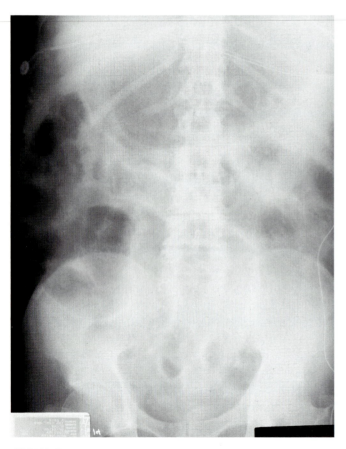

FIGURE 6-3.

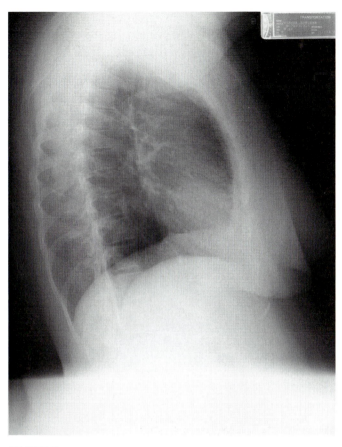

FIGURE 6-5.

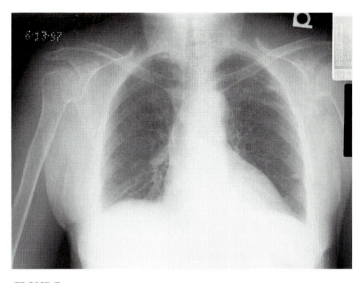

FIGURE 6-6.

111. In relation to the lateral cuneiform, the cuboid is:

(A) lateral.
(B) medial.
(C) posterior.
(D) anterior.

112. Which of the following views best demonstrates the radial head?

(A) AP
(B) PA
(C) Medial oblique
(D) Lateral oblique

113. Which of the following projections demonstrates the olecranon process within the olecranon fossa?

(A) AP, partial flexion
(B) Lateral oblique
(C) Medial oblique
(D) Lateral

114. Which of the following views would be used for suspected fracture of the pisiform if standard projections failed to yield the desired diagnostic information?

(A) Ulnar flexion PA
(B) Radial flexion PA
(C) AP oblique
(D) Cross-table lateral

115. The abnormality in the superior lateral portion of the left lower lobe (LLL) of the radiograph in **Figure 6-6** most likely represents which of the following?

(A) Pulmonary edema
(B) Pulmonary embolus
(C) Calcified granuloma
(D) Emphysema

116. In relation to the pedicles, the lumbar laminae are best described as:

(A) anterior.
(B) posterior.
(C) anterior and inferior.
(D) posterior and inferior.

117. How many processes project from the vertebral arch?

(A) 7
(B) 6
(C) 5
(D) 4

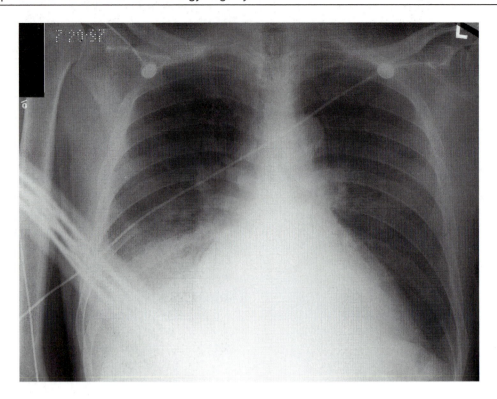

FIGURE 6-7.

118. Which type of fracture is characterized by fractured portions of bone protruding through the skin?

    (A) Greenstick
    (B) Comminuted
    (C) Compound
    (D) Impacted

119. How many lobes does the right lung have?

    (A) 1
    (B) 2
    (C) 3
    (D) 4

120. The density overlying the right lower lobe in **Figure 6-7** most likely represents a (an):

    (A) endotracheal tube.
    (B) central line.
    (C) chest tube.
    (D) x-ray cable.

121. Which projection of the lumbar spine demonstrates the "Scotty dogs"?

    (A) AP
    (B) Oblique
    (C) Lateral
    (D) Flexion and extension lateral

122. Which view of the lumbar spine uses a 5° to 8° caudal angulation?

    (A) AP
    (B) Oblique
    (C) Lateral
    (D) Spot view

123. Of the following, which type of vertebral foramen (foramina) is (are) circular?

    (A) Thoracic
    (B) Cervical
    (C) Lumbar
    (D) Lumbar and thoracic

124. Which of the anatomic descriptions listed below is false concerning the spinal curvatures?

    (A) The cervical and lumbar curvatures are convex anteriorly
    (B) The thoracic and sacral curvatures are convex anteriorly
    (C) The cervical and lumbar curvatures are concave posteriorly
    (D) The thoracic and sacral curvatures are convex posteriorly

125. The correct number of facial bones is:
    (A) 26.
    (B) 14.
    (C) 18.
    (D) 22.

126. A frail, 80-year-old female patient presents for evaluation at the emergency room, having fallen out of bed on her right side. Her right hip is excruciatingly painful. She is unable to move the leg, and her toes are in the externally rotated position. The physician orders a right hip x-ray. Of the following, which is the most correct routine, considering the patient?
    (A) AP right hip, CXR
    (B) AP and frog-leg lateral right hip
    (C) AP and surgical lateral right hip
    (D) AP pelvis, AP and surgical lateral right hip, CXR

127. Which cranial bone forms most of the bony area between the nasal cavity and the orbit?
    (A) Ethmoid
    (B) Sphenoid
    (C) Lacrimal
    (D) Vomer

128. Which of the following describes most correctly the transit of barium on a small bowel follow-through examination?
    (A) Stomach, ileum, jejunum, duodenum
    (B) Duodenum, jejunum, ileum, ileocecal valve
    (C) Ileum, jejunum, duodenum, cecum
    (D) Stomach, GE junction, greater curvature, lesser curvature

129. The anterior two thirds of the hard palate is formed by which bone?
    (A) Maxillae
    (B) Palatine
    (C) Mandible
    (D) Vomer

130. A patient in the supine position is positioned so that the MSP forms a 53° angle with the plane of the film, and the acanthiomeatal line is perpendicular to the film. What view is performed when the CR is directed through the orbit farthest from the film?
    (A) Caldwell
    (B) Jones
    (C) Rhese
    (D) Waters

131. Which view of the sinuses demonstrates all four sinuses?
    (A) Waters
    (B) Caldwell
    (C) SMV
    (D) Lateral

132. The pterygoid process is a part of which bone?
    (A) Ethmoid
    (B) Vomer
    (C) Sphenoid
    (D) Lacrimal

133. Which view of the biliary system is used routinely to demonstrate the biliary tree and gallbladder area free of superimposition from bony structures?
    (A) PA
    (B) RPO
    (C) RAO
    (D) Erect lateral

134. During upper extremity venography, where are tourniquets placed?
    (A) Distal to the wrist
    (B) Distal to the elbow
    (C) Proximal to the wrist
    (D) Proximal to the wrist and elbow

135. Which of the following examinations uses a volumetric injector?
    (A) Hysterosalpingogram
    (B) Venogram
    (C) Arthrogram
    (D) Myelogram

136. Where is contrast medium most commonly introduced during lumbar myelography?
    (A) Subarachnoid space at L3–L4
    (B) Subdural space at L1–L2
    (C) Epidural space at L3–L4
    (D) Pia mater at L1–L2

137. What bone houses the petrous region of the skull?
    (A) Occipital
    (B) Ethmoid
    (C) Temporal
    (D) Sphenoid

138. Which of the following bony landmarks can be described as a thin, sharp, bony projection located slightly inferior to the EAM?
    (A) Zygomatic arch
    (B) Styloid process
    (C) Mastoid process
    (D) Pterygoid process

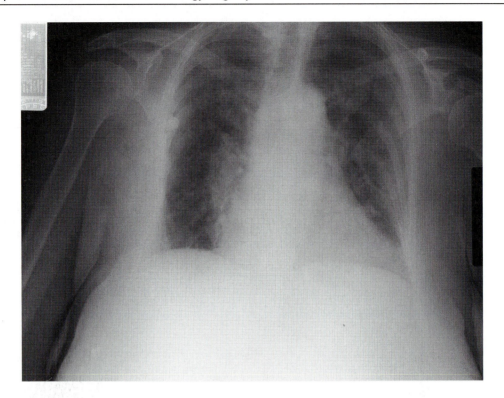

FIGURE 6-8.

139. Examine **Figure 6-8.** The reason this radiograph had to be repeated was:

    (A) motion.
    (B) too light.
    (C) too dark.
    (D) clipping.

140. Which of the following conditions represents the correct diagnosis for the radiograph in **Figure 6-9**?

    (A) Gas gangrene
    (B) Fracture of the distal fifth metatarsal
    (C) Fracture of the middle fifth phalanx
    (D) Fracture of the proximal fifth phalanx

141. Which tangential projection of the patella utilizes cephalic angulation, which varies according to the amount of patellofemoral flexion?

    (A) Homblad
    (B) Settegast
    (C) Camp-Coventry
    (D) Beclere

142. Which of the following methods is (are) used to obtain an axillary view of the glenohumeral articulation?

    (A) inferosuperior
    (B) superoinferior
    (C) rolled film
    (D) all of the above

143. Dilated, tortuous veins directly beneath the esophageal mucosa are known as:

    (A) esophageal varices.
    (B) hiatal hernia.
    (C) ischemic bowel.
    (D) peptic ulcer.

144. The axiolateral position of the mandible utilizing a 25° cephalic angulation entering slightly posterior to the mandibular angle distal from the film best demonstrates which of the following?

    (A) mandibular rami closest to the film
    (B) mandibular rami distal from the film
    (C) mandibular body
    (D) mandibular symphysis

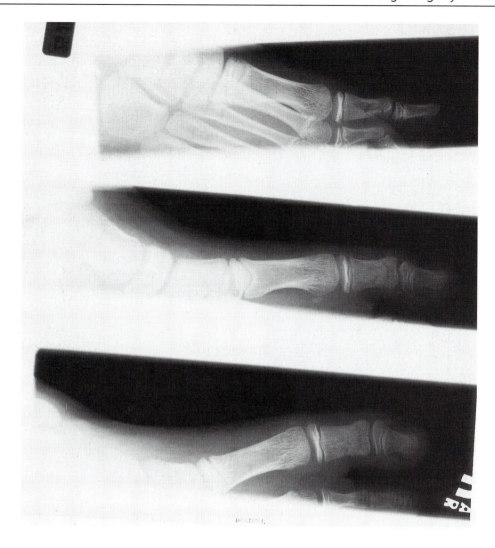

FIGURE 6-9.

145. Which projection of the sternum may utilize a shallow breathing technique?

    (A) AP
    (B) PA
    (C) RAO
    (D) lateral

146. Which of the following bony lower extremity structures is easily palpated and often used as a bony landmark?

    (A) lesser trochanter
    (B) greater trochanter
    (C) acetabulum
    (D) femoral head

147. The distance between the fulcrum levels typically utilized during nephrotomography is:

    (A) 1 mm.
    (B) 0.05 mm.
    (C) 1 cm.
    (D) 5 cm.

148. PA and lateral chest radiographs are performed with the CR directed perpendicularly at the level of:

    (A) T5.
    (B) The SC joints.
    (C) The xiphoid process.
    (D) T7.

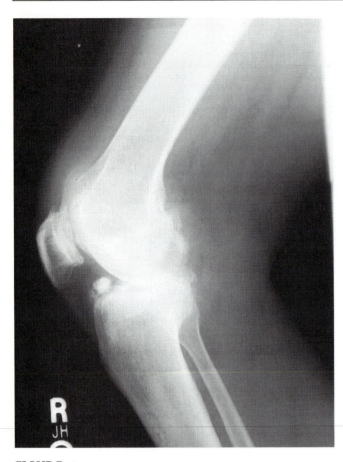

FIGURE 6-10.

149. The radiograph in **Figure 6-10** is an example of which of the following projections?

    (A) AP
    (B) Camp-Coventry
    (C) Lateral
    (D) Settegast

150. The area of increased density on the anterior portion of the tibial plateau in **Figure 6-10** most likely represents:

    (A) sarcoma.
    (B) tibial plateau fracture.
    (C) osteoarthritis.
    (D) gas gangrene.

151. The film shown in **Figure 6-11** is an example of which imaging modality?

    (A) MRI
    (B) Nuclear medicine
    (C) Ultrasound
    (D) Special procedures

152. Which of the following are considered techniques that reduce voluntary patient motion?

    1. explanation of the procedure
    2. short FFD
    3. high kVp and AED

    (A) all of the above
    (B) 3 only
    (C) 2 and 3
    (D) 1 only

153. All of the following conditions are best evaluated with both inspiration and expiration PA chest radiographs except:

    (A) FB.
    (B) respiratory excursion.
    (C) pneumocystosis.
    (D) pneumothorax.

154. If the standard SMV method of imaging the zygomatic arches fails to reveal the arches sufficiently, owing to depressed or flattened arches, each arch can be imaged individually by positioning the patient:

    (A) supine, head rotated toward the area of interest 15°.
    (B) supine, head rotated away from the area of interest 45°.
    (C) prone, head rotated away from the area of interest 45°.
    (D) prone head rotated toward the area of interest 15°.

155. Which of the following demonstrates the correct flow of CSF?

    (A) third ventricle, foramen of Monroe, lateral ventricle, aqueduct of Sylvius, fourth ventricle, foramen of Magendie, subarachnoid space
    (B) subarachnoid space, third ventricle, foramen of Monroe, foramen of Luschka, fourth ventricle, lateral ventricle
    (C) lateral ventricle, foramen of Monroe, third ventricle, aqueduct of Sylvius, fourth ventricle, foramen of Magendie, subarachnoid space
    (D) fourth ventricle, foramen of Luschka, foramen of Magendie, lateral ventricle, third ventricle, subarachnoid space

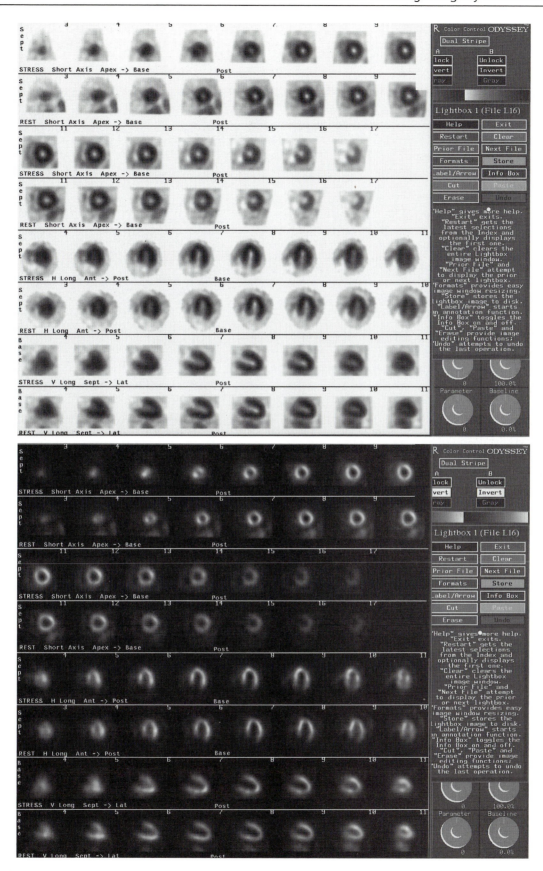

FIGURE 6-11.

156. A suspicious mixed density is noted on a lateral chest radiograph, 10 cm posterior to the sternum. AP tomograms of the chest are ordered to further evaluate the lesion. If the patient measures 40 cm in the lateral dimension and 28 cm in the AP dimension, where should the fulcrum be placed to best demonstrate the area of interest?

    (A) 30 cm
    (B) 18 cm
    (C) 40 cm
    (D) 28 cm

157. Which of the following statements is true concerning the location of the kidneys?

    (A) peritoneum, from T12–L3
    (B) retrogastric, from T8–L1
    (C) retroperitoneum, from T12–L3
    (D) subdiaphragmatic, from T10–L1

158. Which of the following conditions does NOT relate to the importance of obtaining a post-void radiograph during an excretory urogram?

    (A) prostate hypertrophy
    (B) bladder neoplasm
    (C) residual urine
    (D) hydronephrosis

159. During a double-contrast UGI procedure, which position will optimally demonstrate the duodenal bulb and pyloric canal?

    (A) AP
    (B) LPO
    (C) PA
    (D) Right lateral

160. A routine overhead PA view of the stomach on a 10 × 12 cassette is centered approximately at the level of:

    (A) S1
    (B) T10
    (C) L2
    (D) L4

161. Which of the following best describes the position of the esophagus?

    (A) midline, anterior to the trachea, joins the stomach at the cardiac orifice
    (B) slightly left of midline, anterior to the trachea, joins the stomach at the pyloric orifice
    (C) midline, posterior to the trachea, joins the stomach at the cardiac orifice
    (D) midline, posterior to the trachea, joins the duodenum at the sphincter of Oddi

162. Which of the following correctly describes the anatomy that joins to form the common bile duct?

    (A) cystic duct and common hepatic duct
    (B) pancreatic duct and duct of Wirsung
    (C) right and left hepatic ducts and cystic ducts
    (D) sphincter of Oddi and pancreatic duct

163. The most superior midline landmark on the skull is the:

    (A) acanthion.
    (B) glabella.
    (C) outer canthus.
    (D) IOML.

164. Which midline point marks the union of the nose and upper lip?

    (A) outer canthus
    (B) mental symphysis
    (C) IOML
    (D) acanthion

165. The sella turcica is located in which of the following cranial bones?

    (A) sphenoid
    (B) ethmoid
    (C) frontal
    (D) temporal

166. A drop in blood pressure due to extensive blood loss is associated with which of the following?

    (A) cardiac arrest
    (B) respiratory distress
    (C) shock
    (D) head injury

167. Which of these examinations should be performed first?

    (A) SBFT
    (B) IVP
    (C) BE
    (D) UGI

168. A tort is:

    (A) a viral infection.
    (B) a hospital policy.
    (C) an act that results in injury.
    (D) a patient right.

169. The patient has a right to:
     1. a diagnosis from the technologist.
     2. confidentiality.
     3. the lowest reasonable price for treatment.
     4. refuse the examination.

     (A) all of the above.
     (B) none of the above.
     (C) 1 and 3.
     (D) 2 and 4.

170. Look at the structures below and choose the correct numbered sequence representing blood flow through the heart.
     1. left ventricle
     2. left atrium
     3. right atrium
     4. right ventricle
     5. bicuspid or mitral
     6. tricuspid
     7. aortic semilunar
     8. pulmonary semilunar

     (A) 3, 6, 4, 8, 2, 5, 1, 7
     (B) 1, 3, 5, 2, 4, 7, 6, 8
     (C) 3, 4, 6, 2, 8, 1, 5, 7
     (D) 4, 3, 8, 7, 2, 1, 6, 5

171. The portion of the pancreas surrounded by the duodenum is:
     (A) head.
     (B) neck.
     (C) body.
     (D) tail.

172. The best way to support a fractured extremity during a radiologic examination is:
     (A) support the extremity with a pillow.
     (B) support the extremity with a sling.
     (C) support the extremity below the injury site.
     (D) support the extremity above and below the injury site.

173. The type of condition associated with tonic and clonic spasms is:
     (A) HNP.
     (B) grand mal seizure.
     (C) petit mal seizure.
     (D) jacksonian epilepsy.

174. Epistaxis is a term that means:
     (A) partially healed fracture.
     (B) nosebleed.
     (C) vomiting.
     (D) bloody urine.

175. The gauge of a flexible angiocatheter is determined by:
     (A) length.
     (B) diameter.
     (C) degree of rigidity.
     (D) width of aperture.

176. Cyanosis is a term meaning:
     (A) pale, dry skin.
     (B) cold, moist skin.
     (C) blue-tinged skin.
     (D) extreme redness.

177. The ideal location to hang a bag of intravenous solution of D5W is:
     (A) 5 ft above the patient.
     (B) as high as the IV pole will allow.
     (C) 18-24″ above the patient.
     (D) on a level with the IV site.

178. A Foley catheter is used for treatment of:
     (A) incontinence.
     (B) bladder obstruction.
     (C) diarrhea.
     (D) all of the above.

179. All of the following are characteristics of iohexol except:
     (A) approved for intrathecal use.
     (B) HOCM.
     (C) positive media.
     (D) LOCM.

180. The chief drawback to intravenous nonionic contrast material is:
     (A) osmolality.
     (B) osmolarity.
     (C) cost.
     (D) miscibility.

181. Patients are transported to the radiology department in a variety of ways. Which of the following patient conditions would allow the patient to be transported to the radiology department by wheelchair?
     (A) Cheyne-Stokes respiration
     (B) closed head trauma / unknown etiology
     (C) cervical spine injury secondary to recent MVA
     (D) DJD

182. The first step when moving a patient from a wheelchair to the x-ray table is:
    (A) lock the chair
    (B) place a footrest near the table's center
    (C) place arm behind patient's shoulder
    (D) turn the patient's back to the table

183. When administering intravenous contrast, BUN and creatinine tests are performed. Elevated BUN and creatinine levels indicate:
    (A) patient age.
    (B) renal function.
    (C) small bowel obstruction.
    (D) all of the above.

184. Why is an AP projection of the scapula preferable to a PA projection?
    (A) less technique is required
    (B) less OFD occurs
    (C) less FFD is required
    (D) less motion is likely

185. A patient with hypoglycemic shock displays:
    (A) high fever
    (B) dry, hot skin
    (C) sweating and chills
    (D) loss of appetite

186. Which examination would most likely require the patient to sign an allergy history form?
    (A) barium swallow
    (B) Gastrografin enema
    (C) barium enema
    (D) IVP

187. For a patient with suspected esophagobronchial fistula, the most likely choice of contrast in a fluoroscopy-directed examination would be:
    (A) Gastrografin.
    (B) barium sulfate.
    (C) air.
    (D) gadolinium.

188. Which radiographic procedure requires iodized oil as contrast media?
    (A) myelography
    (B) pneumoencephalography
    (C) lymphangiography
    (D) angiography

189. The term extravasation means:
    (A) leakage of intravenous fluids into surrounding tissue.
    (B) presence of air in the peritoneum.
    (C) blood in the stool.
    (D) productive, bloody cough.

190. A contaminated object acting as a source of disease transmission is called:
    (A) vector.
    (B) parasite.
    (C) host.
    (D) fomite.

191. The primary means of hepatitis B transmission is via:
    (A) blood.
    (B) urine.
    (C) feces.
    (D) air.

192. Which of the following procedures utilizes the Sedlinger technique?
    (A) ERCP
    (B) angiography
    (C) PTCA
    (D) TURP

193. A Colles fracture would be diagnosed on which of the following examinations?
    (A) humerus
    (B) elbow
    (C) clavicle
    (D) wrist

194. For which examination must the patient ingest the contrast before arriving in the radiology department?
    (A) small bowel series
    (B) OCG
    (C) hysterosalpingogram
    (D) sialogram

195. Which route for medication does the term parenteral refer to?
    (A) intravenous
    (B) intramuscular
    (C) mucosal
    (D) all of the above

196. The most frequent site of nosocomial infection is:
    (A) urinary tract.
    (B) respiratory tract.
    (C) open wounds.
    (D) digestive tract.

197. Where is the linea aspera is located?
    (A) Anterior femur
    (B) Posterior femur
    (C) Anterior tibia
    (D) Posterior tibia

198. Which of the following correctly describes characteristics of the atlas?

    (A) An odontoid process
    (B) Prominent spinous process
    (C) Articulation with true ribs
    (D) Concave superior articular facets

199. The humeroulnar joint is formed by which of the following?

    (A) Trochlea of the humerus and trochlear notch of the ulna
    (B) Epicondyles of the humerus and ulnar styloid
    (C) Trochlea of the humerus and olecranon process of the ulna
    (D) Epicondyles of the humerus and olecranon process of the ulna

200. Increasing OFD most significantly decreases which of the following factors?

    (A) Magnification
    (B) Density
    (C) Contrast
    (D) Detail

▶▶▶ ANSWERS

1. The answer is (C). SSD must be at least 12″, preferably 15″ during fluoroscopy with fixed fluoroscopic equipment. SSD must not be less than 12″ for all other procedures except dental radiography. 36″, 40″, and 72″ are all examples of commonly used focal film distances (FFD).

2. The answer is (D). The eyes, gonads, and blood-forming organs are especially radiosensitive, having an annual occupational dose limit of 5 rem (50 mSv); however, the hands and feet may safely receive 75 rem (750 mSv) per annum.

3. The answer is (A). Fluoroscopic dose is calculated by using 2 rad · min · mA. Therefore, 2 · 4 · 1.25 = 10 rad.

4. The answer is (B). The film badge is the most widely used occupational monitoring device. Pocket dosimeters are used primarily when large amounts of radiation are likely to be encountered. The thermoluminescent dosimeter is more precise than the film badge, but it is read on a quarterly basis. The cutie pie is a radiation survey device.

5. The answer is (A). The NCRP recommends personnel monitoring for individuals likely to receive 25% of the occupational dose equivalent of 5 rem or 50mSv/ yr. Therefore, occupational dose is expressed by Sv or rem. Rem is the acronym for "radiation equivalent man"; the sievert (Sv) is the SI (international standards) equivalent for rem. Rad (Gy) is the acronym for "radiation absorbed dose." As radiation passes through biologic matter, energy is deposited. Absorbed dose is the amount of energy deposited per unit of mass. LET, linear energy transfer, is a measure of the rate at which energy is transferred from ionizing radiation to biologic matter. It is another means of expressing radiation quality. Rem uses the information collected for rad, but incorporates a quality factor (QF) to help predict biologic effects from radiation exposure. Roentgen or exposure rate (coulombs/kg) is the unit of measurement for exposure in air.

6. The answer is (D). Radiation causes certain materials, notably calcium tungstate and rare earth materials, to luminesce—that is, to glow in the dark. Radiation also causes the thermoluminescent effect, which is the conversion of light in crystals after heating. This is the principle on which the TLD operates. The photographic effect is induced by radiation, causing changes in photographic emulsion so that it may be chemically developed.

7. The answer is (B). Of the various types of interactions between x-rays and matter, the photoelectric effect is the predominant interaction relative to energy absorption in the diagnostic range from 30 to 140 kVp. Photoelectric absorption is four to six times greater in bone than in an equal mass of soft tissue; therefore, this type of interaction is responsible for much of the radiologic contrast, which is manifested by differences in film darkness on the radiograph. The Compton effect is associated primarily with scatter radiation resulting from interaction with tissue, the radiographic table, the cassette, and so on. Scatter radiation comprises 80% to 90% of the beam in soft tissue. Neither coherent scatter nor pair production are associated with the diagnostic range of beam energy.

8. The answer is (A). Tube current, measured in mA, governs the amount of electrons per second produced at the target. As tube current increases, more electrons at the target are produced, and hence exposure rate increases proportionally. Tube potential (kVp), filtration, and distance all affect exposure rate, but not at a directly proportional rate.

9. The answer is (A). Linear energy transfer (LET) may be described as the amount of energy deposited per unit of photon travel, whereas the relative biologic effectiveness (RBE) provides a comparison of the biologic effects from equal doses of different types of radiation. Alpha particles, for example, have a high LET, depositing a high amount of energy over a small area, resulting in a significant biologic effect. On the other hand, an equal dose of high-energy x-ray has a low LET, because the x-ray photon spreads its energy over a greater distance, reducing the biologic effect.

10. The answer is (B). Increasing kVp results in a more penetrating beam, thus reducing patient dose. An increase in the FFD reduces patient dose according to the inverse square law, which states that beam intensity is inversely proportional to the square of the distance from the source.

11. The answer is (C). If fetal irradiation occurs in the first 2 weeks after fertilization, an all-or-none response occurs. In other words, either a spontaneous abortion will take place, or no fetal damage will result. The fetus is most radiosensitive during the first trimester after the initial 2-week period because it is the period of most intensive growth.

12. The answer is (D). X-radiation is created by sudden deceleration of high-speed electrons in an x-ray tube, whereas gamma radiation is emitted from the nucleus of radioactive elements. Both x- and gamma rays travel at the speed of light in a vacuum, can cause biologic change in matter, and have no mass—that is, they are nonparticulate.

13. The answer is (D). The 10-day rule relates to the optimum time period in which to perform elective radiography procedures on women of reproductive age. Because the 10-day period after the onset of menses is the period when unsuspected pregnancy is least likely, elective radiography procedures, particularly those of the abdomen, should be performed during this time.

14. The answer is (B). Filtration in the x-ray tube increases the average energy of the beam by removing low-energy photons, which have little contributory effect toward image production, but which increase patient dose.

15. The answer is (A). The patient is the primary source of scatter in a typical radiographic procedure because he or she is the first object encountered by the radiation emitted by the x-ray tube.

The primary type of interaction produced is Compton scatter, which is nearly as energetic as the primary beam itself. However, distance has a profound effect on scattered beam intensity because scattered beam intensity at 1 m from the patient is 0.1% that of the primary beam.

16. The answer is (C). The roentgen is the unit of measurement that expresses exposure in air. The SI equivalent of roentgen is the exposure rate, expressed in coulombs/ kg.

17. The answer is (D). The Compton effect is the predominant type of x-ray interaction at energy levels greater than 70 kVp.

18. The answer is (D). Acute radiation syndromes arise from acute whole-body exposures in the range from 100 to 1000 R. A supralethal exposure in the range of 600 to 1000 R causes gastrointestinal syndrome, consisting of nausea, vomiting, intractable diarrhea, and profound drop in white blood cells. Unless treated with intensive blood transfusions, bone marrow transplants, antibiotics, and fluids, death from this dose range occurs from sepsis within 2 weeks. A midlethal exposure occurs in the range of 450 R, with one half of the exposed population dying within a month from pancytopenia; this is otherwise known as the bone marrow form of acute radiation syndrome. A sublethal exposure occurs in the range from 100 to 300 R, carrying with it less severe symptoms, although in many exposed people cataracts develop within 2 to 6 years after exposure.

19. The answer is (B). Object–film distance is a geometric factor primarily affecting magnification, distortion, and detail. It has no effect on patient dose. FFD is inversely proportional to patient dose, as defined by the inverse square law. Filtration increases the overall average energy level of the primary beam, thus reducing patient dose.

20. The answer is (C). When available mechanical restraining devices fail to support the patient in a manner that permits obtaining a diagnostic examination, a relative or friend accompanying the patient is the best choice to assist with the examination because their lifetime radiation exposure is likely to be extremely low. As a last resort, other hospital personnel may be used to assist the patient, but radiology personnel should never be used. When using another person in this manner is necessary, protective apparel is provided, and the holder is carefully positioned and instructed so as to avoid exposure to the primary beam.

21. The answer is (A). Bergonie and Tribondeau determined that immature cells (i.e., undifferentiated, stem, or precursor cells, such as those found in bone marrow) or highly mitotic cells (i.e., highly proliferative cells, such as those found in the gonads, or lens of the eye) are most radiosensitive. Myocytes, or muscle cells, are mature, differentiated cells, and therefore fairly radioresistant.

22. The answer is (C). Human cells are classified as either germ cells, which are involved with reproduction, or as somatic cells. Cell division of germ cells is called meiosis. Mitosis (somatic cell division) may be divided into four stages: prophase, metaphase, anaphase, and telophase. Interphase is a resting cycle. Cells are most radiosensitive during the period when chromosomes line up along the nuclear equator—metaphase.

23. The answer is (A). kVp is the exposure factor that controls quality (penetrating ability) of the x-ray beam. As kVp increases, overall energy and frequency of the beam increase, whereas wavelength decreases. Higher kVp technique delivers a smaller absorbed dose to the patient because higher-energy photons tend to pass through the body unchanged to expose the film. Therefore, technique (A), which produces the lowest quantity of photons with the highest penetrating ability, will produce the lowest absorbed dose.

24. The answer is (C). Shadow shields are attached to the x-ray tube itself, and therefore are the best choice for any procedure involving a sterile field. The shadow shield can be accurately directed to protect the gonadal area.

25. The answer is (A). GI examinations usually are performed using barium sulfate, a highly dense material that necessitates exposures be made in excess of 100 kVp to penetrate the material adequately. Therefore, according to NCRP guidelines, the filtration requirements for such a room must exceed 2.5 mm Al equivalent.

26. The answer is (C). Radiation emanating from the tube housing in a different direction from the useful beam is considered leakage radiation. NCRP guidelines state leakage radiation may not exceed 100 mR/hour at a distance of 1 m from the x-ray tube.

27. The answer is (D). The use of immobilization devices, when needed, reduces the need for repeat exposures, thereby reducing unnecessary exposure to the patient. Added filtration increases the overall penetrating ability of the beam, also reducing patient dose. Increased FFD (SID) reduces dose according to the inverse square law; however, to produce technically comparable radiographs with increased SID requires an increase in exposure factors. High-kVp, low-mA technique, with the fastest practical speed, is recommended for lowest patient dose.

28. The answer is (C). During routine radiography, the technologist using only one badge for monitoring should wear the badge at the waist. During fluoroscopy, however, the answer is not as clear for departments using only one badge. If the technologist wears the badge above the apron, his or her head and neck are monitored, and it is assumed the abdomen receives a lower dose because of protection from the lead apron. If the badge is worn below the apron, the measured dose will be less, but the head and neck will be unmonitored. The ideal solution is a two-badge system, but except for monitoring of pregnant women, the use of two badges is not common.

29. The answer is (D). According to the inverse square law,

$$\frac{I_o}{I_n} = \frac{D_n^2}{D_0^2},$$

Therefore, to solve,

$$50/x = 80^2/40^2; \ 6400x = 80,000; \ x = 12.5$$

30. The answer is (C). NCRP regulations stipulate that lead aprons must consist of material equal to 0.50 mm Pb equivalent. Lead gloves must be 0.25 Pb equivalent.

31. The answer is (C). Electrons are produced in the x-ray tube by heating of the thoriated tungsten filament of the cathode, causing it to liberate valence electrons in a process known as thermionic emission.

32. The answer is (A). The smallest target angle and largest actual focal spot permit the greatest heat-loading capacity. Decreasing target angle (making it steeper) increases the effective focal spot. However, recall that steeper target angles also increase the anode heel effect, making FFD and film size an issue.

33. The answer is (C). The autotransformer is a variable transformer that operates on alternating current on the low-voltage x-ray circuit. The kVp selector on the control panel corresponds with a movable contact that selects the appropriate number of coils on the autotransformer.

34. The answer is (C). A double-focus x-ray tube has two filaments and two focal spots. When the small focal spot is selected at the control panel, the small filament is heated and electrons are driven across to a smaller portion of the anode focal track. Conversely, when the operator selects a large focal spot, the large filament is heated, and electrons are driven to a large portion of the focal track.

35. The answer is (B). The key to this problem is understanding that the prefix "milli" refers to thousandths and "kilo" refers to thousands. Multiplying known values in this problem yields the following:

    500 × 0.001 = 0.5 amp,
    and 80 × 1000 = 80,000 volts.

36. The answer is (A). The star pattern resolution object is a grid that is radiographed, demonstrating a focused area on film. The star pattern also demonstrates resolution, the smallest area between two objects, of the focal spot. The focused area is measured; the width and length are representative of the focal spot size.

37. The answer is (A). The phototimer automatically terminates the exposure once a known, predetermined amount of exposure has occurred. The synchronous and electronic timers are older types of timers that were not as accurate, particularly with short exposure times. The type of x-ray device that reciprocates is a reciprocating bucky; there is no reciprocating timer.

38. The answer is (D). Single-phase rectification results in a 100% voltage ripple because it uses the entire waveform. The current fluctuates from zero to peak potential and back to zero. Three-phase current uses the peaks of 3 out-of-phase currents, with 3-phase, 6-pulse producing a 13% voltage ripple, and 3-phase, 12-pulse producing only a 3.5% drop between peaks.

39. The answer is (B). Mutual induction occurs when an alternating current in the primary coil of the transformer links with the secondary coil, inducing in it an alternating, or opposing, current by electromagnetic induction. Because the AC in the secondary coil also induces an opposing current in the primary coil, the process is known as mutual induction.

40. The answer is (D). A rectifier modifies AC to pulsating DC. DC current is unidirectional, ensuring the flow of electrons from cathode to anode. If true AC were applied to the x-ray tube, the filament would be destroyed as polarity changed and electrons rushed back in the other direction. A diode operates by reversing the polarity of the transformer secondary, rendering it nonconductive.

41. The answer is (A). Simple fluoroscopic monitoring of the patient occurs at very low exposure rates, usually in the range of 1-5 mA. When the image is to be recorded, however, the mA must be increased to levels consistent with conventional radiographs, usually in the range of 200 to 400 mA.

42. The answer is (C). The beam-splitting mirror permits continued monitoring of the patient on the TV monitor while a permanent record of the examination is obtained on film. Eighty-five to 95% of the available light is used to expose the film, with the remainder of the light used for the monitor.

43. The answer is (A). To solve, recall the formulas: input screen diameter/output screen diameter^2 = minification gain, and brightness gain = flux gain × minification gain. Therefore :

$$\frac{10^2}{1} \times 60 = 6000$$

44. The answer is (C). The AED is programmed to terminate the exposure once a predetermined exposure level has been attained. The device automatically compensates for decreased exposure factors; however, if screen speed were to be decreased, the resulting radiograph would be underexposed if no changes were made to the AED programming.

45. The answer is (B). Franklin units are a well-known variety of radiography equipment designed to produce high-quality radiographs of the skull, sinuses, and facial bones. In it, the patient is seated upright at a bucky, and the tube arm swings in a wide arc about the patient, allowing a wide variety of views to be obtained in relatively easy fashion. Head units are used infrequently today, however, because CT and MRI provide superior diagnostic information relative to the skull and brain.

46. The answer is (B). mR/mA is the expression used for calibration of mA stations, and is determined by dividing exposure output in mR by the mA. In this instance,

    50 *mR*/500 *mA*(0.02 sec) = 25 *mR/mA*

47. The answer is (A). NCRP Report 102 requires a positive variable beam-limiting device (a collimator) to work in conjunction with the bucky

tray to ensure the light field does not exceed $\pm 2\%$ FFD. Most equipment today includes a function that automatically performs collimation to film or receptor size, but it may be deselected because there are many cases in which the technologist wants the beam to be less than the film size used. In any case, it is vital for the technologist to ensure the field of radiation never exceeds that of the actual film size being used.

48. The answer is (C). When the film and screen are not properly in contact, areas of blur may occur on the developed radiograph. Therefore, another significant source of artifact is poor screen contact. Screen contact is tested with a wire mesh device. To perform the test, a cassette is placed on the x-ray tabletop and the wire mesh device rests on top of the cassette. A typical extremity-type exposure is then made, and the developed film examined. Blurred areas on the film demonstrate areas of poor screen contact. These screens should either be discarded or sent for repair.

49. The answer is (D). I is the variable associated with current in equations. Letter A represents the equation used for transformer law; letters B and C are invalid. Letter D is the variant of transformer law used to determine current on the secondary side of a step-up transformer.

50. The answer is (B). Selection A is the formula for HU produced by a single-phase unit, selection C is the formula for HU produced by a 3-phase, 12-pulse unit, and selection D is the inverse square law.

51. The answer is (D). Most modern x-ray equipment is dual focused, meaning there are two filament sizes to choose from. When the smaller filament is selected, the smaller focal spot is selected, and less area on the disk is bombarded by electrons.

52. The answer is (D). The machine is rated at 200,000 HU. If the remainder of the films you need to take will generate 140,000 HU, you must wait at least 4 minutes until the anode cools to 60,000.

53. The answer is (C). The greater the focal spot size, the greater the head loading capacity. Also, as target angle decreases, actual focal spot size increases while maintaining small effective focal spot size.

54. The answer is (A). Exposure rate at any point in the primary beam varies according to distance and the angle of the rays relative to the target.

The variation of exposure rate according to the angle of ray emission is called the anode heel effect. The smaller (steeper) the angle, the greater the effect. The effect is made more pronounced by short FFDs and larger film sizes.

55. The answer is (D). Focal track is the area on the anode where electrons are directed. Space charge, thermionic emission, and filament current all relate to the production of negatively charged electrons around the cathode.

56. The answer is (B). The step-down transformer is located in the x-ray filament circuit. Its function is to regulate the voltage and current supplied to the filament circuit. When current and voltage from the step-down transformer are applied to the filament, thermionic emission occurs. The x-ray tube current depends on the filament current, because changing mA stations corresponds to changing taps of the filament step-down transformer.

57. The answer is (D). Decreasing the field size reduces the number of interactions between x-ray photons and matter; hence, there is less Compton scatter, and photoelectric interactions will occur. Although the collimator assembly does contribute to added filtration, it does not significantly harden the beam, nor does it focus it.

58. The answer is (B). Roughening of the focal track, localized anode meltdown, and cracking of the anode disk reduce x-ray output because photons must penetrate the uneven surface of the anode.

59. The answer is (A). During radiography of some small parts, or during examinations on extremely thin patients, the required exposure may be less than the minimum exposure time. To compensate, the technologist may consider decreasing kVp, or manually selecting an appropriate technique.

60. The answer is (D). The interaction of photons on the screen material has no effect on screen durability. Poor screen contact is caused by improper handling and maintenance of the screens.

61. The answer is (B). Selection (B) will produce the least amount of heat units over the largest area of the anode; therefore, it represents the least danger. X-ray tube manufacturers provide buyers with tube rating charts that should be consulted before making any questionable exposure. In addition, the manufacturer supplies proper techniques for tube warm-up procedures that should be followed to prevent anode damage.

62. The answer is (D). The HVL is defined as that amount of filtration material that reduces the exposure rate by half. Because initial filtration of the beam increases its overall energy level, a second HVL must be greater than the first.
63. The answer is (B). Sodium carbonate is found in the developer solution; it is an activator. It maintains an alkaline environment (pH of 10–11.5), enhances the action of the reducing agents, and softens and swells the film emulsion so the emulsion can work on deeper lying silver halide crystals.
64. The answer is (A). The answer is obtained using the distance maintenance formula derived from the inverse square law as follows:

$$\frac{I_1}{I_2} = \frac{D_1^2}{D_2^2}$$

Therefore,

$$\frac{10}{x} = \frac{5184}{1600}$$

$$x = 32.4 \ mA.$$

65. The answer is (C). To avoid artifact caused by less-than-optimum storage, film boxes should always be stored vertically in a cool, dry area of between 50°F to 70°F and 40% to 60% relative humidity, away from ionizing radiation. Pressure artifact is a direct result of stacking boxes directly on top of each other.
66. The answer is (A). A focused grid has lead lines that tilt more as they move away from the center of the grid so that they are in alignment with the x-ray source. The process of tilting the lead strips is known as "canting." The grid radius is the focal point in space at which imaginary lines drawn from the lead strips converge. Because there is some room for error, most grid radii are listed in a range; 36″–42″ and 66″–74″ are the most common ranges.
67. The answer is (B). A 400-speed system is approximately twice as fast as a 200-speed system; therefore, only half as much mA as was originally used is required to produce radiographs of the same density.
68. The answer is (A). Light emission by an intensifying screen excited by radiation is known as luminescence. It is the property that allows intensifying screens to play an effective role in x-ray image production. Continued emission of light after exposure to x-ray energy is terminated is known as phosphorescence, screen lag, or afterglow. Crossover is light that passes from one side of the film emulsion to the other through the film base, causing scattering of light and distortion.
69. The answer is (A). A densitometer reading of the unexposed portion of a processed radiograph is called base plus fog. The reading should not exceed 0.2. Base plus fog is the sum of the density of the film base, environmental exposure received during the manufacturing process, and density resulting from film processing.
70. The answer is (C). Because of the wide divergence of densities demonstrated on a single film with a one-view scoliosis survey, gradient screens are often used to provide a more homogeneous density over the length of the film. The screens are arrayed inside the cassette in a series of ascending speeds, with the high-speed end used for the thickest body part, such as the lumbosacral portion of the spine, or, if the leg is examined, the femur portion, and the low-speed end positioned nearest the thinnest body part. Optimally, these cassettes should be wall mounted and labeled as to which screen is where, so that no confusion arises about screen placement during the examination. Obviously, placing the cassette upside down will result in a film too dark at one end and too light at the other.
71. The answer is (C). In a focused grid, the process of tilting the lead strips so that they are aligned toward the focal spot of the x-ray tube is known as canting. Grid radius is the distance from the grid at which lines drawn from the lead strips converge toward the focal spot. Most grid radii occur in a range that allows some room for error. Because most examinations are performed at either 40″ or 72″, grid radius ranges are found from approximately 36″ to 42″ and 66″ to 74″. The lines in a parallel grid are not canted, and therefore parallel grids have a radius of infinity—as distance from the grid is increased, the beam remains parallel.
72. The answer is (A). The greater the grid ratio, the more accurate must be the positioning to avoid grid cutoff. A 12:1 grid would require a greater patient dose than a 6:1 grid, but would be superior in cleanup ability. Selectivity is the ratio of transmitted primary radiation to transmitted scatter radiation, and is related to the lead content of the grid. Two grids may be of the same ratio but have differing lead content. In general, heavier grids have high selectivity and high-contrast improvement factors.

73. The answer is (A). Use the following formula to solve:

$$\frac{mA_1}{mA_2} = \frac{\text{bucky factor}_1}{\text{bucky factor}_2}$$

Substituting,

$$\frac{5}{x} = \frac{1}{5}$$

$$x = 25 \ mA.$$

74. The answer is (B). Scatter radiation is created after the x-ray beam exits the x-ray tube, on its interaction with another object such as the x-ray table or the patient. Filtration, either added or inherent, is associated with the tube itself; its purpose is to increase the overall energy level of the beam by filtering out low-energy photons.

75. The answer is (C). Osteoporosis is a demineralizing condition of the bone found in elderly people, primarily among women. Because of the sometimes quite dramatic loss of density in the bone, a downward adjustment in technique is required during radiography of these patients.

76. The answer is (B). Because of the increase in dense fluid associated with congestive heart failure, patients with this condition require an increase in technical factors to produce a diagnostic radiograph. The possibility of required repeat exposures on such patients highlights the importance of learning the patient's pertinent medical history before the examination.

77. The answer is (B). The bucky factor grid conversion method uses a table of conversion factors. The bucky factor for a 10:1 grid is 5; therefore, when converting from grid to nongrid, the correct technical adjustment is to divide the mA by 5. The kVp is not adjusted.

78. The answer is (C). If the x-ray tube is positioned off-center in relation to the bucky, the result will be a loss of density on the side of the radiograph away from the tube. In the example, the tube is positioned toward the right side of the patient, so grid cutoff occurs on the left.

79. The answer is (D). AEDs work on the principle of preset values equaling exposure values. Whenever the predetermined charge (in the case of a phototimer) has been reached, or level of ionization reached (as with an ionization chamber), the exposure terminates. The AED accounts for part thickness, distance, and density-increasing or -decreasing patient pathology; however, improper positioning over the AED sensor results in an under- or overexposed radiograph.

80. The answer is (A). Undeveloped silver is removed from the film emulsion by the fixer solution. The silver may be removed from solution by a metallic replacement cartridge or by the process of electrolytic plating. Used film is also sold for its silver content.

81. The answer is (C). All of the factors listed have the potential to affect detail: improper grid ratio, exposure time, and kVp would primarily affect density and scale of contrast, however, whereas screen speed is directly related to recorded detail. As screen speed increases, detail decreases.

82. The answer is (C). Although using short exposure times and fast screens reduces the likelihood of involuntary motion producing motion artifact, clear, concise patient instructions are the most important factor in the technologist's ability to reduce voluntary motion.

83. The answer is (B). Elongation and foreshortening occur when the plane of the object and the plane of the image are not parallel. Inclining a tubular, flattened, or wedge-shaped object at a steeper angle in relation to the film while maintaining beam and film alignment results in a foreshortened image, whereas inclining the same types of objects and angling the tube so as to place the beam perpendicular to the long axis of the object produces an elongated image.

84. The answer is (B). Decreasing field size decreases scatter production, producing a shorter scale of contrast. A skilled technologist can dramatically improve radiographic contrast with the conscientious application of collimation.

85. The answer is (B). The radiographic result of differential radiation absorption by varying anatomic tissue types is termed scale of contrast. Because the body's attenuation properties are varying, so is the emerging remnant radiation as it interacts with the intensifying screen and film emulsion. This varying interaction produces a heterogeneity of densities unique to the combinant energies that produced it.

86. The answer is (B). As film enters the automatic processor, a microswitch is activated. Once activated, replenishment solution is added until the microswitch senses the end of the film. This arrangement necessitates that film be placed in the correct orientation as it enters the machine because placing it incorrectly may lead to inadequate replenishment.

87. The answer is (A). Changes in quality of radiation used in a given exposure are made by varying kVp. Therefore, a fixed-mA, variable-kVp technique chart is based on this methodology.

88. The answer is (B). For many years, intensifying screens were composed primarily of calcium tungstate or lead barium sulfate. Because of their superior light-conversion capabilities, however, rare earth materials are more widely used for intensifying screen construction.

89. The answer is (C). As focal film distance increases, the part under examination is exposed to less divergent, more perpendicular rays, resulting in decreased penumbral blurring and magnification. Using FFD as a controlling factor in detail is impractical, however, for two primary reasons: first, increasing FFD also requires an increase in exposure factors, resulting in increased patient dose; second, many grids have an optimal focusing distance, and exceeding this distance results in unwanted grid cutoff.

90. The answer is (A). A fractional x-ray tube is one that uses a comparatively steep target angle of 7° to 10°, which increases detail by reduction of the effective focal spot while maintaining a fairly large actual focal spot. The small effective focal spot reduces penumbra, whereas the large focal spot permits greater heat loading. A negative factor associated with such tubes is an increase in the anode heel effect and associated decrease in film coverage ability.

91. The answer is (D). Although there are instances where the three-dimensional shape of the part being examined relative to the tube and film alignment contributes to elongation of the part, the most likely cause of any appreciable radiographic elongation is tube angulation. Improper OID and FFD are factors that relate to magnification (size) distortion. Grid cutoff is manifested as unilateral loss of density.

92. The answer is (C). A blue tint is added to the film base by the manufacturer to alleviate eyestrain. This tint has a small density. Along with environmental exposure during manufacturing, film is shipped with an inherent density called base fog. An additional density, approximately equal to that of base fog, is added during processing. The sum of the factors equals base plus fog. Base plus fog should not exceed 0.2 by sensitometric measurement.

93. The answer is (D). For any given phosphor, the greater the number of crystals, the greater the capacity for light absorption. Therefore, as long

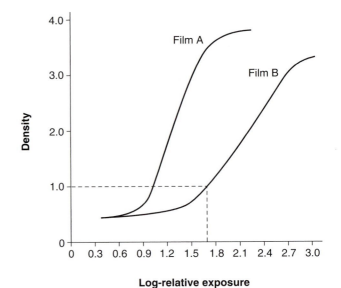

FIGURE 6-12.

as the ratio of crystals per unit of size remains constant, as screen thickness increases, screen speed increases.

94. The answer is (D). The faster the film and screen speed, the more likely quantum mottle will appear. Quantum mottle is the result of the random fashion in which x-ray photons interact with the image receptor. It exists to some degree with all screen/film systems, but it is more likely to become pronounced when the image is produced with relatively few x-ray photons. Because the phenomenon is related to the quantity of photons, it is a function of mA. For a given radiograph, quantum mottle can be reduced by increasing mA and decreasing kVp, or by decreasing screen speed and increasing technique.

95. The answer is (B). Film A, which is positioned to the left of film B, requires less exposure to produce a given density than film B. Therefore film A is faster. However, film B responds to a wider range of exposures than film A, and therefore has greater exposure latitude.

96. The answer is (A). Film contrast is equal to the slope of the straight-line portion of the characteristic curve. Because the slope of film A is greater than the slope of film B, it has greater contrast. The higher the contrast, the shorter the scale of contrast, and the less the exposure latitude.

97. The answer is (C). Look at the dotted line portion of the revised H&D curve in **Figure 6-12.** Remember that an increase in log-relative expo-

sure of 0.3 results in doubling the exposure. Film A produces a density with a value of 1 when a log-relative exposure of approximately 1.0 is applied. Film B produces the same density when a log-relative exposure of approximately 1.6 is applied. The 0.6 log-relative exposure increase that film B requires to produce the same density as film A represents a 4 × increase in exposure.

98. The answer is (B). The straight-line portion of the H&D curve represents the useful density range. The toe represents base plus fog, or D min, whereas the shoulder describes maximum density, or D max. The area past the shoulder describes the solarization point, at which further exposure causes image reversal.

99. The answer is (C). If the x-ray tube is positioned off center in relation to the bucky, the result will be a loss of density on the side of the radiograph away from the tube. In the example, the tube is positioned toward the right side of the patient, therefore grid cutoff occurs on the left.

100. The answer is (A). The RAO projection is most commonly associated with a barium-filled esophagus. The patient is positioned in the right prone oblique position, with the left hand holding a cup of barium and the drinking straw placed in the patient's mouth. The patient is instructed to drink continuously, and a high-kVp, low-mA exposure is made as the patient swallows the barium.

101. The answer is (B). Using the 50/15 rule, choices (A) and (B) are roughly equivalent; however, choice (B) would produce greater density on the finished radiograph because (A) uses a 10:1 grid, which would absorb more of the primary beam than the 8:1 used by (B). Choices (C) and (D) both use a 72″ FFD, which would result in much less density on the radiographs than with a 40″ FFD.

102. The answer is (C). Extremity radiography using this type of film screen combination is typically performed in the range between 45 and 60 kVp. 50 kVp and 1 mA is the most representative choice from those given. If a detail cassette were to be substituted, kVp would remain constant and mA would be increased to maintain short scale of contrast.

103. The answer is (D). Choices (B), (C), and (D) are permutations of choice (A), using the 50/15 rule for density maintenance. Because the grid ratio is constant for all, the radiograph produced using the highest kVp will produce the longest scale of contrast.

104. The answer is (A). Involuntary motion such as peristalsis or cardiac motion cannot be controlled by the patient. Therefore, the most effective means of limiting its effects is reduction of time. According to the reciprocity law, mA and time have an inversely proportional relationship. Therefore, by increasing mA, the technologist can reduce time and reduce the radiographic effects of involuntary motion.

105. The answer is (D). Orthochromatic film is spectrally matched with green light-emitting, rare earth intensifying screens, and should be used only with a safelight that emits the darkest red portion of the light spectrum. Blue-violet light is emitted by calcium tungstate screens, and amber light is fine for use with this type of film.

106. The answer is (C). Humidity must be maintained between 40% and 60% to maintain film supplies free of image-degrading artifact. If humidity falls below 40%, the likelihood of static artifact increases, whereas humidity over 60% is likely to lead to increased fog levels. The Wratten 6B safelight filter is used with film exposed by calcium tungstate screens, whereas film illumination even by proper safe lighting will lead to film fog if the film is held under it too long. White light leaks lead to gross blackening wherever it falls on film.

107. The answer is (B). Dust and lint on the screen itself will produce pinhole artifacts, which are minute, specklike areas of minus density on the radiograph. Pinhole artifacts are easily eliminated by regular cleaning of intensifying screens with a commercially prepared solution.

108. The answer is (C). Although the radiograph is grossly underexposed, enough density is present to determine that the patient is correctly positioned for a KUB examination. Incorrect positioning can cause underexposure with an AED, but because that is not the case in this situation, the most likely of the listed causes of this underexposure is insufficient mA. Incorrect patient instructions may adversely affect the radiograph, resulting in motion or incorrect diaphragm position, but it would not result in an underexposure of this type. Insufficient distance would result in a too-dark radiograph.

109. The answer is (A). Figure 6-4 is a retrograde pyelogram examination. The examination is performed either on a modified cystography table or a standard radiography table, and therefore a 72″ FFD could not be used. The examination uses water-soluble iodinated contrast; hence,

techniques above 70 kVp should not be used to avoid contrast "burnout."

110. The answer is (B). Figure 6-5 is an example of a poorly positioned lateral chest; it is extremely rotated posteriorly. A well-positioned lateral chest should demonstrate the ribs superimposed posteriorly.

111. The answer is (A). The cuboid and cuneiforms occupy the distal row of tarsals, articulating with the metatarsals anteriorly. The cuneiforms, named medial, middle, and lateral, are located medial to the cuboid; therefore, the cuboid is lateral to the lateral cuneiform.

112. The answer is (D). The lateral oblique position of the elbow demonstrates the radial head, neck, and tuberosity free of superimposition from the ulna.

113. The answer is (C). The medial oblique position of the elbow demonstrates the olecranon process within the olecranon fossa. The radial head and neck are superimposed on this view.

114. The answer is (C). The AP oblique projection demonstrates the carpals on the medial side of the wrist, and in particular the pisiform, free of superimposition. The Gaynor-Hart, or carpal canal view, is also useful for unobstructed demonstration of the pisiform.

115. The answer is (C). The circular density in the LLL of Figure 6-6 most likely represents a calcified granuloma or nipple. In this situation, the radiologist would likely order a subsequent chest examination with nipple markers to evaluate the patient further. Calcified granulomas are a mass of nodular granulation tissue resulting from inflammation, infection, or trauma. They may resolve spontaneously, become gangrenous, spread, or remain as a focus of infection.

116. The answer is (D). The vertebral arch is an aggregate structure formed by two laminae and two pedicles. The short bony projections projecting from the lumbar bodies are the pedicles, which complete the sides of the vertebral arch. The laminae are flattened plates, fused in the median plane, and complete the arch posteriorly and inferiorly.

117. The answer is (A). Seven processes project from the vertebral arch: the single posterior spinous process, and the paired transverse, superior articulating, and inferior articulating processes.

118. The answer is (C). A compound fracture is more serious than a simple fracture; it is distinguished from other fracture types by broken portions of bone protruding through the skin. It may result

in osteomyelitis, a serious bone infection requiring massive doses of intravenous antibiotics. A comminuted fracture is one in which the bones are fragmented into many pieces, whereas an impacted fracture is characterized by the broken ends of bones forced into each other. The greenstick fracture is an incomplete fracture common among children, so called because the bone fractures much in the same way as a green twig breaks.

119. The answer is (C). The right lung has three lobes. The upper and middle lobe are separated by the horizontal fissure, whereas the lower and middle lobe are divided by the right oblique fissure. The left lung has two lobes, separated into upper and lower lobes by the left oblique fissure.

120. The answer is (D). Figure 6-7 is a carelessly performed portable AP chest radiograph. The radiographer neglected to remove one of the portable unit's cables from in front of the tube head, projecting its image over the chest.

121. The answer is (B). If performed correctly, the standard posterior oblique view of the lumbar spine demonstrates the apophyseal articulations, commonly said to resemble "Scotty dogs." The Scotty's ear corresponds with the superior articular process, the nose with the transverse process, the neck with the pars interarticularis, the body with the lamina, and the front foot with the inferior articular process.

122. The answer is (D). To visualize the open L5–S1 articulation, a 5° to 8° caudal angulation is used for the spot view, with the CR directed 1.5″ inferior to the iliac crest.

123. The answer is (A). The thoracic vertebrae are the type that most closely resembles a "typical" vertebra. Their size increases as they descend inferiorly, with the upper thoracic vertebrae resembling the cervical spine, and the lower thoracic vertebrae resembling the lumbar spine. Their vertebral foramina are circular; whereas the vertebral foramina of the cervical and lumbar spine are approximately triangular.

124. The answer is (B). When viewed laterally, the four spinal curvatures give the spine its distinctive "S" shape, lending strength, resilience, and flexibility to the spine. The cervical and lumbar spines are convex anteriorly and concave posteriorly, whereas the thoracic and sacral spines are concave anteriorly and convex posteriorly.

125. The answer is (B). The facial skeleton consists of 14 bones, of which only the mandible and vomer are unpaired. The remaining bones are

the paired maxillae, zygomata, nasals, lacrimals, palatines, and inferior conchae.

126. The answer is (D). A single view of the hip is insufficient because there is no means of determining anterior or posterior displacement if a fracture is present. The frog-leg hip view should never be used in conjunction with trauma; it may worsen a fracture or dislocation if one is present. The shoot-through, or surgical lateral view, is the desired lateral projection with trauma cases because it yields the desired information without further insult to the affected area. An AP chest x-ray usually is obtained on patients with a fractured hip because they are often taken to surgery quickly after their initial evaluation, and the chest view is needed by the anesthesiologist to evaluate the patient's cardiac and respiratory status.

127. The answer is (A). The complex-shaped ethmoid bone is situated between the sphenoid and nasal bones and forms most of the bony surface between the orbit and nasal cavity.

128. The answer is (B). A small bowel follow-through examination traces the transit of barium through the small bowel tract, beginning with its most proximal portion, the duodenum, and ending with its distal portion, the ileocecal valve.

129. The answer is (B). The anterior two thirds of the hard palate or roof of the oral cavity is formed by the palatine processes of the maxillae. The hard palate is completed posteriorly by the horizontal plates of the palatine bone.

130. The answer is (C). The described position is the oblique projection of the orbit and optic canal, or Rhese method. The optic foramen is demonstrated in the inferior lateral portion of the orbit using this method.

131. The answer is (D). Although the sphenoidal sinus is of primary concern, all four sinuses are demonstrated on the lateral view. The Waters view demonstrates the maxillary and frontal sinuses, the Caldwell view demonstrates the frontal and ethmoid, and the SMV chiefly demonstrates the sphenoid and ethmoid sinuses.

132. The answer is (C). The sphenoid bone somewhat resembles a bat, with two sets of wings, the greater and lesser, projecting laterally from its body, and two processes, the pterygoid processes, extending inferiorly from the body. The sphenoid articulates with all the cranial bones, and its fragile-appearing body is bound firmly together by them.

133. The answer is (B). The RPO projection is most often used to evaluate the hepatopancreatic ampulla and biliary tree for evidence of calculi or other obstructive pathology.

134. The answer is (D). To facilitate filling of the deep venous system, including the basilic, cephalic, and subclavian veins, tourniquets are placed proximal to the wrist and elbow. AP projections, with the hand supinated, are most often used.

135. The answer is (B). During venography, injection of the contrast is done by hand or with the use of a volumetric pressure injector, which delivers a bolus injection at a predetermined rate. Modern injectors can be programmed for multiple-phase injections, precisely delivering contrast to desired areas, and usually resulting in greater diagnostic accuracy and a decrease in the amount of contrast medium required.

136. The answer is (A). The subarachnoid space is continuous with the ventricular system and communicates with it by the foramen of Magendie and the foramina of Luschka, located between the cisterna magna and the fourth ventricle. Although the cisterna magna is sometimes used as a point of entry to the subarachnoid space, in general the L3–L4 interspace, localized by fluoroscopy, is used for introduction of contrast media because there is no danger of damage to the spinal cord, which terminates at the conus medullaris at the level of L1–L2 in adults.

137. The answer is (C). The petrous region of the temporal bone is seen as a dense wedge between the occipital bone posteriorly and the sphenoid bone anteriorly. The petrous portion houses the middle and inner ear cavities, which contain the sensory receptors for hearing and equilibrium.

138. The answer is (B). Located slightly inferior to the EAM on the inferior aspect of the temporal bone, the styloid process is a needle-like projection that forms an attachment point for the important stylohyoid muscles and ligaments, which secure the hyoid bone.

139. The answer is (D). The radiograph in Figure 6-8 is incorrectly positioned; the centering is too low, resulting in "clipping," or eliminating from view, the left chest apices.

140. The answer is (D). The fifth digit of the foot consists of a proximal and distal phalanx with two expanded articular ends, while the remaining four digits consist of proximal, middle, and distal phalanges. The lucent area in the middle portion of the proximal phalanx on this film, best seen on the oblique projection, represents a frac-

ture of the proximal phalanx. Gas gangrene is radiographically appreciated in the soft tissue of the affected area.

141. The answer is (B). The Settegast view is a tangential projection of the patellofemoral articulation. The CR is directed perpendicularly through the joint space; the degree of cephalic angulation is dependent on the degree of knee flexion.

142. The answer is (D). The CR may be directed in a number of ways to obtain an axial view of the shoulder joint. The method chosen by the radiographer should depend on the patient's ability to abduct the arm at a near right angle to the torso. The rolled film, or Cleaves method, is perhaps the safest, if the modified type of cassette is available.

143. The answer is (A). Esophageal varices constitute a complex of longitudinal, tortuous veins directly beneath the distal esophageal mucosa, which are enlarged as a result of portal hypertension. The vessels are susceptible to hemorrhage, and often the associated portal hypertension is secondary to alcoholic cirrhosis.

144. The answer is (A). The manner in which a lateral mandible is performed depends on the area of interest. When the patient is positioned laterally with the chin extended along with a 25° cephalic angulation entering slightly posterior to the angle of the mandible, the ramus closest to the film is best demonstrated. The body is best seen when the patient's head is rotated approximately 30° toward the image receptor, using the same 25° cephalic tube angulation. Patient rotation of approximately 45° toward the film will produce an optimal image of the mandibular symphysis.

145. The answer is (C). Routine views of the sternum include RAO and lateral views. The sternum is not well visualized using AP or PA patient orientation. The lateral view of the sternum requires suspended respiration; however, the RAO view may use a shallow breathing technique in order to blur the pulmonary markings.

146. The answer is (B). The greater trochanter is an easily palpable, somewhat rectangular bony landmark that can be located on the body surface on the proximal lateral aspect of the thigh. It is particularly useful when other familiar landmarks (e.g., the iliac crest or the symphysis pubis) cannot be located easily because of patient obesity. For example, using the greater trochanter as an orienting landmark, the technolo-

gist knows that the femoral head is slightly superior and medial to it and that the symphysis pubis lies inferomedially approximately 1–1½".

147. The answer is (C). Nephrotomography is tomographic evaluation of the kidney parenchyma in conjunction with excretory urography. Since the kidneys are approximately 3 cm thick, three cuts through the kidneys 1 cm apart are usually sufficient to demonstrate the area of interest. The kidneys lie in an oblique plane in the retroperitoneum, with the upper poles located more posteriorly than the lower poles.

148. The answer is (D). With the exception of lordotic views, chest radiography is performed with a perpendicular CR directed to the level of the seventh thoracic vertebrae. T7 may be localized by measuring approximately 7" inferior from C7 on female patients and 8" inferior from C7 on male patients.

149. The answer is (C). Figure 6-10 is an example of a lateral projection of the right knee. On this view, the patient is placed in the lateral position, with the unaffected knee placed anterior to the affected side. The unaffected knee is flexed so that it is out of the area of the collimated beam, and the affected knee is flexed 30 to 45 degrees, depending on the area of interest. The femoral condyles are superimposed on a correctly positioned radiograph.

150. The answer is (C). The described area on the Figure 6-10 radiograph most likely represents osteophyte formation, or bony outgrowth, on the anterior portion of the tibial plateau. Osteophyte formation is a common manifestation of osteoarthritis.

151. The answer is (B). Figure 6-11 is an example of a rest/stress myocardial perfusion scan using Tc99m sestamibi. The procedure may also use the isotope thallium (Tl-201). With this procedure, the patient is given intravenous injections of low-dose radioisotopes, and single photon emission computed tomography (SPECT) images are obtained, both with the patient at rest and following exercise, usually on a treadmill.

152. The answer is (D). Voluntary motion is motion that the patient can control. The best method of reducing voluntary motion is to give an explanation of the procedure. With a good explanation of the examination and clear instructions to the patient, such as cessation of breathing and movement for the duration of the exposure, voluntary motion can be reduced greatly or eliminated entirely. Use of the short-

est possible exposure time is also a helpful technique with both voluntary and involuntary motion, but the shortest exposure time will not always produce the best diagnostic information. In this case, the requirements of the examination should be weighed against the physical limitations of the patient and the likelihood of the patient's cooperation.

153. The answer is (C). Pneumocystosis is infection with the parasite *Pneumocystis carinii,* which is sometimes found in infants. In recent years, pneumocystosis has become one of the hallmark conditions associated with HIV and AIDS patients. The condition is well demonstrated on standard PA and lateral chest radiographs.

154. The answer is (A). The tangential projection of a single zygomatic arch may be obtained in either the prone or supine method when the MSP is placed at a 15° angle with the image receptor. The prone method demonstrates the side remote from the film, whereas the supine method demonstrates the side closest to the film.

155. The answer is (C). The CSF originates in the choroid plexus, primarily in the lateral ventricles. The flow represented by choice C is correct. Once in the subarachnoid space, the CSF circulates around the cerebrum, cerebellum, and spinal cord.

156. The answer is (B). The zero level of the fulcrum on a tomographic unit is at the tabletop, with ascending increments. Therefore, with the patient supine, a fulcrum level of 18 cm would best demonstrate the lesion in question.

157. The answer is (C). The kidneys are two bean-shaped organs located in the retroperitoneum and embedded in adipose tissue. Their superior border begins approximately at the level of T12 and extends to the transverse process of L3. The right kidney is located slightly more inferiorly than the left kidney because of the large space occupied by the liver.

158. The answer is (D). Hydronephrosis is a condition whereby urine is backed up to the kidney tissue and exerts pressure on it. If this condition is left untreated, it may lead to necrosis and renal failure. It may occur secondarily to a number of conditions; renal calculus or a kink in the ureter secondary to renal ptosis being prominent among them. The presence of residual urine on a post micturition (post-void) radiograph may indicate the presence of a tumor (neoplasm) or prostatic enlargement (hypertrophy).

159. The answer is (B). With a double-contrast UGI examination, the LPO position demonstrates a barium-filled fundus; the duodenal bulb and pyloric canal are seen without superimposition of structures. The projection is important because the duodenum is frequently the site of peptic ulcer disease, which is typified by a sharply circumscribed area of mucous membrane loss. In the LPO position, gravity drains some of the barium from the pylorus and duodenum, yielding a double-contrast projection of the area. The PA projection demonstrates the size, shape, and contour of the barium-filled stomach, and the AP view shows a barium-coated, air-filled body and antrum. The retrogastric area of the duodenum and proximal jejunum can be seen through the air-filled stomach on this projection. Lateral views show a barium-filled duodenum and pyloric canal. These views are obtained primarily to demonstrate the anterior and posterior surfaces of the stomach and to further interrogate the retrogastric space.

160. The answer is (C). Although the location of the stomach varies widely according to body type, of the listed responses, choice C is most correct. L2 may be located by locating the point midway between the xiphoid tip (T10) and the umbilicus (L4).

161. The answer is (C). The esophagus is a collapsed, muscular tube beginning at the level of C6, with its upper one-fifth in the neck and its lower four-fifths in the thorax. It lies posterior to the trachea and moves slightly to the left at its distal end, joining the stomach at the cardiac orifice.

162. The answer is (A). The cystic duct descends from the gallbladder to join the common hepatic duct, which in turn emanates from the right and left hepatic ducts from the liver, to form the common bile duct. The common bile duct later joins the pancreatic duct at the sphincter of Oddi, where it pours bile into the duodenum. The sphincter remains closed, forcing bile from the hepatic ducts to back up into the cystic duct and gallbladder until, during a meal, the gallbladder contracts, relaxing the sphincter, and allowing bile into the duodenum.

163. The answer is (B). External landmarks are used as positioning aids in radiography of the skull, sinuses, and facial bones. The most superior midline landmark on the skull is the glabella, which is located on the inferior portion of the frontal bone.

164. The answer is (D). The union of the nose and

the upper lip is known as the acanthion. A line drawn from it to the EAM is known as the acanthomeatal line and is used as a guide for cranial views, most notably the Waters projection.

165. The answer is (A). The sella turcica, or Turk's saddle, contains the pituitary gland. It is found within the sphenoid bone 1½" anterior and superior to the EAM.

166. The answer is (C). The symptoms of shock include a drastic drop in blood pressure, tachycardia, and inadequate blood flow to the body's peripheral tissues, which results in an insufficient oxygen supply. Causal factors of shock include trauma, hemorrhage, vomiting, diarrhea, inadequate fluid intake, and renal insufficiency.

167. The answer is (B). The correct sequence is IVP, BE, UGI, SBFT. The IVP, BE, UGI, and small bowel series must be scheduled in a specific order. The IVP is done first, because water-soluble contrast media is rapidly excreted. The barium enema is done next. These two examinations are often performed on the same day. Lastly, the UGI tract may be studied. If these three examinations are performed in close proximity, generally a 1-day lapse between the IVP and BE and the UGI is required, and the patient is given a mild laxative in the interim. Any residual barium from the BE will generally not interfere with imaging the esophagus, stomach, and proximal small bowel, although in this case an abdominal film is generally taken before the examination. Although the above sequence is generally accepted as the correct sequencing protocol, it is important to note that some authors have advocated performing the UGI examination first. Supporters of this approach note the direct relationship between the effectiveness of preparation of the colon and the accuracy of the diagnosis. Fecal material may not be appreciated on a routine abdominal scout view, while the lack of residual contrast found on a scout film obtained subsequent to the UGI examination is an obvious indicator of colon cleanliness.

168. The answer is (C). The tort is an act, intentional or unintentional, which results in an injury.

169. The answer is (D). The patient bill of rights includes the right to: refuse treatment to the extent permitted by law, confidentiality of records and communication, informed consent, privacy, respectful care, access to personal records, refusal to participate in research, explanation of hospital charges, and continuing care.

170. The answer is (A). The heart can be considered functionally as two side-by-side pumps. The right side serves the pulmonary circuit; that is, its function is to collect the blood that returns to the heart from the body and to send it to the lungs for oxygenation. The left side is the systemic circuit pump, supplying the body with oxygenated blood from the lungs. The pathway of blood through the heart is as follows: Carbon-dioxide rich and oxygen-poor blood enters the heart through three veins: the superior vena cava (SVC), the inferior vena cava (IVC), and the coronary sinus, which collects oxygen-depleted blood from the myocardium. The blood passes through the tricuspid (right atrioventricular valve) into the right ventricle. When the right ventricle contracts, blood passes through the pulmonary semilunar valve into the pulmonary trunk (right and left pulmonary arteries) and continues into the lungs for gas exchange. Oxygenated blood returns to the left atrium of the heart via the right and left pulmonary veins. Blood passes from the left atrium through the mitral or bicuspid valve into the left ventricle. The left ventricle is the largest and strongest chamber of the heart. From it, blood flows through the aortic semilunar valve into the aorta and is distributed to the body.

171. The answer is (A). The pancreas is an elongated gland located in the epigastric and left hypochondriac region. It has three main portions: the tail, the body, and the head, which is lodged in the curved portion of the duodenum.

172. The answer is (D). While using a pillow as a support device is considered good practice, the main principle to recall when performing radiography of an injured or fractured extremity is to provide support of the limb above and below the site of the injury.

173. The answer is (B). During a grand mal seizure, the patient may experience an aura or warning, consisting of nausea or peculiar sensations anywhere in the body, including odd sounds or flashes of light. The patient may cry out suddenly. Following the aura, the patient falls unconscious, and the muscles become completely rigid. The skin becomes pale and then cyanotic; the pupils are fixed and dilated. The patient may become incontinent. This is known as the tonic phase of the seizure; lasting from 10–20 seconds. The clonic phase follows. This phase is characterized by alternate contracting and relaxing of all the body muscles. The patient's tongue may fall between his teeth, and he may

bite it. The patient may also froth at the mouth. The clonic phase lasts from 2–3 minutes, after which the patient falls into a deep sleep.

174. The answer is (B). The correct medical term for nosebleed is epistaxis. Patients with high blood pressure and nasal irritations commonly experience this condition, which is treated with an erect posture, the head tilted slightly posteriorly, and cold compresses over the nose.

175. The answer is (B). IV needles and catheters are sized according to their diameter. The measurement of diameter is referred to as the gauge. As the diameter of the needle or catheter increases, the gauge decreases; thus, a 23-gauge needle is smaller than an 18-gauge needle.

176. The answer is (C). Cyanosis is a bluish discoloration of the skin and mucous membranes caused by the presence of deoxygenated hemoglobin in the blood. A cyanotic patient is not receiving enough oxygen.

177. The answer is (C). The ideal height is 18–24″ above the IV site.

178. The answer is (D). Although used primarily in conjunction with treatment of the urinary tract, Foley catheters may also be used as a rectal tube.

179. The answer is (B). Osmolality refers to the number of particles in solution. In general, ionic contrast agents are high osmolality contrast media (HOCM), and nonionic agents are low osmolality contrast media (LOCM). Iohexol is a low osmolality contrast agent.

180. The answer is (C). The primary drawback for use of nonionic contrast material is that it is much more expensive than traditional ionic contrast.

181. The answer is (D). Of the conditions listed, the patient with degenerative joint disease, or osteoarthritis, would be the most likely candidate to be transported via a wheelchair. Patients with spine or head injuries who have yet to be evaluated must never be moved by a single person on a stretcher and certainly never in a wheelchair. Cheyne-Stokes breathing is symptomatic of serious underlying neurologic dysfunction; a patient with this condition would not be suited to wheelchair transport.

182. The answer is (B). The procedure for moving a patient from a wheelchair to the table is as follows: place a footrest in close proximity to the wheelchair, near the center of the x-ray table. Maneuver the chair so that the footrest of the chair is adjacent to the table footrest. Raise the footstool on the chair and bring the chair forward, placing the patient's feet on the table foot-

stool. Lock the chair. Place an arm behind the patient's back for support and assist the patient to an erect position. Ask the patient to turn so that his back is to the table, and instruct him to sit on the edge and then slide backward. Instruct the patient to lean backward and hold the edge of the table for support while lifting the patient's legs into position. Support the patient's head and neck while assisting him to a supine position.

183. The answer is (B). BUN and creatinine are markers of renal function. In patients with elevated levels, the possibility of limiting dosage or not performing the examination is considered.

184. The answer is (B). Except in rare instances when a part is intentionally magnified, the rule of thumb is to perform the examination in the projection that places the part closest to the film. In the case of the scapula, the AP projection is preferred.

185. The answer is (C). Hypoglycemic shock may be caused by decreased food intake, insulin overdose, or excessive exercise. Its hallmarks are sweating and chills, nervousness, irritability, hallucinations, numbness, and pallor. Without treatment, it may progress to convulsions and death. Treatment requires an immediate dosage of glucose.

186. The answer is (D). Patients generally sign an allergy history form when undergoing examinations that involve iodinated contrast media.

187. The answer is (B). While Gastrografin aspiration may lead to pulmonary edema, the small amount of barium aspiration necessary to demonstrate the fistula is generally not harmful to the patient.

188. The answer is (C). A lymphangiogram is a radiographic study of the lymphatic system accomplished with the slow introduction of iodized oils into the small lymphatic vessels of the foot. The study takes place over the course of several days, because the contrast media is not absorbed quickly by the body.

189. The answer is (A). Extravasation is a term that means leakage of fluid into the tissue surrounding an injection site. The technologist must be on guard against any appearance of localized swelling or pain at the site. If extravasation does occur, the needle or catheter should be removed and warm, moist compresses should be applied.

190. The answer is (D). Any object, such as an x-ray table or accessory that transmits an infectious organism, is known as a fomite. Other common

fomites include sinks, catheters, IV materials, bedpans, and so on.

191. The answer is (A). The Centers for Disease Control and Prevention (CDC) classify the hepatitis B virus (HBV) as a blood-borne pathogen, meaning that it is transmitted primarily via direct contact with a contaminated blood source, such as needles, IV equipment, transfusions, or wounds. OSHA regulations stipulate that health care workers with direct patient contact must be vaccinated against HBV. The worker may elect not to receive the vaccinations but must sign documentation indicating that immunization was made available and that he or she refused it.

192. The answer is (B). During angiography, the Sedlinger technique is employed for catheterization of blood vessels, usually the femoral artery. The procedure is as follows: A compound needle with inner stylet is used to pierce both walls of the selected vessel. The needle is then carefully withdrawn until steady blood return occurs. The stylet is then removed, and a flexible guidewire is inserted. The needle is withdrawn and a catheter is placed over the guidewire, carefully inserting it into the vessel. The guidewire is then removed, and the vessel is catheterized.

193. The answer is (D). A Colles fracture is a common fracture of the distal radius within 1" of the radiocarpal articulation. The injury generally occurs when a patient attempts to break a fall with an outstretched hand.

194. The answer is (B). The patient ingests the Telepaque approximately 14 hours prior to examination for oral cholecystography.

195. The answer is (D). The term parenteral refers to the administration of medication via any route other than the alimentary canal. These routes include intravenous, intramuscular, and mucosal, as in the conjunctivae of the eye.

196. The answer is (A). A nosocomial infection is acquired in the hospital. The most frequent site of infection is the urinary tract, most likely attributable to the high number of elderly, somewhat immunocompromised patients who are treated with urinary catheterization.

197. The answer is (B). The linea aspera is a pronounced ridge along the posterior aspect of the femur, which provides a location for muscle attachment.

198. The answer is (D). The first cervical vertebrae, or atlas, possess large, concave, superior articular facets that articulate with the occipital condyles. The atlanto-occipital joint permits flexion/extension of this region; hence, it is the joint which permits us to nod "yes." The atlas has neither a true body nor a spinous process.

199. The answer is (A). The humeroulnar joint is formed by the articulation of trochlea of the humerus and trochlear notch of the ulna. The joint permits movement in one direction: flexion/extension in a transverse axis about the trochlea.

200. The answer is (D). Increasing object-film distance (OFD) on an image *most significantly decreases* recorded detail. The primary effect of increasing OFD is an increase in magnification; as images become increasingly magnified, geometric blur also increases, but recorded detail decreases. It should also be noted that increasing OFD causes a decrease in density, because fewer scattered photons reach the image receptor in comparison to an exposure made using little or no OFD (this principle is utilized to advantage with the air gap technique). Loss of density resulting from increased OFD, however, is far less noticeable on the finished radiograph than the loss of recorded detail.

Bibliography

Anderson LE: Anaphylactic shock. In *Mosby's Medical and Nursing Dictionary.* St. Louis, Mosby, 1983.

Anderson LE: Palpation. In *Mosby's Medical and Nursing Dictionary.* St. Louis, Mosby, 1983.

Ballinger PW: *Merrill's Atlas of Radiographic Positions and Radiologic Procedures,* 7th ed. 3 vols. St. Louis, Mosby, 1991.

Basmajian JV: *Primary Anatomy,* 8th ed. Baltimore, Williams & Wilkins, 1982.

Bushong SC: *Radiologic Science for Technologists,* 4th ed. St. Louis, Mosby, 1988.

Carroll QB: *Fuch's Principles of Radiographic Exposure, Processing, and Quality Control,* 3rd ed. Springfield, IL, Charles C. Thomas, 1985.

Chesney MO, Chesney N: *Care of the Patient in Diagnostic Radiography,* 6th ed. St. Louis, Mosby, 1986.

Cullinan AM, Cullinan JE: *Producing Quality Radiographs,* 2nd ed. Philadelphia, JB Lippincott, 1994.

Downey RM: *Radiologic Technology,* AFR 160-30, 2nd ed. Washington, DC, Department of the Air Force, the Army, and the Navy, 1983.

Erlich RA: *Patient Care in Radiography.* St. Louis, Mosby, 1981.

Greulich WW, Pyle SI: *Radiographic Atlas of Skeletal Development of the Hand and Wrist,* 2nd ed. Stanford, CA, Stanford University Press, 1959.

Gunn C: *Guidelines on Patient Care in Radiography.* Edinburgh, Churchill Livingstone, 1982.

Katzenberg RW: *The Contrast Media Manual.* Baltimore, Williams & Wilkins, 1992.

Leonard W: *Radiography Examination Review,* 6th ed. New York, Elsevier Science, 1988.

Marieb EN: *Human Anatomy and Physiology.* Redwood City, CA, Benjamin / Cummings, 1989.

Saia DA: *Radiography: Program Review and Exam Preparation,* 2nd ed. Norwalk, CT, Appleton & Lange, 1996.

Saia DA: *Review for the Radiography Examination,* 2nd ed. Norwalk, CT, Appleton & Lange, 1993.

Selman J: *The Fundamentals of X-ray and Radium Physics,* 7th ed. Springfield, IL, Charles C. Thomas, 1985.

Skucas J: *Radiographic Contrast Agents,* 2nd ed. Rockville, MD, Aspen Publishers, 1989.

Tanner JM, Whitehouse RH, Cameron N et al.: *Assessment of Skeletal Maturation and Prediction of Adult Height.* New York, Academic Press, 1975.

Taylor MC: *Fundamentals of Nursing.* Philadelphia, JB Lippincott, 1989.

Upton AC, et al.: *Health Effects of Exposure to Low Levels of Ionizing Radiation* (BIER V). Washington, DC, National Academy Press, 1990.

Appendix A
Commonly Encountered Medical Abbreviations for the Radiographer

Abbreviation	Meaning	Abbreviation	Meaning
AAS	acute abdomen series	H & H	hematocrit and hemoglobin
ABG	arterial blood gas	Hb	hemoglobin
a.c.	before meals	HDL	high-density lipoprotein
ASAP	as soon as possible	HMO	health maintenance organization
ASIS	anterior superior iliac spine	H.S.	at night
BE	barium enema	Hx	history
b.i.d.	twice a day	IABP	intra-aortic balloon pump
BP	blood pressure	IC	iliac crest
BPH	benign prostate hypertrophy	ICU	intensive care unit
BRP	bathroom privileges	IM	intravascular
BUN	blood urea nitrogen	IOML	infraorbitomeatal line
c̄	with	IP	inpatient
CABG	coronary artery bypass graft	IV	intravascular
cc	cubic centimeter	IVP	intravenous pyelogram
CHF	congestive heart failure	K	potassium
CS	central supply	kg	kilogram
CXR	chest x-ray	KUB	kidneys, ureter, bladder
DC	discontinue	LAB	laboratory
DM	diabetes mellitus	LBP	lower back pain
DMOC	diabetes mellitus out of control	LDL	low-density lipoprotein
EENT	eye, ear, nose, throat	LLL	left lower lobe
ER	emergency room	LLQ	left lower quadrant
ESI	epidural steroid injection	LOC	loss of consciousness
ESRD	end-stage renal disease	LOS	length of stay
F & U	flat and upright	LP	lumbar puncture
g	gram	lt.	left
GB	gallbladder	LUL	left upper lobe
GYN	gynecology	LUQ	left upper quadrant
H or hrs.	hour, hours	MICU	medical intensive care unit

Abbreviation	Meaning
mm	millimeter
MPD	maximum permissible dose
mR	milliroentgen
MRI	magnetic resonance imaging
MRSA	methicillin-resistant *Staphylococcus aureus*
MS	multiple sclerosis
NICU	neonatal intensive care unit
NM	nuclear medicine
noct.	at night
NPO	nothing by mouth (nihil per os)
OB	obstetrics
OML	orbitomeatal line
OP	outpatient
OR	operating room
ORIF	open reduction and internal fixation
OT	occupational therapy
p̄	after
PAL	posterior-anterior and lateral
p.c.	after meals
PE	pulmonary embolus
PFT	pulmonary function test
PO	by mouth
ppm	parts per million
PPO	preferred provider organization
PPV	positive-pressure ventilation
PRN	as needed
PT	physical therapy
PT	prothrombin time
q.2h	every 2 hours
q.4h	every 4 hours
q.8h	every 8 hours
QA	quality assurance
q.d.	every day
QF	quality factor

Abbreviation	Meaning
q.h.	every hour
q.s.	sufficient quantity
RAD	radiology
RAI	radioactive iodine
RAIU	radioactive iodine uptake
RBC	red blood cell
RLL	right lower lobe
RLQ	right lower quadrant
RML	right middle lobe
Rn	radon
rout.	routine
rt.	right
RT	respiratory therapy
RUL	right upper lobe
RUQ	right upper quadrant
Rx	prescription, therapy
s̄	without
SICU	surgical intensive care unit
SNF	skilled nursing facility
SOB	shortness of breath
stat	at once
THR	total hip replacement
t.i.d.	three times a day
TKR	total knee replacement
TSH	thyroid-stimulating hormone
TSR	total shoulder replacement
TUR	transurethral resection
Tx	treatment
UGI	upper gastrointestinal
UR	utililzation review
URI	upper respiratory infection
US	ultrasound
UTI	urinary tract infection
VRE	vancomycin-resistant entero-coccus
WBC	white blood cell

Appendix B

Radiology Websites

Organizations

http://www.rsna.org/—*Radiological Society of North America*

http://www.acr.org/—*American College of Radiology*

http://theabr.org/—*The American Board of Radiology*

http://www.asrt.org/—*American Society for Radiologic Technologists*

Departments

http://cpmcnet.columbia.edu/dept/radiology/ TUTORIAL/—*Uroradiology Tutorial, Columbia University*

http://www.radweb.mc.duke.edu/—*Department of Radiology, Duke University*

http://www.med.harvard.edu/BWHRad/ —*BrighamRAD, Radiology from Harvard University*

http://www.xray.hmc.psu.edu:80/ home.html—*Radiology at Penn State*

http://www.med.umn.edu/radiology/ —*Department of Radiology, University of Minnesota*

http://www.rad.upenn.edu/ —Radiology—*University of Pennsylvania*

http://nuc-med-read.uthscsa.edu/—*Department of Radiology, University of Texas Health Science Center at San Antonio*

http://rpisun1.mdacc.tmc.edu/di/—*Division of Diagnostic Imaging, University of Texas MD Anderson*

http://www.rad.washington.edu/—*Radiology Webserver, University of Washington*

http://chorus.rad.mcw.edu/ chorus.html—*CHORUS, University of Wisconsin*

http://www.mir.wustl.edu /—*The Mallinckrodt Institute of Radiology, Washington University*

http://info.med.yale.edu/diagrad/—*Department of Diagnostic Radiology, Yale University*

General Interest Radiology

http://www.giradiology.com/—*GI Radiology*

http://www-sci.lib.uci.edu/ ~ martindale/ MedicalRad.html—*The Virtual Radiology Center*

http://www.radiologist.com/—*Radiologist.Com, an Internet resource for physicians in radiology*

http://members.aol.com/garyrad/ radcent.htm—*Radiology Central*

Index

Note: Page numbers in *italics* indicate illustrations; those followed by t indicate tables. Q and A denote questions and answers.